Paediatrics

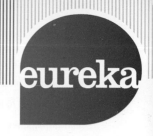

Paediatrics

Sian Foulkes MBBCh BSc MRCPCH
Specialty Registrar in Paediatrics and
Child Health
Abertawe Bro Morgannwg University
Health Board
Swansea, UK

Gemma Trays MBBCh MRCPCH
Specialty Registrar in Paediatrics and
Child Health
Abertawe Bro Morgannwg University
Health Board
Swansea, UK

Carol Sullivan BM BCh MA MRCP
FRCPCH
Consultant in Neonatal and Respiratory
Paediatrics
Abertawe Bro Morgannwg University
Health Board
Swansea, UK

Series Editors

Janine Henderson MRCPsych
MClinEd
MB BS Programme Director
Hull York Medical School
York, UK

David Oliveira PhD FRCP
Professor of Renal Medicine
St George's, University of London
London, UK

Stephen Parker BSc MS DipMedEd
FRCS
Consultant Breast and General
Paediatric Surgeon
St Mary's Hospital
Newport, UK

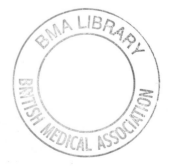

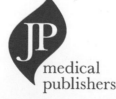

JP
medical
publishers

London • New Delhi • Panama City

© 2018 JP Medical Ltd.

Published by JP Medical Ltd, 83 Victoria Street, London, SW1H 0HW, UK

Tel: +44 (0)20 3170 8910   Fax: +44 (0)20 3008 6180

Email: info@jpmedpub.com   www.jpmedpub.com, www.eurekamedicine.com

ISBN: 978-1-907816-73-4

British Library Cataloguing in Publication Data
A catalogue record for this book is available from the British Library

Library of Congress Cataloging in Publication Data
A catalog record for this book is available from the Library of Congress

Publisher:	Richard Furn
Development Editors:	Thomas Banister-Fletcher, Paul Mayhew, Alison Whitehouse
Editorial Assistants:	Katie Pattullo, Adam Rajah
Copy Editor:	Kim Howell
Graphic narratives:	James Pollitt
Cover design:	Forbes Design
Page design:	Designers Collective Ltd

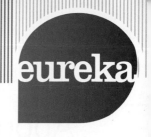

Series Editors' Foreword

Today's medical students need to know a great deal to be effective as tomorrow's doctors. This knowledge includes core science and clinical skills, from understanding biochemical pathways to communicating with patients. Modern medical school curricula integrate this teaching, thereby emphasising how learning in one area can support and reinforce another. At the same time students must acquire sound clinical reasoning skills, working with complex information to understand each individual's unique medical problems.

The *Eureka* series is designed to cover all aspects of today's medical curricula and reinforce this integrated approach. Each book can be used from first year through to qualification. Core biomedical principles are introduced but given relevant clinical context: the authors have always asked themselves, 'why does the aspiring clinician need to know this'?

Each clinical title in the series is grounded in the relevant core science, which is introduced at the start of each book. Each core science title integrates and emphasises clinical relevance throughout. Medical and surgical approaches are included to provide a complete and integrated view of the patient management options available to the clinician. Clinical insights highlight key facts and principles drawn from medical practice. Cases featuring unique graphic narratives are presented with clear explanations that show how experienced clinicians think, enabling students to develop their own clinical reasoning and decision making. Clinical SBAs help with exam revision while Starter questions are a unique learning tool designed to stimulate interest in the subject.

Having biomedical principles and clinical applications together in one book will make their connections more explicit and easier to remember. Alongside repeated exposure to patients and practice of clinical and communication skills, we hope *Eureka* will equip medical students for a lifetime of successful clinical practice.

Janine Henderson, David Oliveira, Stephen Parker

About the Series Editors

Janine Henderson is the MB BS undergraduate Programme Director at Hull York Medical School (HYMS). After medical school at the University of Oxford and clinical training in psychiatry, she combined her work as a consultant with postgraduate teaching roles, moving to the new Hull York Medical School in 2004. She has a particular interest in modern educational methods, curriculum design and clinical reasoning.

David Oliveira is Professor of Renal Medicine at St George's, University of London (SGUL), where he served as the MBBS Course Director between 2007 and 2013. Having trained at Cambridge University and the Westminster Hospital he obtained a PhD in cellular immunology and worked as a renal physician before being appointed as Foundation Chair of Renal Medicine at SGUL.

Stephen Parker is a Consultant Breast & General Paediatric Surgeon at St Mary's Hospital, Isle of Wight. He trained at St George's, University of London, and after service in the Royal Navy was appointed as Consultant Surgeon at University Hospital Coventry. He has a particular interest in e-learning and the use of multimedia platforms in medical education.

About the Authors

Sian Foulkes is a Specialty Registrar in Paediatrics and Child Health. She regularly teaches both undergraduate medical students and junior paediatric trainees. She also has an interest in health education and completed an intercalated degree in Public Health.

Gemma Trays is a Specialty Registrar in Paediatrics and Child Health, with a special interest in community paediatrics. She is actively involved in both undergraduate and postgraduate education, teaching clinical skills and preparing trainees for membership exams.

Carol Sullivan is a Consultant in Neonatal and Respiratory Paediatrics. She has 20 years' experience teaching medical students and trainees in clinics and in lectures, as well as setting undergraduate and postgraduate examinations. She has a Postgraduate Certificate in Medical Education and is a Fellow of the Higher Education Academy.

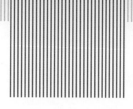

Preface

Paediatrics is the care of children from birth to adulthood, encompassing every clinical specialty from cardiology to palliative care. It is highly rewarding, but not without its challenges: young patients often cannot, or do not want to, communicate their symptoms.

The practice of paediatrics is not the sole preserve of paediatricians: one third of patients seen by general practitioners are children, and specialists in other disciplines will all be required to treat children at some point. All clinicians should therefore have a basic knowledge of childhood diseases and how to safeguard children.

Eureka Paediatrics provides you with an understanding of common paediatric conditions and the science behind them. Chapter 1 explains the physiology and anatomy that underlie normal growth and development, while chapter 2 describes the clinical assessment of children and management of paediatric conditions. Subsequent chapters cover disorders of individual body systems and emergency and community care, supplemented by explanatory case examples, artworks and graphic narratives. Finally, a self-assessment chapter is included to help you with exam revision.

We hope *Eureka Paediatrics* reflects the fascinating and fun career of paediatrics, and provides the knowledge you need to be confident when managing children in every clinical setting.

Sian Foulkes, Gemma Trays, Carol Sullivan
July 2017

Contents

Chapter 13 Skin disorders

Chapter 14 Haematological disorders

Chapter 15 Childhood cancer

Chapter 16 Emergencies

Chapter 17 Community paediatrics and integrated care

Chapter 18 Self-assessment

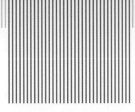

Glossary

ACTH	adrenocorticotrophic hormone	HDU	high-dependency unit
ADHD	attention deficit hyperactivity disorder	Hib	*Haemophilus influenzae* type B
ALP	alkaline phosphatase	HLA	human leucocyte antigen
ALT	alanine transaminase	HPV	human papilloma virus vaccine (cervical cancer vaccine)
ASD	atrial septal defect		
AST	aspartate aminotransferase	Ig	immunoglobulin
ATP	adenosine triphosphate	IGF	insulin-like growth factor
AVSD	atrioventricular septal defect	IO	Intraosseous
BCG	bacillus Calmette–Guérin	IUGR	intrauterine growth restriction
BMI	body mass index	IVC	inferior vena cava
BP	blood pressure	JIA	juvenile idiopathic arthritis
CGH	comparative genomic hybridisation	LH	luteinising hormone
CNS	central nervous system	LLSE	lower left sternal edge
CPAP	continuous positive airway pressure	MAG3	mercaptoacetyltriglycine
CPR	cardiopulmonary resuscitation	MCADD	medium-chain acyl-coenzyme A dehydrogenase deficiency
CT	computerised tomography		
CTFR	cystic fibrosis conductance transmembrane regulator	Men	meningitis vaccine
		MMR	measles, mumps and rubella vaccine
DA	ductus arteriosus	MRI	magnetic resonance imaging
DC	direct current	NSAID	non-steroidal anti-inflammatory drug
DMSA	dimercaptosuccinic acid	PDA	patent ductus arteriosus
DTaP/IPV	four-in-one diphtheria, tetanus, acellular pertussis and polio vaccine	PEFR	peak expiratory flow rate
		PICU	paediatric intensive care unit
DtaP/IPV/Hib	five-in-one diphtheria, tetanus, acellular pertussis, polio and *Haemophilus influenzae* type B vaccine	PPHN	persistent pulmonary hypertension of the newborn
		SD	standard deviation
DTPA	diethylenetriaminepenta-acetic acid	SIDS	sudden infant death syndrome
DV	ductus venosus	SUDI	sudden unexpected death in infancy
ECG	electrocardiography	SVC	superior vena cava
EEG	electroencephalography	SVT	supraventricular tachycardia
FEV_1	forced expiratory volume in 1 s	T_3	tri-iodothyronine
FGM	female genital mutilation	T_4	thyroxine
FISH	fluorescence in situ hybridisation	Td/IPV	three-in-one tetanus, diphtheria and polio
FSH	follicle-stimulating hormone		
FVC	forced vital capacity	TOF	tracheo-oesophageal fistula
G6PD	glucose 6-phosphate dehydrogenase	TRH	thyrotrophin-releasing hormone
GBS	group B *Streptococcus*	TSH	thyroid-stimulating hormone
GHRH	growth hormone–releasing hormone	ULSE	upper left sternal edge
GP	general practitioner	VSD	ventricular septal defect

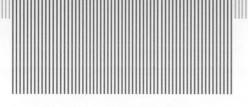

Acknowledgements

We would like to acknowledge the help and support from Howard Whitehead, Medical Photographer, and the medical illustration department of Abertawe Bro Morgannwg University Health Board.

Many thanks to all the patients and parents who gave us permission to include their photographs.

We are grateful to the following people for providing images for use in this book: Steven Allen, Sujoy Banerjee, Dana Beasley, Sharon Blackford, Philip Connor, Tania Davis, Michelle James-Ellison, Dewi Evans, Rachel Evans, Sally Meecham-Jones, David Laws, Maha Mansour, Lucinda Perkins.

SF, GT, CS

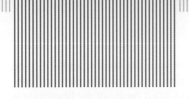

Chapter 1
First principles

Starter questions

Answers to the following questions are on page 46.

1. Why does smoking during pregnancy reduce the baby's lung capacity?
2. Can mothers be given X-rays while pregnant?
3. Why do some people get appendicitis on the left side of the body, rather than the right?

Prenatal development

The creation of a human is a complex process. It starts at conception with the fusion of genetic material from the egg and sperm, and continues throughout the prenatal period to culminate in the birth of a neonate capable of life outside the uterus. Disruption of normal prenatal development results in congenital anomalies.

Prenatal development is divided into two periods.

- In the **embryonic period** (from fertilisation to day 56, i.e. the end of week 8), the unicellular fertilised egg undergoes rapid cell growth (a series of cell divisions) and cellular differentiation to form a multicellular embryo containing the precursors of the major organ systems – a process called embryogenesis

- The **fetal period** (weeks 9–38) begins 8 weeks after fertilisation, from which point the embryo is termed a fetus; growth and development continue throughout this period as the organ systems mature in preparation for birth

Fetal, embryonic and gestational ages

Throughout this book, fetal age is given in terms of embryonic age, not gestational age, unless otherwise specified. Gestational age is calculated from the first day of the mother's last menstrual period, which falls, on average, 2 weeks before ovulation. Embryonic age is the time from conception, day 0 is taken as is the day of fertilisation. Therefore, embryonic age is gestational age minus 2 weeks. By the end of a normal pregnancy, the gestational age of the fetus is 40 weeks, and its embryonic age is 38 weeks.

> **'Embryo' is the term for an organism in the early stages of prenatal development (generally up to the end of week 8).** It is variously applied to the entity created by fertilisation either from conception (as in this chapter) or from implantation onwards, until it is termed a fetus (generally at the start of week 9).

Embryonic period

In the first period of embryonic development, embryogenesis leads to formation of a complex multicellular entity with rudimentary organ systems and a human appearance, measuring almost 20 mm in length. The process occurs in several phases:

1. fertilisation and blastocyst formation
2. implantation
3. formation of germ cell layers
4. early organogenesis

Each of these is a critical phase in prenatal development. Disruption of any of the processes that occur in these phases can lead to miscarriage or congenital anomalies in the neonate.

Days 0–5: fertilisation and blastocyst formation

Figure 1.1 shows events that occur in the first week of embryogenesis. Fertilisation takes place in a fallopian tube, when a single sperm penetrates the egg and their genetic material, 23 chromosomes in each cell, combines. This union results in a single cell, the zygote, which contains 46 chromosomes in 23 pairs. The zygote starts travelling down the fallopian tube to the uterus.

On its journey down the fallopian tube, the zygote undergoes a rapid series of cell divisions (cleavage). By day 3, cleavage has resulted in formation of a ball of 16 cells called the morula.

At day 5, the morula develops a fluid-filled cavity; it is now termed a blastocyst (**Figure 1.2**). The fluid-filled centre of the blastocyst is the blastocoel; this is surrounded by a layer of cells called trophoblasts. A collection of cells pushed by fluid to one pole of the blastocyst is called the inner cell mass.

The inner cell mass forms the basis of the early germ cell layers, from which, via cellular differentiation, the organ systems are developed.

Day 6: implantation

On day 6, the trophoblast layer of the blastocyst implants into the uterine wall (see **Figure 1.1**). This enables the blastocyst to obtain energy for cell growth and differentiation by infiltrating the maternal circulation through the uterine wall. The trophoblasts eventually become the placenta.

Days 7–18: formation of germ cell layers

The next phase of embryogenesis is the formation of the three germ cell layers – endoderm, mesoderm and ectoderm – that form the basis of all organs and tissues of the body. These arise from the inner cell mass of the blastocyst.

Bilaminar embryonic disc

The inner cell mass first forms a bilaminar (two-layer) structure called the embryonic disc (**Figure 1.3**).

- **Dorsal layer:** cells of this layer differentiate into epiblast cells; the amniotic sac originates from this epiblast layer
- **Ventral layer:** cells of this layer become hypoblast cells; the yolk sac originates from this hypoblast layer

The amniotic sac fills with amniotic fluid, thereby protecting the growing embryo (and later fetus) from external forces. The yolk sac gives rise to the linings of the digestive system.

Trilaminar embryonic disc

At about day 16, gastrulation occurs. In this process, a population of epiblasts migrate

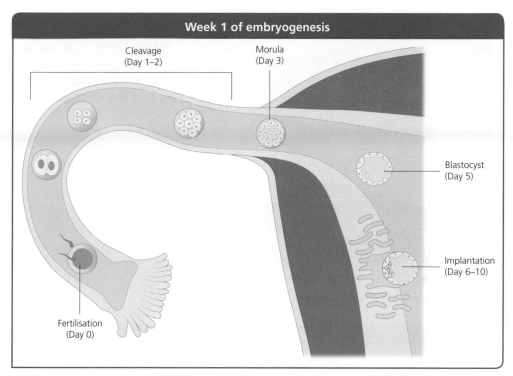

Figure 1.1 Week 1 of embryogenesis: fertilisation of the egg through to development of the blastocyst, which implants into the uterus.

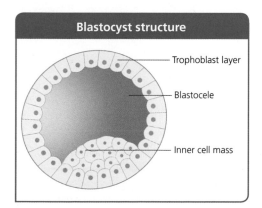

Figure 1.2 Structure of a blastocyst on day 5. The inner cell mass is forming on the inner surface of one of its poles.

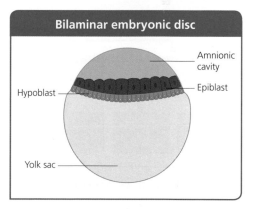

Figure 1.3 The bilaminar embryonic disc. The amniotic cavity and yolk sacs are forming.

medially through a groove-like structure, known as the primitive streak, which forms on the epiblast layer (**Figure 1.4**).

The migrating epiblasts form a new germ cell layer called the mesoderm, thereby trans-

forming the bilaminar embryonic disc into a trilaminar (three-layer) structure. The epiblasts remaining in the epiblast layer form the ectoderm layer, and the hypoblasts form the endoderm.

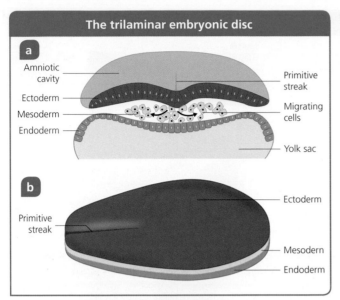

Figure 1.4 Transverse (a) and 3D (b) images of the migration of epiblasts through the primitive streak to form the trilaminar embryonic disc, comprising the three germ cell layers (endoderm, ectoderm and mesoderm).

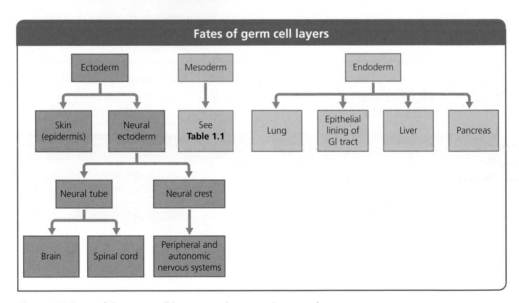

Figure 1.5 Fates of the germ cell layers as embryogenesis proceeds.

Fates of the germ cell layers

All tissues and organs of the body develop from the germ cell layers: the ectoderm, the endoderm and the mesoderm (**Figure 1.5**). The embryo assumes its three-dimensional shape as a result of lateral folding (rolling up along its sides): the three germ cell layers migrate laterally and ventrally, i.e. towards underside of body. As the embryo grows in length it forms a 'C' shape in a rostral to caudal direction (**Figure 1.6**).

Ectoderm

Cells of the most superficial layer of the ectoderm differentiate to form the skin, sebaceous glands, hair and nails, thereby forming the outer tissue of the body. The inner layer of the ectoderm develops into the nervous system.

Endoderm

The endoderm migrates laterally and ventrally and meets to form the primitive gut tube, with the foregut at the rostral end, the hindgut at the caudal end and the midgut between the two (**Figure 1.7**). Endoderm forming the primitive gut tube develops into the epithelial lining of the gastrointestinal tract and forms the liver, pancreas, lungs and bladder.

Mesoderm

The mesoderm layer grows laterally. The most lateral mesoderm is termed the lateral plate mesoderm; the most medial mesoderm, the paraxial mesoderm; and the mesoderm between the two, the intermediate mesoderm (**Table 1.1** and **Figure 1.7**).

- The **lateral plate mesoderm** splits into the somatic (dorsal) and splanchnic (ventral) mesoderm with small cavities between them. As lateral folding occurs the layers meet in the midline and the cavities merge to form the intraembryonic coelom (**Figure 1.7**). The intraembryonic coelom forms the pericardial, pleural and peritoneal cavities

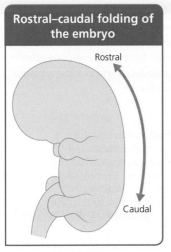

Rostral–caudal folding of the embryo

Rostral

Caudal

Figure 1.6 Rostral–caudal folding at the head and tail ends of the embryo, respectively, starts at the beginning of the 4th week, causing the embryo to form a 'C'-shaped structure

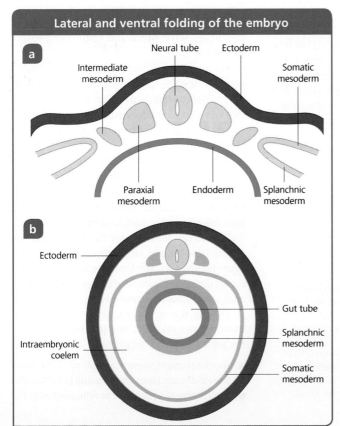

Lateral and ventral folding of the embryo

a

Intermediate mesoderm

Neural tube

Ectoderm

Somatic mesoderm

Paraxial mesoderm

Endoderm

Splanchnic mesoderm

b

Ectoderm

Gut tube

Splanchnic mesoderm

Intraembryonic coelem

Somatic mesoderm

Figure 1.7 Lateral and ventral folding of the embryo. (a) During lateral folding the germ cell layers grow laterally and ventrally, and meet in the midline along the underside of the embryo. (b) This results in the gut and the intraembryonic coelomic cavity being formed, which give rise to the abdominal and thoracic cavities.

Fate of the mesoderm		
Mesoderm	Subdivision	Derived structures
Lateral plate	Somatic mesoderm	Bones
		Blood vessels
		Connective tissue
	Splanchnic mesoderm	Heart
		Smooth muscle of gastrointestinal tract
Intermediate	–	Urogenital system
Paraxial	Somites	Musculoskeletal system (i.e. bone, cartilage, muscle, ligaments)

Table 1.1 Fate of the mesoderm

- The **intermediate mesoderm** develops into the urogenital system
- The **paraxial mesoderm** develops into paired segments called somites on either side of the neural tube

Days 19–56: early organogenesis

Organogenesis (organ formation) occurs from day 19, once the germ cell layers have formed and the basic structure of the embryo is in place, and continues into the fetal period. Most structures develop from two tubes: the neural tube and the primative gut tube.

The organ systems and structures are discussed here in turn:

- nervous system
- gastrointestinal tract
- respiratory system
- cardiovascular system
- head and neck
- musculoskeletal system
- urogenital system

Teratogens are agents that disrupt the development of the embryo, e.g. certain drugs and viruses. They interfere with the differentiation of tissues and organs, causing birth defects or intrauterine deaths. Thalidomide was a teratogen that caused limb deformities in thousands of babies in the 1950s and 1960s.

Nervous system

The nervous system comprises:

- the **central nervous system**, i.e. the brain and spinal cord
- the **peripheral nervous system**, which relays information between the brain and spinal cord and the peripheral nerves (motor and sensory)
- the **autonomic nervous system**, which acts independently of conscious control to regulate the function of smooth muscle (stomach, intestines and bladder), cardiac muscle and glands

Use of recreational drugs and consumption of alcohol during pregnancy has negative effects on neurodevelopment. They increase the incidence of intellectual and behavioural difficulties later in life.

Brain and spinal cord development

The central nervous system is the first organ system to develop when the neural tube, the precursor of the brain and spinal cord, forms in week 3.

Formation of the neural tube (neurulation) begins when the specialised mesodermal cells of the notochord, a rod-like structure in the midline of the embryo, induce the ectodermal tissue above it to thicken, thereby forming the neural plate.

The neural plate develops a furrow along its midline. This is termed the neural groove; its upper edges are the neural folds. As the groove deepens, the neural folds come together and fuse, initially in the middle of the tube then cranially and caudally. By day 26, this process has produced a tubular structure called the neural tube (**Figure 1.8**). The brain forms at the cranial end of the neural tube, and the spinal cord forms along rest of the tube towards the caudal end.

During the 4th week, the brain develops from the neural tube. The process starts with the formation of three primary vesicles:

- the forebrain (prosencephalon)
- the midbrain (mesencephalon)
- the hindbrain (rhombencephalon)

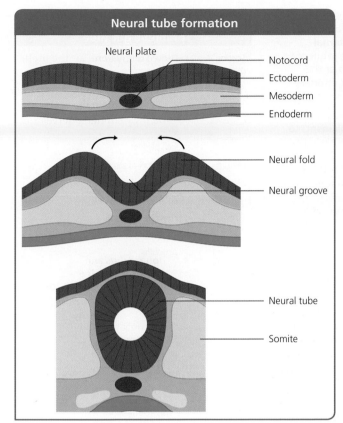

Neural tube formation

Neural plate

Notocord

Ectoderm

Mesoderm

Endoderm

Neural fold

Neural groove

Neural tube

Somite

Figure 1.8 Formation of the neural tube. Folding of the neural plate at the neural groove causes the neural folds to become higher and eventually join to form the neural tube, which ultimately develops into the central nervous system. Cells not incorporated into the neural tube are known as neural crest cells and migrate to form other neural and non-neural tissue.

Neural tube defects are caused by failure of the neural tube to close completely.

- If this occurs at the cranial end of the tube, the result is anencephaly (failure of brain development), which is incompatible with life

- If it occurs at the caudal end of the tube, the result is spina bifida, which is associated with hydrocephalus, urinary incontinence and lack of sensation in the limbs

As the embryo grows, further cell division and differentiation lead to formation of five secondary vesicles (telencephalon, diencephalon, mesencephalon, metencephalon, myelencephalon) during the 5th week, and development of the central nervous system continues throughout prenatal life to eventually result in formation of the final structures of the brain and spinal cord (**Table 1.2**).

Embryological origins of the central nervous system

Embryological structure	Final CNS component
Forebrain (prosencephalon)	Cerebral hemispheres
	Thalamus
	Hypothalamus
	Retina
Midbrain (mesencephalon)	Midbrain
Hindbrain (rhombencephalon)	Pons
	Cerebellum
	Medulla
Spinal cord	Spinal cord

Table 1.2 Embryological origins of components of the central nervous system (CNS)

The ventricles of the brain form from the lumen of the neural tube.

Neural tube defects are associated with low levels of folate in the maternal serum. Folate deficiency is the result of low dietary intake of folic acid or the use of antiepileptic drugs that interfere with folate metabolism.

Women who are trying to conceive are advised to take folic acid supplements to decrease the risk of their baby having a neural tube defect. A higher daily dose of folic acid is recommended for those taking antiepileptic drugs, and their medication is reviewed to minimise the risk of other malformations associated with the use of these drugs.

Peripheral nervous system

The peripheral nervous system develops from neural crest cells. These are the cells of the neural folds that are not incorporated into the neural tube during neurulation. Instead, they migrate and differentiate into many different cell types, including those of bone, muscle and nervous systems other than the central nervous system.

A population of neural crest cells migrate from the midline to the peripheries. Here, they differentiate into the motor neurones and dorsal root ganglia of the peripheral sensory nerves, including the cranial nerves.

Autonomic nervous system

The autonomic nervous system is also formed from migrating neural crest cells. This occurs at about 5 weeks.

- The **sympathetic nervous system** starts to form when neural crest cells migrate from their origin to behind the aorta; they then form a sympathetic chain (a series of ganglia connected by nerve fibres) on each side of the spine
- The **parasympathetic nervous system** forms from neural crest cells that migrate to in front of the aorta

Gastrointestinal tract

The primitive gut is the result of lateral and ventral folding of the endoderm to form a tube. The tube has a distinct foregut, midgut and hindgut (**Table 1.3**) from the 4th week of

GI structures deriving from the primitive gut tube	
Section	Derived structures
Foregut	Oesophagus
	Stomach
	Proximal half of the duodenum
	Liver
	Gall bladder
Midgut	Distal half of the duodenum
	Pancreas
	Ileum
	Jejunum
	Caecum
	Appendix
	Ascending colon
	Proximal third of the transverse colon
Hindgut	Distal two thirds of the transverse colon
	Descending colon
	Sigmoid colon
	Rectum
	Upper part of the anal canal

Table 1.3 The primitive gut gives rise to the structures of the gastrointestinal system, and structures of other organ systems

embryogenesis. The terms 'foregut', 'midgut' and 'hindgut' are also applied to the regions of the definitive gastrointestinal tract.

The primitive gut tube gives rise to the digestive system, i.e. the organs of the gastrointestinal tract, the liver, the pancreas, etc., as well as many other organ systems, including the respiratory and urogenital systems. Organs originating from the primitive gut tube develop from buds produced by outpouching of the primitive gut tube (**Figure 1.9**).

Foregut

The foregut section of the primitive gut develops into the length of gastrointestinal tract extending from the oesophagus to the proximal half of the duodenum. The liver and respiratory tract arise as outpouchings of the foregut.

Midgut

The primitive midgut is the region of the gastrointestinal tract bounded by the duodenum and the splenic flexure of the colon.

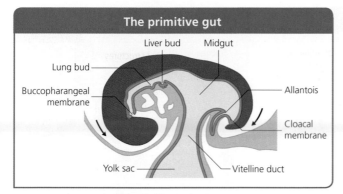

The primitive gut

Liver bud   Midgut

Lung bud

Buccopharangeal
membrane

Allantois

Cloacal
membrane

Yolk sac

Vitelline duct

Figure 1.9 The primitive gut and structures that arise from it. The cloacal membrane covers the cloaca, a structure produced early in development of the urogenital system.

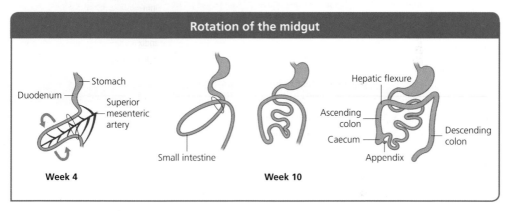

Rotation of the midgut

Stomach

Duodenum

Superior
mesenteric
artery

Small intestine

Week 4

Hepatic flexure

Ascending
colon

Caecum

Appendix

Descending
colon

Week 10

Figure 1.10 Rotation of the midgut occurs outside the abdominal cavity during week 4 and the midgut returns inside at week 10.

The pancreas also develops from the midgut, from outpouching of its duodenal part.

As a consequence of rapid growth of the midgut including the liver, the abdominal cavity becomes too small to contain them. This causes the developing gut to herniate (protrude) through the vitalline duct into the yolk sac during the 4th week of embryogenesis. At the same time, the gut rotates 90° anticlockwise around an axis of the superior mesenteric artery (**Figure 1.10**). During the 10th week of embryogenesis, the midgut returns to the abdominal cavity, rotating a further 180°, in an anticlockwise direction, to a total of 270°.

Hindgut

This section of the primitive gut develops into the descending colon and rectum.

During embryonic development, the large intestine grows lengthwise. However, because it is shorter it does not coil like the midgut structures.

Failure of the intestines to return to the abdominal cavity results in a condition called exomphalos. At birth, the baby's gut lies outside the abdomen, encased in a membranous sac protruding through the umbilicus (omphalocoele). Urgent surgery is required to position the gut in the abdominal cavity.

Respiratory system

The respiratory system starts to develop at week 4 of embryogenesis. A diverticulum (blind-ending pouch) forms from the ventral wall of the foregut (**Figure 1.11**). The diverticulum elongates to form the tracheal bud and from the distal end of this branch the bronchial buds, precursors of the trachea and bronchi, respectively.

The bronchi divide into smaller and smaller bronchioli until sacs called alveoli form at the

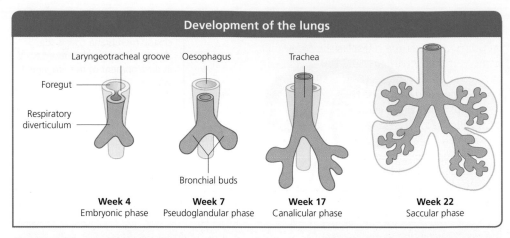

Figure 1.11 Stages of lung development. The lungs continue to develop beyond the fetal period and in to childhood.

Lung development		
Stage	Embryonic age (weeks)	Development
Embryonic	4–5	Respiratory buds develop as outpouchings of the ventral foregut
Pseudoglandular	5–17	Bronchi and segmental bronchi are formed
Canalicular	17–24	Bronchioli continuously divide into smaller canals, and capillaries form close to their epithelium. Surfactant synthesis begins
Saccular	24–36	Primitive alveolar sacs develop
Alveolar	36 onwards*	Alveoli continue to grow and develop throughout childhood
*Continues to age of 8 years.		

Table 1.4 Phases of lung development and maturation

ends of the smallest brochioli. Gas exchange occurs at the surface of the alveoli when the baby is born (**Table 1.4**). Thus the alveoli take on functions previously carried out by the umbilical cord, namely the provision of oxygen and removal of carbon dioxide. The development and maturation of the lungs continue beyond the fetal period and into childhood.

Surfactant

Specialist lung cells called type 2 pneumocytes start to develop in the alveoli at 24 weeks embryological age. They secrete surfactant, a substance that reduces surface tension at the air–alveolar interface, keeping the alveoli open and thereby preventing the lungs from collapsing.

The amount of surfactant produced increases as the lungs mature during the fetal period. The first few cries at birth cause amniotic fluid in the alveolar sacs to be absorbed into the neonate's bloodstream and lymphatic system. Surfactant remains as a thin layer lining the surface of the alveoli.

Premature babies may require direct administration of artificial surfactant into the lungs via a breathing tube. Their lungs are immature and they have lower levels of type 2 pneumocytes, so they may have insufficient surfactant to prevent lung collapse. This can lead to a condition known as respiratory distress syndrome.

Cardiovascular system

The heart starts to develop at about day 20, when two endocardial heart tubes develop from the mesoderm. By the end of week 3, they merge to form a single endocardial tube. At this point, the tube contains the common atria, ventricles, truncus arteriosus, bulbus cordis and sinus venosus. The heart begins to pump blood at day 22. The tube folds, bulges and loops to form the basic structure of the heart (**Figure 1.12**).

Between days 27 and 37, the cardiac septum develops from structures called endocardial cushions. Cardiac valves and major vessels also develop. The heart is fully formed by week 7.

> **Ventricular septal defect is one of the commonest congenital heart anomalies (5 per 1000 live births).** It is caused by improper formation of the wall between the two ventricles. Small ventricular septal defects are often asymptomatic and may go undetected. Large defects result in heart failure, with symptoms including breathlessness, poor feeding and failure to gain weight.

Head and neck

The structures of the head and neck develop from five pairs of pharyngeal arches (1st, 2nd, 3rd, 4th and 6th), which appear early in the 4th week and are located on the lateral walls of the pharynx (**Figure 1.13**). They are symmetrical, located on either side of the pharynx, and grow ventrally to meet medially.

> **The 5th pharyngeal arch is a transient structure.** It regresses and does not form any permanent structures.

The pharyngeal arches consist of a mesoderm core lined externally with ectoderm and internally with endoderm. The arches are separated by deep pouches. Each pharyngeal arch develops its own blood vessels, nerves, muscle and cartilage from the neural crest cells that migrate into it, resulting in formation of specific structures for each pharyngeal arch (**Table 1.5**).

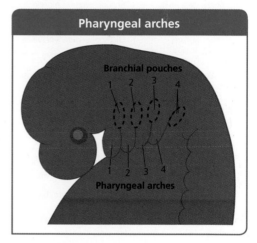

Figure 1.13 Location of pharyngeal arches, which form structures of the head and neck. Arch 6 is not visible on the external surface of the embryo.

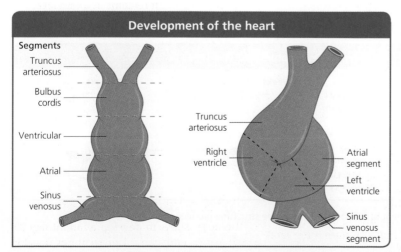

Figure 1.12 Looping and folding of the endocardial tube during development of the heart.

Fates of pharyngeal structures	
Pharyngeal structure	Derived structures
1st pharyngeal arch	Upper and lower jaw
	Palate
	Small bones of ear
	Trigeminal nerve
	Muscles of mastication
1st pharyngeal pouch	Middle ear
	Eustachian tube
2nd pharyngeal arch	Hyoid bone
	Muscles of facial expression
	Facial nerve
2nd pharyngeal pouch	Supratonsillar fossa
3rd pharyngeal arch	Stylopharyngeus muscle
	Part of hyoid bone
	Glossopharyngeal nerve
	Internal carotid artery
3rd pharyngeal pouch	Inferior parathyroid glands
	Thymus gland
4th and 6th pharyngeal arches	Right subclavian artery
	Aorta
	Vagus nerve
	Muscles and cartilage of the pharynx and larynx
4th pharyngeal pouch	Superior parathyroid glands

Table 1.5 Fates of the pharyngeal arches and pouches

Face

The face is formed between the 4th and 8th weeks (**Figure 1.14**). It arises from:

- the **frontonasal prominence**, which arises from neural crest cells
- the **maxillary and mandibular prominences**, which arise from the 1st pharyngeal arch

The nose forms from swellings and pits that form on the frontonasal prominence.

The frontonasal prominence forms the bridge of the nose, the forehead and the frontal and nasal bones. The maxillary prominences form the upper lip and cheeks, maxilla, zygomatic bone and palate. The mandibular processes form the chin, lower lips and lower cheek and mandible. The stomodeum is a depression that becomes the mouth.

Musculoskeletal system

The musculoskeletal system comprises muscle, cartilage and bone, which arise from the mesoderm layer of germ cells. Somites, segments of paraxial mesoderm that develop in week 3 along the length of the embryo in a rostral to caudal direction, differentiate into:

- **dermatomyotomes**, which form the skeletal muscle of the trunk and limbs, the cartilage and the skin
- **sclerotomes**, which form the spine and ribs

The limbs grow from limb buds, which develop from somites, and appear at week 4. The limb buds elongate to form primitive fingers and toes, which are present by about day 40 (**Figure 1.15**). The spaces between each finger or toe form by apoptosis (programmed cell

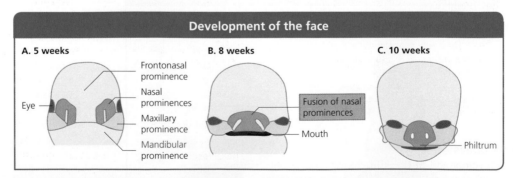

Development of the face

A. 5 weeks

Eye

Frontonasal prominence

Nasal prominences

Maxillary prominence

Mandibular prominence

B. 8 weeks

Fusion of nasal prominences

Mouth

C. 10 weeks

Philtrum

Figure 1.14 Development of the face from the three structural prominences.

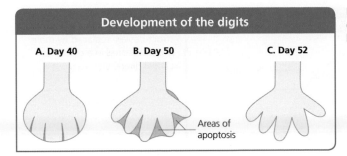

Development of the digits

A. Day 40   **B. Day 50**   **C. Day 52**

Areas of
apoptosis

Figure 1.15 Development of the
digits, which grow from limb
buds.

death), leaving individual digits by the end of
the 8th week.

> **Failure of apoptosis between the digits
> results in webbing between adjacent
> fingers or toes.** This condition is called
> syndactyly.

Urogenital system

The formation and development of the urinary system and the genital system are closely associated. They develop from intermediate mesoderm forming a urogenital ridge on either side of the aorta. They are close in proximity and briefly share a common excretory duct (cloaca).

Urinary system

This is made up of the kidneys, ureters, bladder and urethra. The kidneys appear to 'migrate' upwards from the pelvis to their final position in the lumbar area around week 8. This is the consequence of elongation of the lumbar area and loss of the 'c' shape folding as the embryo grows, giving the illusion of movement.

> **Failure of a kidney to ascend results
> in the kidney being located in the
> pelvis, i.e. a pelvic kidney.** This is often
> an incidental finding because it has
> no impact on the kidneys' ability to
> function.

Kidneys

Development of the kidneys starts with formation of tubular nephric structures, the primitive kidneys, from the urogenital ridge. Development proceeds in three successive stages: pronephros, mesonephros and metanephros. These structures form in a cranial to caudal direction, with one replacing the other as the kidney becomes more advanced and capable of function (**Figure 1.16**). The definitive kidney becomes functional during the 12th week. The urine it produces is excreted into the amniotic fluid.

Pronephros The pronephros is the first stage of renal development. The pair of pronephri form at the start of the 4th week, in the cervical region. They are essentially early renal tubules that are non-functioning and disappear by week 5.

Mesonephros The next stage is the mesonephros. The mesonephri develop later in week 4, in the thoracolumbar area of the embryo. The mesonephros forms a mesonephric duct (also known as the Wolffian duct) and mesonephric tubules. The mesonephric tubules form renal corpuscles and begin to filter blood, and the filtrate drains into the mesonephric duct. The mesonephric tubules regress, but the mesonephric duct persists and opens into the cloaca at the tail of the embryo.

Metanephros The metanephros is the final stage of kidney development; it gives rise to the definitive adult kidney. The metanephros forms at week 5 from an outgrowth of the mesonephric duct called the ureteric bud and intermediate mesoderm termed metanephric blastema. The metanephric blastema develops into the renal corpuscles and tubules. The ureteric bud develops to form the collecting system of the ureter, renal pelvis, calyces and collecting tubules.

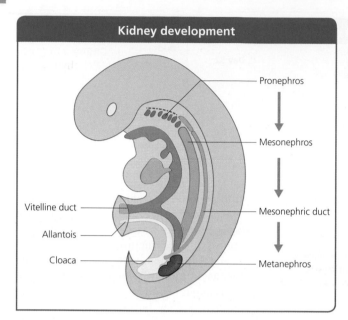

Kidney development

Pronephros

Mesonephros

Mesonephric duct

Metanephros

Vitelline duct

Allantois

Cloaca

Figure 1.16 The stages of kidney development. The primitive structures are replaced by more advanced ones in a cranial to caudal direction.

Bladder and urethra

The endoderm of the hindgut forms the epithelium of the urinary bladder and most of the urethra. During the 4th to 7th week, the urogenital septum divides the cloaca into the anorectal canal and the primitive urogenital sinus. The bladder forms from the urogenital sinus and the surrounding mesoderm, as does the female urethra and most of the male urethra.

Genital system

The genital system, consisting of the internal and external sex organs, does not start to differentiate into male or female organs until week 7. Before this, the gonads and reproductive tracts are undifferentiated.

The **earliest that a baby's sex can be determined** on an antenatal US scan is at 16 weeks' gestation.

Internal genitalia

Primitive gonads develop, from intermediate mesoderm, at the rostral end of the mesonephric duct during the 5th week of embryonic life. At about day 46, a paramesonephric (Müllerian) duct forms parallel to the mesonephric duct.

Testes-determining factor, a protein located on the Y chromosome, initiates male differentiation. The absence of expression of this protein means that female genitalia will develop.

Male genitalia In males, at about 7 weeks, the primitive gonads develop into testicles and the mesonephric duct forms the vas deferens. The paramesonephric duct regresses.

Female genitalia In females, at about 7 weeks, the ovaries develop from the primitive gonads, the mesonephric duct regresses, and the paramesonephric ducts become the uterus and fallopian tubes.

The testes descend from their abdominal location into the scrotum through the inguinal canal, at about 33 weeks. Checking whether both testes have descended into the scrotum is part of the standard examination of newborn babies.

External genitalia

The penis and clitoris develop from the genital tubercle in males and females, respectively. The lateral genital swellings form the scrotum in males and labia majora in females; these structures start to form at 6 weeks.

- In males, dihydrotestosterone produced by the testes stimulates growth of the penis and scrotum at about 11 weeks
- In females, oestrogen produced by the ovaries stimulates the labia and clitoris to develop at about 11 weeks

Other structures of the external genitalia develop from the cloaca, the common opening of the digestive, urinary and, in females, the genital tracts. A urorectal septum develops to separate the rectum on the dorsal side from the bladder, urethra and, in females, the lower part of the vagina on the ventral side (**Figure 1.17**).

Fetal period

The second period of prenatal development begins at 9 weeks, the point at which the embryo is now termed the fetus. Throughout this period, which culminates in birth at about 38 weeks, the organ systems formed in the embryonic period continue to grow and mature. The focus is on growth of the fetus, in both length and weight, along with the laying down of fat stores to provide the neonate with an energy reserve for use after birth.

> **The age at which a fetus is considered viable varies between countries. In the UK it is 23 weeks' gestation (embryonic age, 21 weeks)**. Resuscitation is not attempted for babies born before this.

The placenta

The placenta is the temporary organ of pregnancy that attaches the fetus to the uterine wall. This arrangement enables the exchange of gases between the maternal and fetal circulations: oxygen to the fetus, and carbon dioxide to the mother. Nutrients pass from mother to fetus via the placenta, and waste products pass from fetus to mother.

Maternal antibodies cross the placenta, thereby giving the fetus immunity to diseases to which the mother is immune without encountering them itself (passive immunity). The placenta also secretes several hormones, including human chorionic gonadotrophin, oestrogen and progesterone, which maintain the pregnancy (preventing miscarriage) and promote changes in the mother's body in preparation for birth, for example softening of pelvic ligaments and growth of breast tissue.

> **A small number of fetal cells enter the maternal circulation** via microscopic breaks in the placental membrane. These cells can be isolated from maternal blood and used for prenatal testing for genetic conditions such as Edwards' syndrome. This is known as non-invasive prenatal testing.

Development of the placenta

The placenta develops from the trophoblast layer of the blastocyst. During week 2, the trophoblasts form finger-like projections

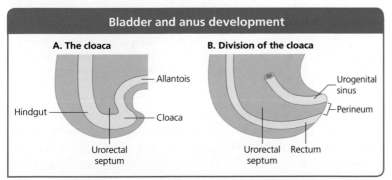

Bladder and anus development

A. The cloaca

Hindgut

Allantois

Cloaca

Urorectal septum

B. Division of the cloaca

Urogenital sinus

Perineum

Urorectal septum   Rectum

Figure 1.17
Development of the bladder and anus. (a) The cloaca. (b) The cloaca divides to form the rectum and urogenital sinus.

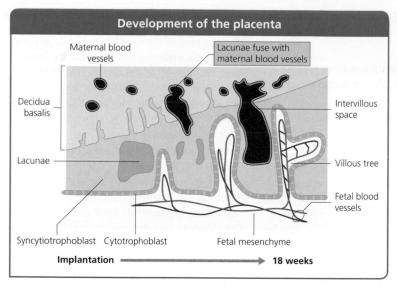

Development of the placenta

Maternal blood vessels

Lacunae fuse with maternal blood vessels

Decidua basalis

Intervillous space

Lacunae

Villous tree

Fetal blood vessels

Syncytiotrophoblast   Cytotrophoblast   Fetal mesenchyme

Implantation ⟶ **18 weeks**

Figure 1.18 The development of the placenta from implantation to 18 weeks.

(villi) extending into the endometrium (the mucous membrane lining the uterus) (**Figure 1.18**). The space surrounding the villi are filled with blood from the maternal uterine arteries, and gas exchange between the maternal and fetal circulations occurs by the 4th week. Nutrients, waste products and gases diffuse across the placental membrane between the blood vessels of the mother and those of the fetus, but the maternal and fetal blood do not mix.

> **An excess of amniotic fluid is termed polyhydramnios.** It is associated with several conditions, including oesophageal atresia, in which the fetus is unable to swallow the fluid, which therefore accumulates.

Amnion and amniotic fluid

The embryo is surrounded by two fluid-filled sacs produced when the blastocyst forms in the very early stages of pregnancy. These are the amniotic sac, which contains the amniotic fluid, and the yolk sac. The amnion is the membrane that fills with amniotic fluid. The fetus is suspended in the amniotic sac by the umbilical cord.

The functions of amniotic fluid are to:

- protect the fetus by acting as a shock absorber
- allow fetal movements, which are necessary for normal musculoskeletal development
- aid lung development, by expanding the lungs thereby preventing hypoplasia
- provide basic nutrients, i.e. water, electrolytes and proteins, to help the fetus grow

Adaptations at birth

Starter questions

Answers to the following questions are on page 46.

4. Why do babies cry at birth?
5. Why do many newborn babies have an audible murmur in the first few hours which is not there the next day?
6. Are elective caesarean sections risk-free?

In the uterus, the fetus relies on the umbilical cord and placenta for gas exchange, the provision of nutrients and the elimination of waste. At birth, clamping of the umbilical cord causes loss of oxygenation from the placenta, which results in changes to the baby's circulation. In addition, the baby's first cry aerates the lungs. This, and the baby's subsequent breathing, enables oxygenation from the baby's lungs rather than the placenta. These changes are described separately below but occur simultaneously immediately after birth.

> **Although the walls of the umbilical vein come together to stem bleeding, it remains patent (open) for the first few days after birth.** This means that it is possible to insert a large central venous catheter into the lumen of the umbilical vein for long enough for it to be used as a route of IV access in the sick neonate. This is also true for the umbilical arteries. The umbilical vein eventually becomes the ligamentum teres, passing from the umbilicus to the porta hepatis.

Cardiovascular system

The path of circulation of blood in the fetus is very different to that in the newborn baby (**Figure 1.19**). Oxygenated blood supplied to the fetus originates from the placenta, whereas a baby's blood is oxygenated by the lungs. Three structures have roles in the transitional circulation:

- the ductus venosus
- the foramen ovale
- the ductus arteriosus

Fetal circulation

Blood flows directly across the fetal heart, directed by the relatively high resistance to flow through the lungs compared with the lower resistance across the atrial septal opening, the foramen ovale, in the heart. In addition, in fetal life the ductus arteriosus diverts blood from the right ventricle and pulmonary artery into the descending aorta, so that it further bypasses the lungs and left side of the heart; this results in right-to-left flow. In the fetus, half most of the blood blood from the umbilical vein flows directly into the inferior vena cava via the ductus venosus, thereby bypassing the liver. A smaller volume of blood from the umbilical vein flows into the sinusoids (small blood vessels) of the liver before entering the inferior vena cava.

Circulatory changes at birth

At delivery, the ductus venosus constricts so that all blood passes through the liver into the inferior vena cava. The ductus venosus becomes the remnant called the ligamentum venosum, which passes through the liver from the portal vein to the inferior vena cava.

At birth, the baby takes its first breath, which increases blood flow to and from the lungs. Also, the placental circulation is removed by clamping of the umbilical cord, which increases systemic vascular resistance (see **Figure 1.19b**). This leads to:

- closure of the ductus arteriosus by muscular contraction of its wall, which dramatically increases blood flow through the lungs,

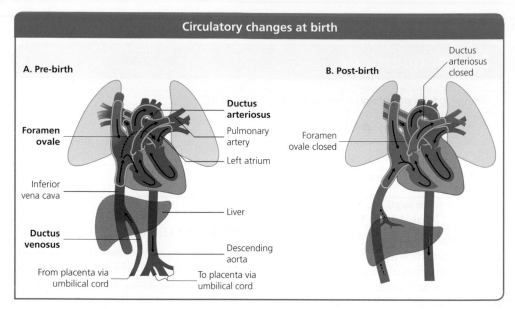

Figure 1.19 The circulatory changes that occur at birth. (a) The circulation before birth. The dashed arrows show flow from the inferior vena cava, through the foramen ovale, into the left atrium. (b) The circulation after birth.

leading to increased pressure in the left atrium compared with the right atrium

- closure of the foramen ovale as the difference between left and right atrial pressures forces a flap of tissue called the septum primum against the atrial septum

The foramen ovale usually closes functionally at birth. However, anatomical closure, which is achieved by tissue proliferation and adhesion, takes many months. Similarly, functional closure of the ductus arteriosus usually occurs in the first few days after birth, but anatomical closure, resulting in formation of the ligamentum arteriosum, is not complete until 12 weeks of age.

At birth, the right ventricular wall is similar in thickness to the left ventricular wall, reflecting the equal resistance to flow and therefore the equal work of the heart muscles of both ventricles in utero. In the first few months after birth, the right ventricle wall gradually thins and the left ventricular wall thickens, because the right ventricle has to pump only against the relatively low resistance in the pulmonary artery, and the left ventricle has to pump against the higher pressure in the aorta.

Patent ductus arteriosus is the consequence of failure of the ductus arteriosus to close after birth. Because the ductus arteriosus remains open, it allows blood to flow from the aorta to the pulmonary artery (left-to-right flow) after birth. The ductus arteriosus may close in the first few weeks, especially in the preterm baby. However, patent ductus arteriosus that persists after a few months usually requires surgical intervention to achieve closure.

Respiratory system

Prenatally, the fetal lungs are filled with fluid and the pulmonary vessels are vasoconstricted. At birth, the baby takes deep breaths, which promotes the absorption of this fluid from the alveoli into the lymphatics and bloodstream. A small amount of fluid is also expelled via the bronchi and trachea. With respiration, air enters the lungs, which expand to fill the pleural cavity.

Persistent pulmonary hypertension of the newborn is a life-threatening condition caused by failure of the normal adaptations at birth. The condition is usually triggered by underlying lung pathology such as meconium aspiration, congenital pneumonia or lung hypoplasia.

Pulmonary vascular resistance is increased in the fetus, which causes the circulating blood to pass through the heart bypassing the lungs (**Figure 1.19a**). This is a consequence of two main factors. First, in utero there is relative hypoxia (low oxygen levels in the blood), which is a potent vasoconstrictor. Second, the fetal lungs are not fully expanded, being full of fluid rather than air, and this causes mechanical compression of the vessels. When the neonate takes its first few breaths at birth, the consequent removal of lung fluid and aeration of the lungs leads to:

- straightening of mechanically compressed vessels and thinning of the muscular walls of the pulmonary arteries by stretching of the lungs, thereby decreasing pulmonary vascular resistance and markedly increasing pulmonary blood flow
- increasing levels of oxygen in the alveoli, resulting in oxygenation of the blood

Normal growth

Starter questions

Answers to the following questions are on page 46.

7.   Why is a child's length longer than their height?
8.   Why are wrist X-rays used to estimate a child's age?
9.   Why are teenagers often described as being 'all hands and feet'?
10. Why do teenagers develop body odour?

A child's growth is the progressive increase in body mass over time – the child becomes larger. The term 'growth' is also applied to physical development, such as the many changes that occur at puberty. Growth in height occurs through lengthening of the long bones and spine, and is accompanied by corresponding increases in the volume of muscle mass, internal organs and tissues.

Maternal nutrition and the intrauterine environment are the primary influences on the size of the baby at birth and in the first month. Infant nutrition is the main determinant of growth in the first year, and genetic influences have more effect thereafter.

Most healthy children grow in a predictable pattern. Normal growth is pulsatile, with periods of rapid growth ('growth spurts') interspersed with periods of no measurable growth. It is also seasonal, with increased growth in spring and summer.

Different terms are used to describe children at different ages:

- neonate, birth to 28 days
- infant, 28 days to 1 year
- child, 1–10 years
- toddler, 1–3 years
- young child, 4–6 years
- older child, 7–10 years
- adolescent, 11–17 years

Growth variables

At regular assessments of child health and development (see Chapter 2), the growth variables that are measured are:

- weight
- height, or length if under 2 years of age, and
- head circumference

The results are compared against normal ranges on centile charts (**Figure 1.20**). These are derived from population studies in large numbers of children, and there are separate male and female charts, and charts for specific populations.

Within a given population at a given age, characteristics such as weight and height follow a normal distribution (a Gaussian distribution), as shown in **Figure 1.21**. There is a relationship between this and the centile data:

- centiles correspond to areas under the normal distribution curve
- the 50th centile equals the population mean, i.e. the average (note that it is not an 'ideal')
- the number of children more than 2 standard deviations (SDs) below the mean equals the number who are more than 2 SDs above the mean, and this corresponds approximately to the 3rd and 97th centiles

Assessing growth

A child is judged to have normal growth if they approximately follow a centile line.

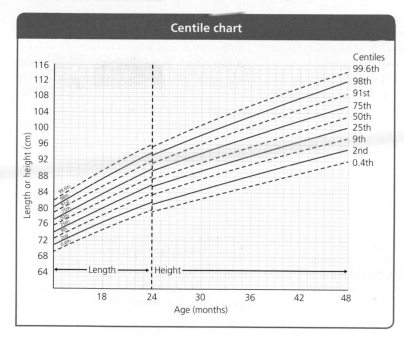

Figure 1.20 A centile chart for height in boys aged 0–4 years.

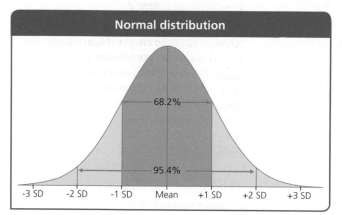

Figure 1.21 A normal (i.e. gaussian) distribution, showing the percentages of the population that fall within 1 standard deviation (SD) and 2 SDs of the mean.

All processes in growth are dynamic, so a single point on a centile chart, unless well outside the 3rd or 97th centiles, must interpreted with caution. For correct interpretation, centiles for more than one variable need to be determined together, for example weight and height. For children younger than 2 years, head circumference is also compared against the normal range. Additionally, body mass index (BMI) can be used to assess children over 2 years of age.

> **Body mass index is the relative proportion between the child's weight (in kilograms) and their height (in metres) squared.** For children over 2 years of age, BMI can be plotted on centile charts to diagnose overweight and obesity, and also to detect cases of undernutrition.

Serial measurements are more useful than single values. They enable assessment of the child's progress over time, which is necessary given the pulsatile and seasonal nature of growth (see below). It is also helpful to obtain measurements of the parents' heights to determine the child's genetic potential. In this way, it is possible to determine whether a child's short stature, for example, is more likely to be familial (as is usual) or caused by an underlying disorder. The further away a child's measurements lie from the population mean and from the midparental target height, the more likely the presence of an underlying pathology.

> When assessing a child's height, midparental target height is considered, as well as population standards. It is the mean of the father's and mother's heights, and therefore the expected height of the child on reaching adulthood.

Weight

In the first week after birth, a baby normally loses about 5–10% of birthweight because of loss of extracellular fluid. However, by about the age of 2 weeks, they have started to gain weight and then grow quickly with their first growth spurt. By the age of 4–6 months, a baby's weight is usually double the birthweight, and treble by 12 months.

Between the ages of 1 and 5 years, the average child gains about 2 kg/year. They continue to grow at a steady pace until a further growth spurt begins at the start of puberty, sometime between the ages of 9 and 15 years.

Height

Postnatal linear growth, i.e. increase in height or length, occurs in three phases:

- infancy (birth to 1 year)
- childhood (from 12 months to onset of puberty)
- puberty

During infancy, nutrition is the main influence on growth, so obesity may correlate with tall stature. During childhood, During

infancy, nutrition is the main influence on growth, so obesity may cause tall stature. During childhood, growth hormone and insulin-like growth factor (IGF 1) are the two main hormones influencing linear growth. During puberty, the sex hormones have a major effect on growth. Therefore normal linear growth reflects the weight in the first year, with length increasing 25 cm/year on average. After it slows to an average growth of about 5 cm/year between the age of 4 years and puberty. Height velocity usually decelerates before the pubertal growth spurt.

> In boys, the onset of the pubertal growth spurt occurs relatively late in puberty compared with the early growth spurt in girls.

Height velocity

This is calculated from differences in height measurements over a period of time. In children older than 2 years measurements are taken at intervals of at least 3 months over a period of at least 1 year.

Height velocities stay much closer to the 50th centile than absolute measurements of height. Growth accelerates during the pubertal growth spurt, but the timing of the peak of this growth spurt varies widely from child to child (**Figure 1.22**).

Head circumference

Head circumference increases in line with the increase in weight in the first year, doubling by 4–6 months of age and trebling by 1 year. Most head growth is complete by 4 years of age.

Phases of growth

Growth occurs in four distinct phases:

- the **intrauterine phase** (8 weeks embryonic age to birth), with physical growth greatest in the third trimester
- **infancy and early childhood** (birth to 18 months), a phase of rapid growth
- **childhood** (18 months to the onset of puberty), a phase of slow, steady growth

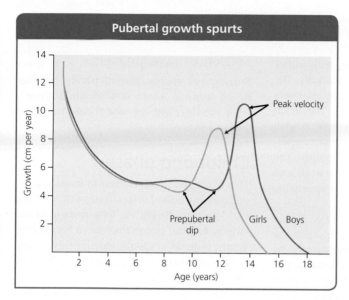

Figure 1.22 Growth spurts of puberty and height velocity.

- **puberty** (from 10 years in girls and 12 years in boys, on average), a phase of rapid growth initially, followed by a gradually slowing down of growth

Intrauterine phase

Intrauterine growth occurs from an embryonic age of about 8 weeks, when the major organs have been formed and continue to increase in size. Growth during this time depends on three sets of factors: maternal, uteroplacental and fetal.

> **Fetal growth is mediated by insulin, insulin-like growth factor (IGF) 1, IGF 2 and maternal nutrition.** It is independent of endogenous growth hormone.

Maternal factors

For optimal intrauterine growth, the mother requires a diet that ensures good nutrition, including intake of a sufficient amount of iron. Pre-existing chronic conditions affecting the mother, including diabetes and cardiac, renal or respiratory conditions, can restrict the growth of the fetus, primarily by their effects on placental function. Fetal growth is also restricted by maternal smoking, which reduces placental blood flow.

> **Iron deficiency anaemia during pregnancy is associated with preterm delivery, low birthweight and infant mortality.** Iron is vital for maternal haemoglobin synthesis and also growth of the fetus and placenta.

Uteroplacental factors

For fetal growth to occur, the placenta must be functioning adequately to deliver nutrients to the fetus, remove waste products and enable the exchange of gases between fetal and maternal blood. If growth falters, placental function is assessed by using Doppler US to measure blood flow in the umbilical arteries. Absent or reversed Doppler blood flow in the umbilical arteries is associated with an abnormal placenta and increased risk of fetal demise. This finding usually triggers urgent delivery, even if this means that the baby will be born before term.

Fetal factors

Intrauterine infection, caused by transfer of an infection (e.g. rubella or cytomegalovirus) from mother to fetus, can cause growth restriction (see page 146). Chromosomal abnormalities can also result in poor growth, e.g. in Down's syndrome or Turner's syndrome.

Infancy and early childhood phase

The proportions of an infant's body differ from those of older children and adults. The head and trunk of the infant are relatively large compared with the limbs. The brain grows rapidly during the first 6 months, with a corresponding increase in head circumference of 8 cm on average. After 6 months, the limbs grow more rapidly than the head and trunk, which results in the limbs appearing longer in proportion.

Growth is slower in infancy than during the fetal period. However, it is still rapid; the average infant is double its birthweight by 5–6 months of age. Growth in infancy and early childhood depends mainly on adequate nutrition, although normal thyroid function is also essential because it contributes to growth during this phase

The body composition of a newborn differs from that of older children, with a higher proportion of body water and lower stores of fat and protein. Therefore, to maintain their rapid growth, babies need more calories per kilogram of weight. Adequate intake of iron is essential for normal neurodevelopment, and vitamin D supplementation is recommended for bone mineralisation in countries in which the population has limited exposure to sunlight, such as the UK.

Neonatal weight loss

Most newborns experience a normal weight loss in the first 3–5 days of life, of up to 5% of their birthweight. This is a consequence of movement of water, by osmosis, from the intracellular to the extracellular compartment, followed by diuresis (elimination of the excess water via urination). The weight loss occurs regardless of the method of feeding, although breastfed babies tend to lose more weight than formula-fed babies (an average of 6–7% of birthweight). This difference probably reflects the fact that breastfed babies consume a much smaller volume of fluid initially, because colostrum (the first milk produced) is much more energy- and nutrient-rich than infant formula (see page 39).

Subsequent weight gain

Subsequent weight gain depends on adequate feeding. About 80% of babies regain their birthweight by the time they are 2 weeks old.

Childhood phase

This phase, which lasts from 18 months until puberty, is a period of steady growth, with the child gaining height via lengthening of the long bones and spine. The rate of increase in height reduces gradually during this phase, from about 9 cm/year to about 5 cm/year by the age of 10 years.

Significant brain growth continues during this phase and as a result the brain reaches almost its adult volume by the age of 5 years. Adequate nutrition remains necessary, but growth during middle childhood depends mostly on hormonal influences. Deficiencies of either result in faltering growth (see pages 63 and 332).

> **Beyond infancy and before puberty, growth of the healthy child progresses in line with the reference centiles.** Obese children will be taller than expected from mid-parental height, and taller than most of their peers at a relatively early age. Chronic illness usually has more of an effect on weight than on height.

Hormones affecting growth

Growth hormone and thyroid hormones are the key determinants of growth during middle childhood.

Growth hormone

Growth hormone is secreted by the anterior pituitary gland in response to growth hormone–releasing hormone (GHRH) released from the hypothalamus. GHRH is secreted in pulses, triggered by multiple stimuli including exercise; secretion peaks after the onset of deep sleep.

Growth hormone acts in two ways (**Figure 1.23**).

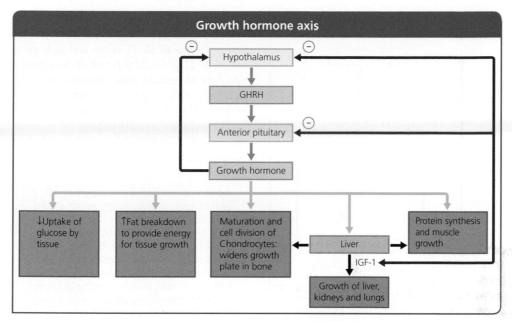

Figure 1.23 The growth hormone axis: growth hormone acts tissues either directly or indirectly via IGF-1. GHRH, growth hormone–releasing hormone; IGF-1, insulin-like growth factor 1.

- It acts by stimulating cell division and maturation of chondrocytes (cartilage-forming cells) in the epiphyseal growth plates; this leads to widening of the growth plate and lengthening of the bone as the cartilaginous material later ossifies
- It acts indirectly by stimulating the liver to release IGF 1, which then stimulates growth of many tissues in the body including muscle, cartilage, bone, liver and nerves

> **Children with isolated growth hormone deficiency have similar weight and length to the normal population at birth. However, by the age of 2 years they are shorter and stockier than their peers.**

Thyroid hormones

The thyroid hormones, i.e. tri-iodothyronine and thyroxine, are necessary for normal growth throughout childhood (they are also essential for the development of the central nervous system in the fetus and infant). The thyroid hormones promote protein synthesis and, along with with growth hormone, promote bone growth. Their release from the thyroid is under the control of the hypothalamus, acting via the pituitary gland (**Figure 1.24**).

> **In malnutrition, growth is impaired by inhibition of the production of IGF 1 as well as the lack of nutrients or substrate necessary for growth.**

Puberty phase

This is the period of transition from childhood to adulthood, when an individual becomes physically and sexually mature and physiologically capable of reproduction. The reproductive organs, which have undergone only minimal growth since infancy, enlarge and mature rapidly during puberty.

Puberty usually follows a predictable sequence of events (**Table 1.6**). One of the first signs of puberty in girls is the pubertal growth spurt, an acceleration of growth in height. Boys also experience a pubertal growth spurt, but it occurs later than in girls.

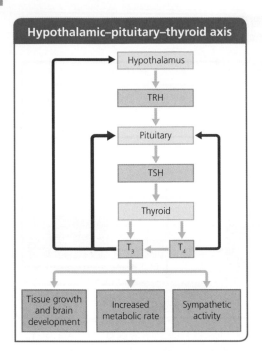

Hypothalamic–pituitary–thyroid axis

Figure 1.24 The hypothalamic–pituitary–thyroid axis. Most of the action and negative feedback is mediated by tri-iodothyronine (T3), formed from the peripheral conversion of thyroxine (T4). TRH, thyrotropin-releasing hormone; TSH, thyroid-stimulating hormone.

The timing of achievement of the various milestones of puberty and the age at which this phase is complete vary between individuals (**Figure 1.25**). On average, girls enter puberty at about 10 years of age and boys about 2 years later. Puberty is completed in girls at about the age of 15–17 years, and in boys at about 16–17 years. This is one of the reasons why men are usually taller than women; boys have more time to grow taller before they experience the pubertal growth spurt, and take longer to reach the end of puberty (after which there is minimal further growth in height), so boys have a longer time to grow overall.

> **Adolescence is the period between 10 and 19 years of age, during which a child becomes an independent adult.** It is a time of emotional, psychological and social maturation. To help them with this transition, adolescents should be treated in a manner that acknowledges their increasing independence and helps them to take responsibility for their own health.

Hormonal control

The exact trigger initiating puberty is unknown. Puberty itself is controlled by hormones of the hypothalamic–pituitary–gonadal axis (**Figure 1.26**). It begins with increasing pulsatile secretion of gonadotrophin-releasing hormone from the hypothalamus. The increasing levels of gonadotrophin-releasing hormone stimulate the release of the gonadotrophins, i.e. follicle-stimulating hormone and luteinising hormone, from the anterior pituitary gland.

Pubertal milestones

Milestone	Definition	Timing
Adrenarche	Activation of the zona reticularis in the adrenal cortex, leading to increased production of adrenal androgens	Before puberty, at 6–8 years of age
Thelarche (girls)	Breast development	2–3 years before menarche
Gonadarche	Increasing testicular volume	About 12 years of age
Pubarche	Appearance of pubic hair	Girls: about 6 months after thelarche (but in a minority, pubic hair is the first sign of puberty) Boys: 1–2 years after initial testicular enlargement
Menarche (girls)	Onset of menstruation	Just under 13 years of age, on average
Spermarche (boys)	Onset of sperm production	13–14 years of age, on average

Table 1.6 Milestones of puberty.

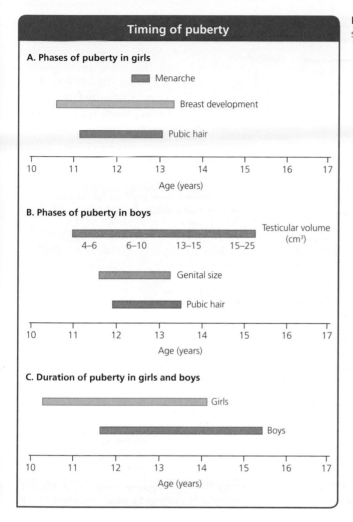

Figure 1.25 Timing of the sequence of events in puberty.

This, in turn, leads to the release of sex hormones: oestrogen from the ovaries and testosterone from the testes.

Adrenarche

The hypothalamic–pituitary–gonadal axis is not the only source of the sex hormones that regulate the changes that occur during puberty. Adrenarche, which occurs a few years before the start of puberty, leads to a slow rise in circulation of weak androgens ('male' steroid hormones). In some children, this is associated with the appearance of pubic and axillary (armpit) hair and the development of sebaceous glands; in others, it is a completely asymptomatic event. The trigger for adrenarche is unknown.

Physical features

The main physical changes during puberty are development of secondary sexual characteristics, i.e. the characteristics that define the male or female sex but are not present at birth or directly part of the reproductive systems.

Both girls and boys undergo a growth spurt during puberty, which accounts for about 17% of their final adult height. It occurs during early puberty in girls and later puberty in boys (see **Figure 1.25**). The main factors promoting this growth are oestrogen and growth hormone, although (as with all other periods of growth) normal thyroid function and adequate nutrition are also essential.

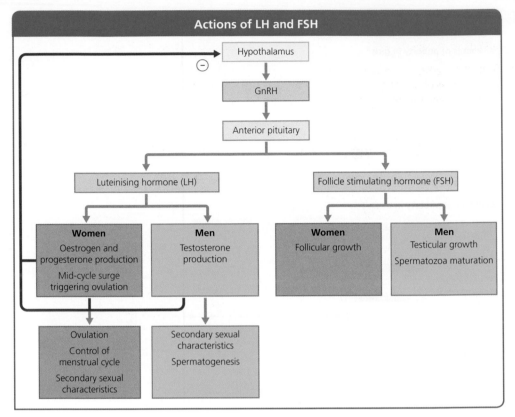

Figure 1.26 Actions of luteinising hormone (LH) and follicle stimulating hormone (FSH) in men and women. GnRH, gonadotrophin-releasing hormone.

Oestrogen promotes bone growth by increasing secretion of growth hormone. This, in turn, increases production of IGF 1, which stimulates growth of many body tissues. Therefore the initial effect of oestrogen is to promote growth. However, at the end of puberty oestrogen is responsible for the maturation of chondrocytes and osteoblasts, which ultimately leads to fusion of the epiphyseal plates, thereby preventing further growth.

Side effects of puberty

The changing hormone levels during puberty have various secondary effects, some of which may be distressing (**Table 1.7**). Increased androgen levels lead to increased production of sebum in the skin, which in excess contributes to the development of acne; this is a very common problem. Most cases of acne can be managed at home with the use of over-the-counter washes and ointments. However, severe cases require referral to a dermatologist (see page 364).

Side effects of puberty and their causes	
Side effect	Cause
Acne	Increased sebum production in the skin
Moodiness	Increase in sex hormone production
Body odour	Bacterial breakdown of sweat produced by apocrine glands
Gynaecomastia (breast tissue enlargement in males)	Oestrogen and testosterone imbalance

Table 1.7 Potentially distressing side effects of puberty and their causes

Another problem related to changing hormone levels during puberty is gynaecomastia (enlargement of male breast tissue); this affects nearly half of boys at some point during puberty. Gynaecomastia is the consequence of several factors that contribute to an imbalance of oestrogens and testosterone. The condition is not pathological, and it resolves spontaneously later in puberty.

Tanner staging

The progress of puberty is assessed in a standardised way by using the Tanner stages. These describe the development of each feature of puberty from the prepubertal stage until adult maturity (**Figures 1.27**).

Changes in girls

The duration of puberty in girls varies between individuals. It is related to the

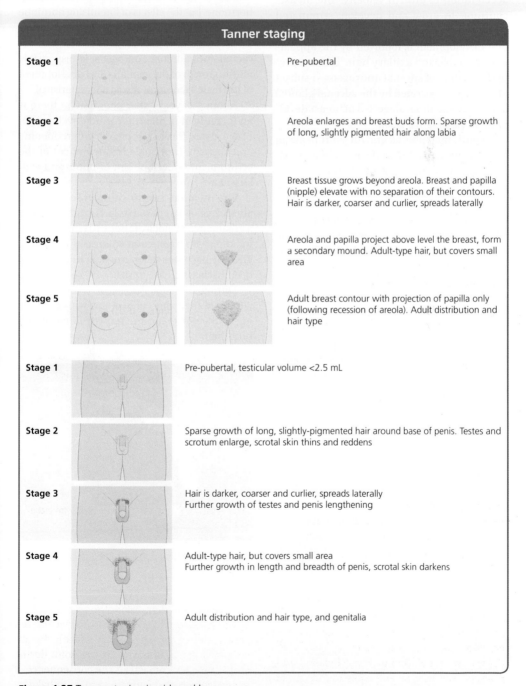

Tanner staging

Stage 1			Pre-pubertal
Stage 2			Areola enlarges and breast buds form. Sparse growth of long, slightly pigmented hair along labia
Stage 3			Breast tissue grows beyond areola. Breast and papilla (nipple) elevate with no separation of their contours. Hair is darker, coarser and curlier, spreads laterally
Stage 4			Areola and papilla project above level the breast, form a secondary mound. Adult-type hair, but covers small area
Stage 5			Adult breast contour with projection of papilla only (following recession of areola). Adult distribution and hair type
Stage 1			Pre-pubertal, testicular volume <2.5 mL
Stage 2			Sparse growth of long, slightly-pigmented hair around base of penis. Testes and scrotum enlarge, scrotal skin thins and reddens
Stage 3			Hair is darker, coarser and curlier, spreads laterally. Further growth of testes and penis lengthening
Stage 4			Adult-type hair, but covers small area. Further growth in length and breadth of penis, scrotal skin darkens
Stage 5			Adult distribution and hair type, and genitalia

Figure 1.27 Tanner staging in girls and boys.

timing of onset; the earlier the onset of puberty, the longer its duration.

Breast bud development The first physical changes apparent in girls is the development of breast buds, i.e. small growths of breast tissue under each nipple and areola, and an acceleration of growth velocity. The breasts continue to grow and develop, stimulated by oestrogen secreted by the ovaries. Breast bud development is followed by the appearance of pubic and axillary hair. This is a secondary effect of adrenal androgens (a subset of androgens secreted by the adrenal glands) and occurs at about stage 2–3 of breast development (see **Figure 1.25a**).

In girls, the pubertal growth spurt peaks at about stage 2–3 of breast development. Maximum growth velocity is about 8–9 cm/year.

Menarche This is the term for the first occurrence of menstruation,which usually occurs at about the age of 13 years, and 2–3 years after the onset of puberty. Oestrogen levels increase steadily from early puberty. One of its effects is enlargement of the uterus, and it also causes the ovaries and follicles to grow and mature. Once oestrogen levels are sustained the endometrium thickens. The effects of oestrogen, along with those of other hormones (including progesterone) and the onset of negative feedback, produce a cyclical pattern of endometrial thickening and loss. Very high mid-cycle levels of oestrogen cause a surge of luteinising hormone, which triggers ovulation; however, ovulatory cycles are often not consistently established until about a year after menarche.

Once menarche has been achieved, there is little subsequent growth in height (only about 5 cm).

Changes in boys
In boys, the first physical sign of puberty is increasing testicular volume (gonadarche) (see **Figure 1.25b**), which occurs at an average of 12 years of age. Testicular volume is measured by comparing the size of the testicles with the size of the 'beads' of an orchidometer (**Figure 1.28**). A boy has officially entered puberty when his testicular volume reaches 4 mL.

The increase in testicular size is mainly secondary to the secretion of follicle-stimulating hormone, but the effects of luteinising hormone also contribute. In turn, the testes begin to secrete testosterone and this, combined with the secretion of adrenal androgens, is responsible for the growth of the genitalia and development of the male secondary sexual characteristics.

About 1–2 years after gonadarche there is an increase in penile length and development of the glans. This is associated with reddening and rugosity (a wrinkled appearance) of the scrotum, and development of pubic and axillary hair.

The pubertal growth spurt in boys occurs about 2 years later than in girls, and it reaches a greater peak velocity (about 10 cm/year), coinciding with a testicular volume of 10–12 mL. The boy becomes taller and also broader, and his muscles increase in size.

During the final stages of puberty, boys complete their masculinisation with deepening of the voice and the growth of facial and body hair.

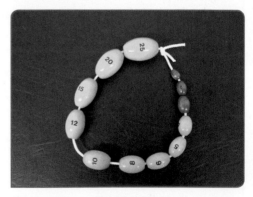

Figure 1.28 An orchidometer, used to measure testicular size.

Normal development

Starter questions

Answers to the following questions are on page 47.

11. When do children develop a hand preference?
12. Why should particular attention be paid to the social skills of a child with delayed speech?

Child development refers to how a child develops functional skills to change from being an immobile and fully dependent infant, through childhood, to become a fully functioning and independent young adult. Progress is monitored by noting the achievement of developmental milestones, which mark the acquisition of skills in four domains:

- **gross motor**, i.e. the skills of using large muscle groups such as the limbs and trunk, progressing from rolling to sitting to walking
- **fine motor**, i.e. skills performed by using the smaller muscles, for example manipulation of objects and drawing, achieved by the muscles of the hand
- **communication and language**, i.e. the use of gestures (non-verbal communication), the development of speech and the understanding of language
- **social**, i.e. the skills needed to interact appropriately with others and to carry out self-care activities such as feeding and toileting

Developmental milestones

An individual child's progress is assessed by recording when they have achieved developmental milestones in each of the four domains. The milestones are specific skills that developmentally normal children have attained by a certain age.

The age at which different children achieve each milestone varies widely. In recognition of this, age ranges are used to specify when each milestone would be expected to occur. The median age is the age at which half the population acquire that skill; it serves as a guide to normal development

If a child has an underlying impairment, development in the associated domain will be delayed. For example, a hearing deficit may underlie speech delay. Delay in achieving a particular milestone is often the first indication of underlying condition; for example, delay in walking may indicate Duchenne's muscular dystrophy (see page 261), and delay in acquiring fine motor skills in one hand compared with the other may indicate hemiplegic cerebral palsy. Delay can be in one domain (isolated specific delay) or several (global developmental delay).

Early detection enables prompt treatment of correctable conditions, particularly in cases of hearing or visual impairment, because interventions can be put in place to improve the problem, e.g. glasses or a hearing aid to halt or reverse the delay. It also means that the child can receive support to optimise their potential, including access to ongoing services, such as special schooling for children with complex needs (see page 427).

The term 'potential' is often used to refer to the possibility of a child with a developmental disorder, particularly an intellectual disability, leading a full and enjoyable life both in childhood and continuing into adulthood. Early recognition of any delays in achieving developmental milestones, followed by timely provision of appropriate treatment and support for both the child and their family, helps increase the likelihood of these children fulfilling their potential.

Any individual child will not be at the same stage of development in all domains at the same time. For example, some children advance more rapidly in their gross motor skills than in their speech (in the communication and language domain), and vice versa, even within the same family.

Provided that developmental milestones are achieved within the normal age range, the age of acquisition of developmental milestones does not predict a child's abilities later in life.

Sequence of milestone acquisition

The exact timing of the achievement of milestones varies greatly between individual children. However, within each domain it usually follows a typical and predictable sequence, because a child will be unable to achieve a new milestone until they have mastered the necessary skills for it, which are gained via achievement of the relevant previous milestone. For example, good pincer grasp is a prerequisite for drawing. Similarly, a child will be unable to sit in a stable position until they have engaged their back muscles in rolling, and crawling will not be possible until they are able to support their back in sitting.

Factors affecting milestone acquisition

Development is driven by genetic and environmental factors. A child's genetic make-up determines their potential, and the environment in which they grow up influences the degree to which this potential is fulfilled. For optimal development, the environment needs to meet the child's physical and psychological needs, for example a good diet, appropriate treatment for any illness, and emotional, cognitive and social experiences. The provision of support and encouragement from the parents and wider family when the child is practising new skills is particularly beneficial to their development.

Each child follows an individual developmental path, influenced by the opportunities they are given and the physical and mental stimulation they receive. Chronic ill health

with prolonged periods in hospital may affect development if, for example, the child lacks opportunities to explore; as a result, their development may temporarily plateau. Also, a child who can walk but is not allowed to play outside will be late in acquiring more advanced gross motor skills.

When assessing development, allowances are made if a child was born prematurely. In such cases, development in the first 2 years is assessed at the child's 'corrected gestational age', i.e. the age calculated from their expected date of delivery, rather than their actual 'chronological age'. For example, for a child born 12 weeks early, the '6-month' developmental assessment is carried out at their chronological age of 9 months (6 months' corrected age). After 2 years of age, the few months' difference is of little significance because of the wide age range of ages over which the higher development milestones are acquired.

Developmental domains

The four domains of child development are gross motor, fine motor, communication and language, and social.

Gross motor skills

Gross motor development is the development of skills involving large skeletal muscles. Newborns have various reflex responses to position or movement; these are called primitive reflexes (**Table 1.8**). Primitive reflexes are automatic, do not have to be learned and gradually disappear as secondary (acquired) reflexes develop. The child must lose their primitive reflexes for their development to progress:

- the asymmetrical tonic neck reflex needs to disappear to enable rolling; persistence of this reflex is a frequent finding in infants with cerebral palsy
- balance reactions are necessary for a child to sit in a stable position

Persistence of the primitive reflexes or delay of acquisition of secondary reflexes suggests delayed development.

Primitive and acquired reflexes in infants			
Reflex	How elicited	Response	Age when present
Primitive reflexes			
Moro's reflex	With the baby supine, and their head supported with one hand, the head is suddenly released before the support is quickly restored	Abduction and extension of the arms, with opening of the hands, followed by adduction of the arms and crying	Birth to 5 months
Truncal incurvation reflex (Galant's reflex)	With the baby held in ventral suspension, the examiner's fingertip is used to stimulate down each side of the back	Flexion of the spine to the stimulated side	Birth to 8 months
Palmar grasp reflex	Placement of the examiner's finger onto the palm of the hand or sole of the foot	Flexion of fingers or toes; with testing of the palmar grasp, the strong grasp and contraction of the arm muscles enable the baby to be raised by its hands from supine position	Birth to 5 months
Asymmetrical tonic neck reflex	With the baby supine, turning their head to one side	Extension of the arm and leg on that side, and flexion on the opposite side	6 weeks to 5 months
Acquired reflexes			
Balance reactions	Baby's body displaced to the side when in the sitting position	Extension of the arm to prevent falling	7 months onwards
Parachute reaction	The child is held in a ventral position and rapidly lowered, head first, towards the table	The arms extend to save the child from hitting its head	5 months onwards

Table 1.8 'Primitive' reflexes are inborn and are replaced by acquired (secondary) reflexes

In the first year, development is most noticeable in the domain of gross motor skills, and this development continues throughout childhood. It occurs in a cranial-to-caudal manner. Thus, the child achieves strength in the neck muscles, followed by the back muscles, followed by the legs. The strengthening of muscles in this order provides the child with the abilities needed to achieve subsequent milestones; for example, a child must have good head control before they can sit independently. To be able to sit, they need to have matured from having a curved back to having a lumbar lordosis, which develops from the muscle movements necessary for rolling, and also from developing the righting reflex.

The milestones of gross motor development are typically attained in the following order:

1. head control
2. rolling
3. sitting
4. crawling
5. walking (via pulling themselves up to stand and cruising, i.e. walking while holding on to furniture or other supports)

Infants who get around by 'bottom shuffling' may never crawl. Instead, they progress straight from sitting to pulling to stand. They often start walking later than infants who go through the crawling stage.

Once a child is walking, they are expected to be able to perform more complex motor tasks, for example climbing the stairs, running, practising ball skills (kicking, catching and throwing) and pedalling a tricycle (**Table 1.9**).

Milestones: gross motor skills	
Mean age of acquisition	Gross motor skills
18 months	Walks steadily
	Can squat and carry objects while walking
2 years	Can run and kick a ball
	Walks up and down stairs one step at a time, using two feet per step, while holding on
3 years	Can jump and momentarily stand on one foot
	Can pedal a tricycle
4 years	Can hop and balance on one leg
	Walks up and down stairs, using one foot per step
5 years	Can skip and catch a ball

Table 1.9 Milestones in gross motor development from 18 months of age

Rolling is a very complex motor manoeuvre. It requires coordination of both arms and legs, and both head and trunk. If a child can roll over at an appropriate age (i.e. before 7 months), they are unlikely to have a significant gross motor deficit detected later on.

Fine motor skills

Fine motor skills are those requiring the use of the smaller muscles of the body, predominantly those of the hands and fingers, and include the skills needed to manipulate objects. Development in this domain is supported by visual development, which starts at birth, but most fine motor skills are seen later than the start of the development of gross motor skills. The complex skills of drawing and writing develop from the age of 3 years.

A child's fine motor development cannot be assessed independently of the assessment of vision, because good vision is essential for carrying out fine motor tasks. This is particularly true for more complex fine motor skills, for example using a pincer grip to pick up small objects from the floor. The development of fine motor skills also overlaps with social

Milestones: fine motor skills and vision	
Mean age of acquisition	Observation
4 weeks	Fixes and follows a face through 45°
3 months	Fixes and follows a face or object through 180°
	Watches own hands
4 months	Reaches out for but unable to grasp a cube or similar small object
6 months	Depth perception
	Reaches out for and grasps a cube or similar small object (with a palmar grasp)
	Does not look for an object they have dropped or seen dropped
7 months	Transfers a cube or similar small object from hand to hand (facilitated by the ability to sit)
9 months	Develops an immature pincer grasp
	Looks for toys they have seen fall off a table
	Bangs cubes or other small objects together
12–15 months	Uses a mature pincer grasp to pick up small items such as crumbs
	Releases objects
	Casting: deliberately throws toys and watches as they fall to the ground
18 months	Produces to-and-fro scribbles on paper
	Turns the pages of a book, two or three pages at a time
	Can build a tower of three cubes
2 years	Produces circular scribbles on paper
	Drawing: copies a vertical line
	Turns pages singly
	Can build a tower of six cubes and a 'train' of cubes
3 years	Drawing: copies a circle
	Builds a copy of a bridge of three cubes and a tower of nine cubes
4 years	Drawing: copies a cross and a square
	Draws a person with a head, trunk and legs
	Can builds 'stairs' with six cubes
5 years	Drawing: copies a triangle
	Draws a person with a recognisable face

Table 1.10 Milestones in fine motor and visual development

development, because fine motor skills are required for self-care skills such as feeding oneself.

> **The primitive palmar grasp reflex needs to be lost before voluntary grasping can occur.** Abnormal persistence of the palmar grasp may indicate cerebral damage, as may its absence or asymmetry in the newborn period.

Milestones in the domain of fine motor skills are shown in **Table 1.10** and **Figure 1.29**. The use of one-inch cubes and the ability to build increasingly complex structures with them, such as towers of increasing height to 'trains' and 'stairs', are assessed, as well as drawing skills (see page 95). The development of fine motor skills is particularly dependent not only on normal vision but also appropriate opportunities for learning, via the provision of objects to explore with their hands, stimulation from parents, etc.

Visual development

Milestones in visual development progress from fixing and following a face through to accurate depth perception when reaching for a toy, for example (see **Table 1.10**). The retina and other parts of the eye are relatively mature at birth, but myelination of the optic pathway is incomplete and depends on exposure of the retina to unobstructed light. Therefore the identification and correction of conditions that affect the lens, e.g. cataracts, is vital for normal visual maturation.

Visual acuity is poor at birth; a neonate can detect only light and dark and movements. Visual acuity is considered normal at a reference value called 6/6 vision, i.e. the ability to discern letters at a distance of 6 m. Reference values of 6/6+ indicate vision that is worse than normal. Acuity is 6/18 at 1 year, 6/12 at 2 years and 6/6 at 4 years.

> **Once a baby learns to grasp objects, they learn to bring it to their mouth.** Mouthing adds to their exploration and understanding of objects. Voluntary release of an object occurs several months after the development of voluntary grasp.

Communication and language

The communication and language domain covers the development of skills needed to communicate and interact with others through the use of gesture (non-verbal communication) and speech, and the understanding of language. A child's progress in this domain is assessed alongside hearing, because adequate hearing is needed to develop communication and language skills (**Table 1.11**). The development of speech is monitored, from babbling to the use of single words at first, followed by longer sentences. The understanding of language is manifested by the child's ability to follow instructions, progressing from simple to increasingly complex. Milestones also include the ability to name colours and body parts, and counting.

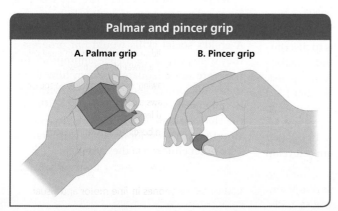

Palmar and pincer grip

A. Palmar grip   B. Pincer grip

Figure 1.29 (a) Palmar grip. The child picks up the object using the whole palm. (b) Pincer grip. The child picks up the object using their thumb and index finger.

Milestones: hearing, and communication and language	
Mean age of acquisition	**Observation**
4–6 weeks	Quietens or cries in response to sound
3 months	Responds to speech
	'Cooing' vocalisation
6 months	Babbling
9 months	Recognises own name
	Two-syllable babble
12 months	Can use two words with meaning (e.g. 'Mum' or 'Dad')
18 months	Understands simple commands
	Uses 6–20 words with meaning
	Can point to parts of body when requested to do so
2 years	Joins two or three words
	Uses 50 words
	Can follow a two-stage command
3 years	Uses at least 200 words
	Can follow two-part directions
	Can answer when asked their name, age and sex
	Uses three- or four-word sentences
	Can name one colour
4 years	Can count to 10
	Can name several colours
	Asks lots of questions
	Uses prepositions, produces elaborate sentences and starts to use the past tense correctly
	Develops memory, with often verbatim knowledge of long stories

Table 1.11 Milestones in the development of hearing, and communication and language

In the first year, an infant learns to discriminate between different sounds and practises them with babble. Vowel sounds develop first, then the back consonants (e.g. the hard 'g') and then the lip and tongue consonants (e.g. 'p'). Some sounds, such as 'th', may not be made until the child is 5 years old. In the first year, comprehension of words must develop before the child is able to use meaningful and expressive language.

> **Language development is related to general intellectual development and the use of language in the home.** In cases of speech delay, non-verbal communication is also assessed to exclude autism spectrum disorder (see page 430); a finding of isolated speech delay makes a neurological disorder unlikely.

The first meaningful words appear on average at 1 year of age, but with a wide range of normal. At 18–24 months, most children are saying simple two-word combinations. Sentences gradually increase in length; adjectives, adverbs and pronouns are introduced; and language is used in play, with the child animating their toys and talking to them.

The normal variation in the age at which developmental skills are acquired is particularly pertinent in the domain of communication and language. Vocabulary varies widely, most noticeably at about the age of 2 years, at which there is a range over 12 months around the mean (i.e. 18 months to 2½ years) for simple word combinations and asking for items with simple names.

Social skills

This domain is concerned with the acquisition of skills required for self-care, positive relationships with others and appropriate social interaction. Stimulating interactions with parents or other caregivers, as well as other people in the child's life, are essential for the development of social skills, as they are for skills in other developmental domains. A child's social skills would not progress if they were provided with age-appropriate toys but were not adequately shown how to use them. Reciprocal social activities with family members, such as playing peep-bo and the shared enjoyment of nursery rhymes, are vital to social development, as is interaction with other children of the same age.

Milestones: social skills	
Mean age of acquisition	**Social skills**
6 weeks	Social smile
3 months	Recognises mother
6 months	Laughs
9 months	Stranger awareness (prefers mother)
	Plays peep-bo
	Feeds self with biscuit
12 months	Imitates gestures such as clapping hands and waving bye-bye
	Finger feeds
	Plays with toys such as stacking beakers but tends to prefer taking items apart rather than putting them together
18 months	Can use a cup and spoon-feed self
	Can remove shoes and socks
	Mimics activities such as cleaning the house, and symbolic play
2 years	Can use a fork
	Plays alone
3 years	Eats with a knife, fork and spoon
	Make-believe play with other children
	Toilet-trained during the day and maybe the night
4 years	Can dress and undress self (apart from shoelaces), brush teeth and use the toilet without help

Table 1.12 Milestones in social development

Milestones in the social skills domain are listed in **Table 1.12**. The age at which the child started smiling and laughing are noted, and progress in the sophistication of their play is assessed, from the use of simple cause-and-effect toys, through pretending (symbolic and imaginative play), to playing with other children rather than in parallel with them. Self-care skills, including feeding oneself, dressing and undressing and toileting skills, are also included in the assessment.

Emotional development is an essential element of social development. It requires understanding emotions and the development of reasoning and appropriate emotional responses. The following underlie healthy emotional development throughout childhood:

- a sense of basic trust, which the child acquires in infancy from having their physical and psychological needs met (e.g. by being fed, and by bonding with parents or caregivers)
- the confidence to exert their own will, most apparent during the 'terrible twos', when they start to assert their independence
- the practice of social behaviour with peers, for example at nursery
- the drive to achieve in the primary school years
- a sense of identity as an adolescent

Feeding and nutrition

Starter questions

Answers to the following questions are on page 47.

13. Why is an excessive milk intake bad for a toddler?
14. Why is breastfeeding encouraged for HIV positive mothers in developing countries, but contraindicated for HIV positive mothers in developed countries?

Good nutrition is vital for the optimal growth, health and well-being of all children. It requires the intake of different types of food in the correct proportions to provide the body with the required macronutrients and micronutrients. Nutritious food should be provided, and a healthy attitude towards food and positive eating habits (e.g. eating at mealtimes and avoiding snacking between meals) should be encouraged from early in the child's life. These are the foundations for healthy dietary choices in adulthood.

Macronutrients

Macronutrients are energy-providing nutrients required in large amounts to maintain body functions and activity. The three macronutrients provide energy in the form of calories:

- carbohydrates provide 4 calories per gram
- proteins provide 4 calories per gram
- lipids provide 9 calories per gram

Micronutrients

Micronutrients are elements required in only small amounts but are essential to enable the body to produce enzymes, hormones and other substances necessary for proper growth and development. As small as the required amounts of micronutrients are, the consequences of a deficiency are severe. Examples of micronutrients include:

- iodine
- vitamin A
- iron

Early feeding

There are two options for the feeding of neonates and infants: breastfeeding or feeding with infant formula, a liquid food based on cows' milk and formulated to resemble breast milk as closely as possible. Human breast milk is the ideal; in addition to meeting the baby's nutritional needs until the age of 6 months, it provides substances not present in infant formula that benefit the immune system. However, despite the superiority of breast milk, breastfeeding rates are not as high as they should be. In the UK, for example, only 70–80% of mothers start breastfeeding at birth and only 20–25% are practising exclusive breastfeeding at 6 weeks, falling to 15% at 3 months of age, though many mothers do combine breastfeeding and formula feeding.

At 6 months of age, solid food should be gradually introduced (known as weaning), while the infant continues to receive milk, ideally still breast milk. At 12 months, normal full-fat pasteurised cows' milk can be given and the child should be on a nutritious and varied diet. Unmodified cows' milk should not be given to babies under 1 year of age, because it contains too much protein, sodium and potassium for their immature kidneys to process.

The World Health Organization recommends exclusive breastfeeding for the first 6 months of life. In several countries it is written in law that employers must provide facilities to enable a woman to express her milk whilst at work.

Breastfeeding

Breast milk provides a complete source of nutrition for full-term newborns. It contains all the protein, lipid, carbohydrate, vitamins, minerals and trace elements necessary for energy and body functions, although in many countries with low levels of sunlight vitamin D supplementation is recommended from the ages of 1 month to 5 years. Also, vitamin K is required in the first few days to prevent haemorrhagic disease of the newborn (see page 217). Breast milk is also the optimal milk for premature infants because it prevents against necrotising enterocolitis.

During pregnancy, the mother's breasts undergo changes that enable milk to be produced after delivery. The breasts usually enlarge as the milk-producing glands mature, and in later pregnancy these glands fill with early milk called colostrum. Breastfeeding should begin within an hour of delivery, with the baby placed on the mother's chest, with skin-to-skin contact. Suckling of the nipple by the baby stimulates the production of the pituitary hormones oxytocin and prolactin, resulting in milk production and release, known as 'let-down' (**Figure 1.30**).

After production of the initial milk, colostrum, further milk production is regulated primarily by the emptying of the breast.

Benefits

In the first day or two, the baby feeds on the colostrum, which contains a high amount of protein and antibodies compared with mature breast milk. It also lines and thereby protects the infant's immature gut.

Breastfeeding has many benefits over formula feeding (**Table 1.13**). The protein in breast milk is more easily digested. Also, breast milk contains proteins (including immunoglobulins) absent from infant formula that act against pathogenic organisms and thereby prevent severe gut inflammation. The presence in breast milk of prebiotics and probiotics, such as lactobacilli, which colonise the baby's bowel, help inhibit the growth of enteropathic bacteria that are responsible for gastroenteritis. Many benefits of breastfeeding continue after breastfeeding is discontinued, e.g. the reduced likelihood of obesity in childhood or heart disease in adulthood.

Difficulties

Some mothers have difficulty establishing breastfeeding, but this is usually resolved with support and advice from breastfeeding advisers. Common problems include the baby not latching on properly, attaching to the nipple alone rather than taking a good mouthful of breast. This can lead to painful

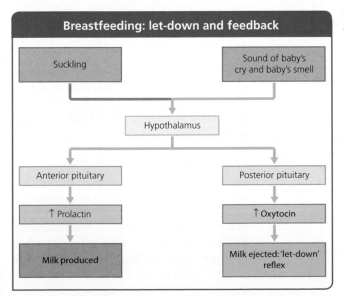

Figure 1.30 Breast milk ejection ('let-down') and feedback.

Benefits of breastfeeding	
Benefits for the child	**Benefits for the mother**
Lower rates of infections such as gastroenteritis, otitis media and lower respiratory tract infections	Reduced blood loss after delivery (the release of oxytocin helps the uterus to contract, thereby reducing uterine bleeding)
Reduced risk of necrotising enterocolitis in premature babies	Reduced risk of breast and ovarian cancer, and cardiovascular disease
Lower risk of developing type 1 diabetes mellitus in childhood	Helps in postnatal weight loss
Lower likelihood of being overweight in childhood	Positive effect on mother–infant bonding
Reduced risk of sudden infant death syndrome	Convenience: milk always readily available and at the right temperature
Reduced risk of childhood cancers	Financial: breast milk is free
Reduced risk of heart disease and hypertension in adulthood	Potentially less anxiety related to illness in the child, and less need for parents to take time off work to care for an ill child, because breastfed babies are less likely to become ill or require hospitalisation

Table 1.13 Benefits of breastfeeding over formula feeding

nipples, which further discourages breast-feeding. Tongue tie (**Figure 1.31**) is common and does not usually affect the ability of the baby to breastfeed, so it does not necessarily require treatment.

Contraindications to breastfeeding are:

- maternal HIV infection
- maternal tuberculosis
- mother receiving chemotherapy drugs or radiation therapy
- herpes simplex lesions on the mother's breasts
- galactosaemia (a metabolic disorder characterised by the inability to metabolise galactose) in the infant

With breastfeeding, it is not possible to measure the volume of milk the infant is taking. They can be assumed to be receiving enough milk if they:

- are content and satisfied after most feeds
- are gaining weight after the first 2 weeks
- have at least six wet nappies a day after the first few days
- are passing at least two yellow stools every day after the first few days

In low- and middle-income countries, infant formula is often contaminated because of poor sanitation and limited access to clean water. In these countries, breastfeeding significantly reduces the incidence of gastrointestinal infections, resulting in improved survival. UNICEF estimates that a formula-fed child living in unhygienic conditions is 6–25 times more likely to die from diarrhoea and 4 times more likely to die from pneumonia than a breastfed child.

Formula feeding

Infant formula is used when breastfeeding is contraindicated or there is a maternal preference for formula feeding over breastfeeding. Infant formula is a modified version of skimmed cows' milk.

Composition of infant formula

The two main proteins present in milk are whey and casein. One of the major differences between human breast milk and unmodified cows' milk is the ratio of whey to casein. Breast milk contains predominantly whey proteins (about 60–70%), whereas cows' milk

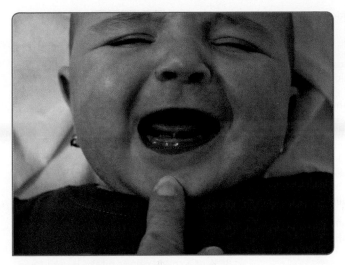

Figure 1.31 Tongue tie is a common finding. It rarely affects breastfeeding so does not require treatment.

contains predominantly casein (80%). The whey:casein ratio of infant formulae is made similar to that of human milk, although some are formulated to be 'whey-dominant' and others 'casein-dominant'.

- Whey is easier to digest than casein, so whey-dominant formula is recommended for younger babies
- Casein-dominant formula is often labelled as being suitable for 'hungrier' babies, because theoretically the longer time needed to digest the casein would lengthen the intervals between feeds

The caloric value of both type of formula is the same. A baby can remain on whey-dominant formula for the whole first year.

Manufacturers of infant formula try to replicate human breast milk. In addition to modification of the whey:casein ratio, infant formula is fortified with:

- vitamins, especially vitamins D and K
- minerals, including iron
- nucleotides, which may enhance the infant immune system (although there is a lack of evidence for this)
- polyunsaturated fatty acids, such as docosahexaenoic acid and arachidonic acid, which are thought to have a role in infant brain development
- prebiotics, which may stimulate the growth of 'good' bacteria in the gut (although there is a lack of evidence for this)

These substances are present naturally in human milk. The mineral content of infant formula is modified to reflect that of human milk. Infection and practicality issues mean that antibodies cannot be added to formula milk.

> Specialised milks are available for feeding babies, not exclusively breastfed, with specific conditions, such as cows' milk protein allergy, galactosaemia and phenylketonuria. Premature babies also receive specialised formulae because of their increased nutritional requirements, or alternatively breast milk fortified with vitamins and iron.

Weaning

Weaning is the introduction of solid food into a baby's diet. The ideal age to start weaning is about 6 months of age, when the baby's gastrointestinal system is mature enough to digest solid food and they are developmentally able to sit upright while eating. Solid food should never be introduced before the baby is 17 weeks' old.

Breastfeeding or formula feeding should continue during weaning and until the infant is 12 months' old, from which point whole cows' milk can be given. As the child's appetite is satiated by food, the volume of milk taken over each 24-h period decreases, but milk continues to contribute a significant proportion of an infant's nutritional requirements until 1 year of age.

> **From 1 year of age, children can drink whole cows' milk.** They should have full-fat dairy products until 2 years of age. From 2 years, provided that they are eating and growing well, they can have semiskimmed milk. From the age of 5 years, 1% fat and skimmed milk are also appropriate.

The first weaning foods are generally:

- mashed or soft-cooked fruit and vegetables
- baby rice or cereal mixed with the infant's usual milk

Finger food, i.e. food that has been cut into pieces big enough for the baby to hold in their fist with a little sticking out, are then introduced; this supports the infant's fine motor development and helps them learn to chew. Once the infant is used to solids, they can move on to soft-cooked meat, boneless fish, pasta, toast and full-fat yoghurts.

From 8–9 months, the infant is given three meals a day. These are given as a mixture of soft finger foods and chopped foods. By 12 months, the child should be eating a wide variety of foods, provided by three meals a day and healthy snacks between meals.

Nutrition

All children need a healthy balanced diet, i.e. a diet consisting of a variety of nutritious foods, in the correct proportions, from all the food groups. Compared with adults, children have a higher calorie requirement for their size to provide them with enough energy to fuel their usually higher levels of activity and fulfil their energy requirement for growth.

A child's calorie requirement is greatest in the first 5 years. Therefore the composition of a young child's diet differs from that of older children and adults; it is a comparatively high-fat and low-fibre diet. As they become older, their diet becomes more like that of an adult's (**Figure 1.32**).

> **A healthy term infant trebles in weight in their first year.** At 4 months of age, 30% of a child's caloric intake is used for growth. Only 5% is used for growth by 1 year, and 2% by 3 years.

Daily calorie requirements for children vary depending on their age, sex and activity levels (**Table 1.14**). Children with an active lifestyle consume a higher number of calories, whereas those with a more sedentary lifestyle consume fewer calories.

A high-fibre diet is unsuitable for young children, because of the small size of their stomachs; it would give them an early feeling of fullness, thereby reducing their appetite before enough food has been consumed to provide the calories they require. The small stomachs of younger children compared with older children also means that they need to be fed more frequently.

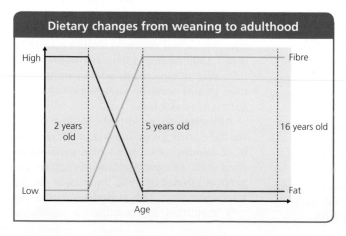

Dietary changes from weaning to adulthood

Figure 1.32 Relative changes in the ideal fat and fibre content of the diet from weaning to adulthood.

Childhood calorie requirements		
Age (years)	Calorie requirement*	
	Girls	Boys
1	717	765
2–3	800–1400	800–1400
4–8	1000–1800	1250–2000
9–13	1500–2200	1600–2600
14–18	1600–2400	1900–3200

*Ranges reflect the differences in calorie requirements between children with the least and most active lifestyles.

Table 1.14 Calorie requirements in childhood

Government schemes help families on a low income to make healthy food choices. The UK scheme is called Healthy Start: women and families with a child under 4 years of age, and who receive certain government benefits, are eligible for vouchers that can be exchanged for fresh fruit and vegetables, infant formula or milk. Education is also provided to encourage healthy eating.

Carbohydrates

Carbohydrates have many functions in the body but are primarily used as a source of energy. They can be metabolised to generate energy in the short term, or stored for energy generation at a later time. In children, they provide the energy needed for growth.

For children older than 1 year, as for adults, carbohydrates should make up 45–65% of daily caloric intake. Food sources rich in carbohydrates include oats, beans, pulses, pasta and rice.

Fats

Fats are molecules made up of glycerol and fatty acids. One gram of fat provides more energy than one gram of carbohydrate, so fats are a better source of energy for the growing child. Furthermore, intestinal absorption of dietary fats enables absorption of fat-soluble vitamins.

In contrast to adults, whose diet should consist of no more than 25–30% fat, 40% of all calories ingested by a child aged 0–4 years, and 35% for older children, should come from fat. However, as with adults, dietary fats should be in unsaturated form; the amount of saturated fat should be limited. Good sources of fat include full-fat milk and cheese, meat and oily fish.

Fat deficiency can result in a lack of energy for growth. In children with conditions causing fat malabsorption, it may also lead to a deficiency of the fat-soluble vitamins.

Protein

Protein is essential for growth and repair. It is also used to generate energy when carbohydrate is unavailable. Proteins are chains of smaller molecules called amino acids.

Essential amino acids, for example phenylalanine, are amino acids that can be obtained from dietary sources only. To avoid deficiency, a child's diet must include these amino acids. Sources of protein include meat, fish, eggs, beans and pulses. Lack of protein results in suboptimal growth, muscle mass and immune function.

Vitamins and minerals

Vitamins and minerals carry out essential functions in biochemical reactions throughout the body (**Table 1.15**). They cannot be synthesised by the body, so adequate amounts must be provided by the diet to avoid the problems associated with deficiencies.

Minerals required by the body include iron, calcium, magnesium, sodium and potassium. Vitamins are divided into two groups: fat-soluble and water-soluble.

- The fat-soluble vitamins are vitamins A, D, E and K
- Water-soluble vitamins include vitamin C and the B group vitamins (including folic acid and vitamin B_1, i.e. thiamine)

Fat-soluble vitamins are stored in the liver and body fat. Water-soluble vitamins are easily absorbed directly from the intestine but are not stored in the body, so regular intake is required.

Vitamins and minerals: roles, sources and deficiency symptoms			
Vitamin	Roles	Sources	Deficiency or symptoms of deficiency
A	Contributes to immune function Required for production of retinal pigments essential for vision in low-light conditions	Liver Oily fish Dairy foods	Impaired immune function Night blindness
B_1 (thiamine)	Coenzyme in carbohydrate metabolism and glucose production	Various foods, including wholegrains, meat, fish, dairy and vegetables	Beriberi (symptoms include muscle weakness, peripheral neuropathy and cardiac failure)
B_9 (folic acid, i.e. folate)	Contributes biochemically to red blood cell formation Contributes biochemically to in DNA formation	Green vegetables Liver Fortified cereals	Macrocytic anaemia Poor weight gain Neural tube defects in the fetus
C (ascorbic acid)	Cofactor in collagen synthesis Contributes to in immune function (exact mechanism unclear) Increases intestinal absorption of iron	Fruit such as oranges and strawberries Vegetables such as broccoli and peppers	Scurvy (impaired collagen synthesis leading to poor wound healing, bone weakness and fragile blood vessels)
D	Maintenance of bone health through regulation of calcium levels	Main source: synthesis in skin exposed to sunlight Oily fish, eggs and fortified cereals	Rickets (leading to poor growth, delayed walking, skeletal deformities and bone pain) Seizures or cardiomyopathy possible in infants
E	Antioxidant, which protects cell membranes	Nuts and seeds Cereals Soya	Ataxia, weakness and peripheral neuropathy (all rare)
K	Role in blood coagulation	Broccoli Spinach Vegetable oils	Bleeding tendency Haemorrhagic disease of the newborn

Table 1.15 Roles, sources and symptoms of deficiency of vitamins and minerals

Children with cystic fibrosis can become deficient in fat-soluble vitamins.
The deficiency is the consequence of pancreatic insufficiency and poor fat absorption.

Healthy term babies are born with a store of iron that is sufficient to meet their requirements for the first 6 months of life. After this time, iron-rich foods should be introduced early into the weaning diet to prevent the development of iron deficiency. Good sources of iron are meat and green vegetables.

Iron

Iron is essential for the production of haemoglobin and normal neurological development in babies and young children. Iron deficiency usually manifests as iron deficiency anaemia (see page 371).

A common cause of iron deficiency in young children is excessive consumption of cows' milk. Cows' milk is low in iron, and the iron that is present is more difficult to absorb than that in breast milk.

Vitamin D

Vitamin D is essential for bone health in children, and there is increasing evidence that it has a role in preventing many other diseases. Vitamin D is present in oily fish, eggs, fortified cereals and infant formula. It is also synthesised in the skin via the conversion of 7-dehydrocholesterol to cholecalciferol (vitamin D_3) on exposure to sunlight.

Vitamin K

Vitamin K is essential for the normal function of many coagulation factors; deficiency results in a bleeding tendency.

Breast milk contains less vitamin K than formula milk; breast-fed babies therefore have a higher risk of vitamin K deficiency bleeding. All newborn children receive vitamin K injections regardless of how the mother intends to feed, meaning mothers can breast feed without risk.

Answers to starter questions

1. Smoking during pregnancy reduces the number of lung branches and alveoli the baby will have at birth. Although the lungs continue growing until about 8 years of age the child will never achieve the same lung capacity as if their mother had not smoked.

2. X-rays are avoided during pregnancy, particularly in the first 12 weeks. This is a critical time for fetal development and any exposure to radiation during this time can result in birth defects.

3. During fetal development the gut herniates into the umbilical cord and rotates anticlockwise through 270 degrees. If this process does not occur correctly the caecum and appendix will remain in a different location, such as the right upper quadrant of the abdomen or the left iliac fossa (in situs inversus). If these individuals develop appendicitis they will feel the pain in the location where their appendix settled.

4. Babies cry at birth due to a variety of stimuli, including the discomfort of being born and exposure to the cold air. This also makes the baby take a deep breath that pushes fluid from the lungs into the lymphatic circulation allowing the lungs to inflate. This reduces the pulmonary vascular resistance and supports the circulatory changes at birth.

5. It is often possible to hear blood flowing through a ductus arteriosus that is still closing in the first few hours after birth. Once the duct has closed no murmur is audible. The disappearance of the murmur needs to be confirmed because in some babies the ductus arteriosus can persist or the murmur could be due to congenital heart disease.

6. If a baby is delivered without the mother going into labour it is not always ready to breathe independently. The baby may not take sufficient deep breaths to clear the lung fluid from its lungs, resulting in a maladjustment of circulation that causes persistent pulmonary hypertension (PPHN). A milder problem is transient tachypnoea of the newborn (TTN), caused by fluid remaining in the lungs.

7. A child's height is measured standing up, while their length is measured lying down. Length is measured up until 2 years of age because young children cannot reliably stand up. There is some compression of the spine when standing that makes the measured height slightly shorter than measured length. This is reflected on growth charts by a small downward shift of the centile lines at 2 years of age.

8. At birth the skeleton consists of 300 different parts, but by adulthood there are 206 bones. Fusion and ossification occur in a predictable sequence as the child grows. Bone age is assessed from an X-ray of the left hand and wrist using a reference atlas; by looking at the presence or absence of ossification centres and the shape and degree of fusion of the epiphyses a child's age can be estimated. However, many conditions affect the ossification process (see Chapter 12).

9. The pubertal growth spurt is not a uniform increase in size: initial growth occurs in the hands, feet and limbs (progressing distally), with truncal growth occurring later. Therefore, in early puberty teenagers can appear clumsy and awkward in their movements.

10. Babies and young children have an odourless, mainly water and salt sweat secreted from the eccrine glands. At puberty, the apocrine glands (mainly found in axillae and genital area) are activated. This sweat contains fatty acids and proteins that produce an odour when degraded by the normal commensal bacteria living on the skin.

Answers *continued*

11. Babies do not develop a hand preference until 18–24 months of age. An early hand preference is a sign of an underlying neurological problem, such as cerebral palsy.

12. Delayed speech and a lack of social skills is an indication of autistic spectrum disorder. Children with isolated delayed speech often have very good social and non-verbal skills that make up for the speech deficit.

13. Full-fat milk is an excellent source of energy and calcium for toddlers, but is low in iron. Toddlers who drink excessive amounts quickly feel full. If they are not hungry at mealtimes they will fail to get the right balance of nutrients, in particular iron-rich foods, which can lead to iron deficiency anaemia.

14. In developed countries HIV positive mothers are advised against breastfeeding due to the small risk of transmission of the HIV virus via breast milk. In developing countries this risk is outweighed by the benefits of breastfeeding, which can be lifesaving. In developing countries bottle feeding has a high risk of contamination from dirty drinking water and frequently leads to gastroenteritis, infections or lethal diarrhoeal illnesses.

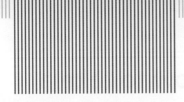

Chapter 2
Clinical essentials

Introduction

The majority of paediatric diagnoses are made on the basis of signs and symptoms elicited as part of the history and examination process.

- Symptoms are features reported by a patient in the history, and provide subjective evidence of disease or disorder
- Signs are features detectable by a health care professional, especially during the examination, and provide objective evidence of disease or disorder

This information is collated with the results of appropriate investigations to determine the most likely diagnosis and decide the best approach to management.

Paediatricians routinely use two examination procedures unique to the specialty:

- the examination of the newborn, a 'top-to-toe' examination to identify any congenital or birth-related problems
- the developmental examination, which assesses the development of the child to determine if it is appropriate for the child's age or delayed

Common symptoms and how to take a history

Starter questions

Answers to the following questions are on page 124.

1. Why might a child's mother have no knowledge of her child's antenatal or family history?
2. Why are mobile phones helpful when taking a history?
3. Why should a description of 'bilious' always be clarified?

Effective history taking allows you to obtain reliable and relevant information about a child's symptoms. Additional skills are needed when taking a paediatric as opposed to an adult medical history.

Children mature at different rates. They vary at different chronological ages not only in their physical abilities but also in their ability to express themselves and to understand and interact appropriately with others (see page 94). Therefore the approach to history taking must be tailored to the individual child, taking into account developmental age and ability to communicate.

Sometimes, it is difficult to obtain a history directly from the child. They may be preverbal or too distressed to answer questions, or they may have a learning disability or other condition (e.g. cerebral palsy) that affects how they communicate. In such instances, it may be necessary to rely on the adult accompanying the child (usually a parent) to supply information.

Listen to the parents; they know their child best. However, be cautious if abuse or fictitious or induced illness is suspected: the history provided could be unreliable and should not override information from the child, assuming they are old enough to provide a history.

Parents may be anxious, tired or distracted by the need to attend to the child and any siblings, which may interfere with history taking. In such cases, a brief and focused history may be more appropriate than a comprehensive one.

Preparation

The consultation should take place in a child-friendly setting, with space for the child to play (**Figure 2.1**). Most paediatric departments and general practitioner (GP) practices are designed to be welcoming to children. Your approach should be friendly to help the child feel at ease.

Address both the child and the adult accompanying them. Greet the child by name, get down to their eye level to introduce yourself, and start with a light-hearted question about their journey or a toy they have bought with them.

The parent or other accompanying adult

The paediatric patient is almost always accompanied by an adult. Establish who this is: in most cases the accompanying adult is a parent, but they may be another relative or

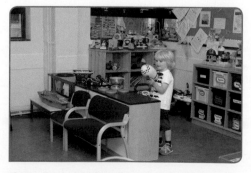

Figure 2.1 A child-friendly environment helps put children and parents at ease.

a family friend, teacher or social worker. The nature of their relationship with the child will determine the extent of their knowledge of the child's past medical history; it also has implications regarding consent to investigation and treatment (see page 436). 'Who have you brought with you today?' is a useful, natural-sounding enquiry that also helps to engage the child's interest.

Adolescents may attend alone. This supports their growing independence, and encourages self-management of chronic conditions such as diabetes.

> **Observe the interaction between parent and child.** Unusual interaction, e.g. the child appearing fearful of the parent, or not going to them for comfort if scared or hurt, are signs of child abuse.

Communicating with the child

Include the child in the consultation as much as possible. This helps younger children feel at ease, thereby making them more likely to cooperate during the subsequent examination. It also helps older children feel respected, and that their concerns are being taken seriously. Furthermore, being included in the consultation gives children with a chronic condition an opportunity to start taking responsibility for its management in preparation for independent adult life.

> **It may be necessary to talk to the child separately from their parents,** for example when enquiring about potentially embarrassing or sensitive subjects such as problems at school or home. The information obtained from the separate interviews is then collated.

Children are generally able to provide some of their own history from the age of 4 years. However, do not assume from a child's age or disability that they are unable to communicate.

> **Although some injuries arise as a consequence of cultural practices,** such as female genital mutilation (see page 439), these are still considered to be deliberate injury to the child.

Taking a history

Paediatric history taking follows a similar structure to history taking in adults. A standardised format is used to gather information in sufficient detail to enable possible causes to be excluded. However, unlike in adult clinical practice, it is often the patient's parent or guardian who provides the history rather than the patient themselves.

Taking a history for an adopted child or a child in care (e.g. living with foster parents or in a residential children's home) may not be straightforward. If the child's guardian is unaware of their past medical history, the relevant information needs to be obtained from a third party, for example a social worker, with access to the child's medical records.

Several components of the history are specific to paediatric medicine: the antenatal, birth, immunisation and development history (**Table 2.1**). Birth history can have significant implications for a child's health and development. For example, a premature baby may have a wheezy chest and developmental delay as a consequence of being born early.

Health promotion and illness prevention are a focus of paediatric medicine. The consultation is an good opportunity to informally screen for developmental problems and check for uncertain or incomplete immunisation status, and then take appropriate action.

Past medical history

The past medical history is discussed to ascertain the patient's health status before the presenting problem arose. Information is gathered about previous medical problems and their management, including details about significant illnesses and hospital admissions.

In paediatrics, the past medical history includes the antenatal and birth history. This

The paediatric history	
History	**Considerations**
General	Any significant illness in the past, including infections such as measles and chickenpox?
	Has the child ever been admitted to hospital or been seen in an outpatient clinic?
	Any common conditions (e.g. eczema) that the parent is unaware are relevant?
Antenatal	Was the mother well during pregnancy?
	Did she take any medications during pregnancy?
	Were the antenatal scans normal? In cases of suspected abnormality, what action was taken?
Birth	Where was the baby born?
	What type of delivery was it? Spontaneous or induced vaginal delivery? Elective or emergency caesarean section?
	Was there premature rupture of membranes? Did the mother receive antibiotics in the peripartum period?
	At what gestation was the baby born?
	What was the birthweight of the child?
	Did they need resuscitation at birth?
	Was the child admitted to the neonatal unit? If so, why, and for how long? What interventions were needed (e.g. therapeutic hypothermia or ventilation)?
Drug, allergy and immunisation	Any allergy to medication?
	What medication (including vitamins) is the child taking? When and why was it started?
	Is the drug treatment being adhered to? Have there been any adverse effects?
	If the child is receiving regular drug treatment, has the dose been adjusted according to their weight?
	Is alternative medicine being used? For example, is the child being given herbal supplements? Some parents are reluctant to divulge that they are trying non-mainstream treatments, or do not think of it as relevant
Social	Who does the child live with? If they are adopted or in care, why is this?
	If the child's parents are separated, does the child have contact with the parent who is not their primary caregiver?
	Is the family known to social services? If so, why?
	If the child is adopted or in care, do they have any contact with their biological parents?
	Are there any smokers at home? If so, do they smoke inside?
	Do the parents work? If so, what do they do?
	What is the home environment like?
Development	Ask a few questions about each developmental domain (see page 53) to ascertain whether the child's development is progressing as expected; a more detailed developmental assessment is necessary if any problems are identified

Table 2.1 Paediatric considerations in history taking

covers any significant complications during the pregnancy, birth or neonatal period that may be relevant to the child's current health status. Questions are asked with the aim of obtaining clues suggesting certain diagnoses or information that can be used to narrow down the list of possible causes.

Questions about antenatal and birth history are not always needed. For example, birth history is relevant for a paediatric patient with wheeze but not for a teenager with a football injury. Clinicians should exercise discretion when deciding which questions can be omitted from the antenatal and birth history.

Antenatal history

Enquiries are made about the mother's pregnancy. Was she healthy? Was she taking any medication or recreational drugs? Was the baby growing normally? Did the mother need to see a consultant obstetrician? If so, why? The information obtained is particularly helpful when treating an unwell neonate, for example a baby undergoing withdrawal from prescription or non-prescription drugs.

Antenatal information is not always readily available if the child is adopted or in care. However, the child's social worker can usually retrieve the information from their records.

Birth history

This gives clues as to particular diagnoses, and is especially useful when treating the unwell neonate. For example, prolonged rupture of membranes may have predisposed the baby to infection. For older children, fetal distress may have led to hypoxia, with consequent developmental delay. Type of delivery is relevant; for example, forceps delivery is associated with bruising and subsequent jaundice.

Family history

The family history documents how the child is related to family members and includes information on any medical conditions known to affect the family. It is particularly relevant if there are concerns about an inherited disease. Recording information about at least two generations is helpful for identifying any hereditary conditions. Ask specifically about the ages of family members, and any illnesses they have. Ask also about unexpected deaths in the family, including sudden infant deaths, which may suggest an undiagnosed metabolic condition.

> **Do not assume that all siblings have the same biological parents.** Siblings with a different biological mother or father may be at risk of different conditions based on that parent's family history. Therefore always clarify whether or not the child's siblings share the same biological mother and father.

Drug, allergy and immunisation history

This component of the history is a record of all medications, both prescribed and purchased over the counter, that the child is receiving, as well as their allergies (if any) and vaccinations. Children tend not to be on regular medication, because chronic disease is less common in the paediatric compared with the adult population. Knowledge of the medication the child is taking and what they might have received in the past, including whether or not the treatment was successful, can contribute to making the diagnosis.

If a parent reports a drug allergy, clarify exactly the type of reaction. Occasionally parents erroneously consider a symptom of an illness or the adverse effect of a drug to be an allergy. This is particularly common when antibiotics have been given; a rash caused by the underlying infection, or a common adverse effect of antibiotics such as loose stools, can be interpreted as an 'allergy'.

Check that the child's vaccinations are up to date. A child who is fully immunised in accordance with the national vaccination schedule is less likely to have the diseases the vaccines protect against. However, if the child has not been vaccinated keep these diseases in mind when considering diagnoses. If the child's immunisation status is incomplete, enquire as to why this is the case. The consultation is a good opportunity to explain the important role of these vaccines in protecting children from preventable diseases, and to encourage uptake (see page 421).

Developmental history

Unless the consultation is specifically for developmental concerns, in which case this component will be lengthy, the developmental history tends to be used as a brief screening tool to assess whether a child is at the appropriate stage of development for their age. Ask a few questions about development that are appropriate to the child's age, covering the four domains of development, i.e. gross motor, fine motor, communication and language, and social (see page 94). A more detailed assessment is carried out if problems are identified (see page 93).

This part of the consultation is a good time to enquire about school. Which school does the child attend? Is their attendance satisfactory? Are there any educational concerns? Ask specifically about bullying, because this is a common cause of school refusal.

Social history

In the social history, the child's family life and home environment are explored to get an overview and understanding of the child and their family. Who is living at home? What support does the family have? Support, for example from grandparents, is particularly valuable when a child has a chronic disease, such as severe cerebral palsy, and a person is needed to look after siblings while a parent takes the child to multiple appointments or cares for them during stays in hospital.

Are the parents employed? Do they have transport? It may feel awkward to ask certain questions in the social history, but the information is necessary to understand any difficulties the child and their family face. For example, lack of money for transport may prevent a family experiencing deprivation from attending appointments.

Enquire about the child's home environment. Do any smokers live with the child? Is there any damp? Smoking, pet dander, and damp and mould exacerbate chest symptoms.

Ask about recent life events such as the death of a relative. The information obtained is particularly useful when assessing a child with unusual symptoms for which there is no medical explanation.

Common symptoms

Common symptoms in patients presenting to the paediatric admissions unit or outpatient clinic include fever, shortness of breath, vomiting and pain at various sites (especially abdominal pain). When taking a pain history for any system, a structured approach based on the mnemonic SOCRATES is used (**Table 2.2**).

Responses to questions asked in the pain history, supplemented by responses to additional questions specific to the system in question, provide a good understanding of the patient's pain to help identify possible causes.

The severity of pain is usually expressed as a score out of 10. However, younger children find this difficult, so visual pain charts can help them rate pain severity (**Figure 2.2**).

Cough

Cough is a reflex response triggered by the stimulation by pulmonary irritants of cough receptors in the lower respiratory tract. This causes a rapid inspiration followed by a forceful expiration against a closed glottis. The glottis then opens, with a consequent rapid expulsion of air. Reduced mucociliary clearance or the presence of excessive mucous results in a cough.

The SOCRATES mnemonic		
Letter	Meaning	Example question(s)
S	Site	'Where does it hurt?'
O	Onset	'When did the pain start?'
C	Character	'Could you describe the pain?'
R	Radiation	'Does the pain move to other areas?'
A	Associated symptoms	'Do you have any other symptoms?'
T	Timing	'How long does the pain last?'
E	Exacerbating and relieving factors	'What makes the pain worse?' 'Does anything make it better?'
S	Severity	'How would you rate the pain on a scale of 1 to 10, with 10 being the worst pain you have ever felt?'

Table 2.2 The SOCRATES mnemonic for taking a history of pain

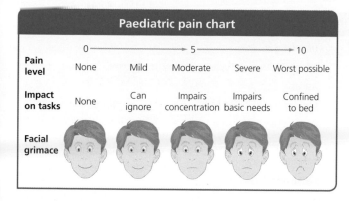

Figure 2.2 A paediatric pain chart for assessment of a child's discomfort.

Cough is often called 'chestiness' or labelled as a 'chest infection' by parents. A chronic cough is one that persists for >6 weeks (**Table 2.3**).

Focused history

The history establishes the nature of the cough, i.e. whether it is dry or productive. Hearing the cough, or being given a good description of it, aids diagnosis (see Figures 4.1 and 4.2). Determine how long the cough has been present, how it started and how it has progressed.

- Did the child have problems in the neonatal period?
- Did the cough start after a viral infection or choking episode?
- Is it present at night?

There may be precipitating factors, such as exercise, a change in the weather, or contact with animals. Their presence provides clues to the diagnoses, as does the presence of any accompanying symptoms (**Table 2.4**). A chronic cough that wakes the child at night is more likely to have a pathological origin rather than a habitual (psychogenic) cough.

> **Parents often use the term 'wheezing' to describe any abnormal respiratory noise.** Always clarify what they mean by 'wheeze'.

> **Primary ciliary dyskinesia** is a condition that causes a productive cough, rhinitis and recurrent middle ear infection. About 50% of patients with primary ciliary dyskinesia have situs inversus (in which major organs are in a mirror image of the usual arrangement). Situs inversus, sinusitis and bronchiectasis, together known as the Kartagener triad, characterise a subtype of primary ciliary dyskinesia called ciliary dyskinesia syndrome (Kartagener's syndrome).

Childhood cough: causes	
Type of cough	Causes
Acute	Acute infection (viral or bacterial, including croup)
	Foreign body (including aspiration)
	Exposure to an irritant
Chronic	Asthma
	Recurrent viral infections
	Post-bronchiolitic wheeze
	Cystic fibrosis or bronchiectasis
	Gastro-oesophageal reflux
	Chronic aspiration or foreign body inhalation
	Pertussis
	Tuberculosis
	Primary ciliary dyskinesia
	Congenital anomaly
	Psychogenic
	Passive smoking
	Cardiac causes

Table 2.3 Causes of acute and chronic childhood cough

Cough: associated symptoms and underlying conditions	
Associated symptom	Underlying condition
Runny nose	Allergic rhinitis or viral upper respiratory tract infection
Wheeze or breathlessness	Asthma
Upper airway noise (stridor)	Croup or inhaled foreign body
Ear infections	Primary ciliary dyskinesia
Faltering growth or loose stools	Cystic fibrosis
Infections elsewhere	Immunodeficiency
Vomiting or dyspepsia	Gastro-oesophageal reflux

Table 2.4 Symptoms associated with cough and possible underlying conditions

Breathlessness

Breathlessness is the sensation of shortness of breath or objective difficulty in breathing. It is normal for respiratory rate and breathing effort to increase with exercise, but this must be proportional to the level of exertion applied. The first indicator of breathlessness in preverbal children is usually breathlessness on feeding.

Focused history

Breathlessness is acute (developing suddenly over minutes or hours) or chronic (developing over weeks or months), and persistent or intermittent. Not all causes of breathlessness are respiratory (**Table 2.5**).

- When did the breathlessness start, and did anything trigger it?
- Is it present all the time?
- Is it getting worse?
- Does it stop the child from doing anything?
- What is their exercise tolerance?
- Does the child make any noises associated with breathlessness?

Sounds audible without a stethoscope include wheeze, stridor, stertor, rattle and grunting (**Table 2.6**).

Listen to the child's description of their symptoms, if they are able to provide one. Chest tightness may occasionally be expressed as 'heaviness'.

Cardiomegaly indicates a cardiac cause of breathlessness. It may be found when a chest radiograph is carried out to investigate a suspected heart condition or respiratory disease.

Causes of breathlessness	
Cause	Clue(s) to diagnosis
Asthma	Wheeze
	Precipitation by exercise, upper respiratory tract infections, allergens
Pneumonia or other chest infection	Cough
Bronchiectasis	Clubbing
Cardiac failure	Enlarged heart on chest radiograph
Metabolic acidosis	Smell of acetone (diabetic ketoacidosis)
Neonatal causes	History of prematurity or problems at birth
Panic attacks	Tingling of fingers
Pain	History (or behaviour in an infant)
Neuromuscular	Muscle wasting or weakness

Table 2.5 Causes of breathlessness in children

Exercise tolerance

When assessing exercise tolerance, for example in cases of suspected asthma, the general rule is that younger children should be able to keep up with their peers when playing. School-age children should be able to take part in a full physical education lesson. It is difficult to evaluate shortness of breath on exercise in overweight children because their decreased exercise tolerance may be a consequence of their increased body weight and lower level of stamina rather than any pathology.

Respiratory sounds	
Term	Description
Wheeze	High-pitched whistling sound caused by obstruction of airflow in intrathoracic airways (lower trachea to small bronchi and large bronchioles); occurs in expiration and occasionally also inspiration
Stridor	Harsh inspiratory noise caused by obstruction of airflow at larynx or extrathoracic trachea; with mild degree of narrowing, stridor is audible only on activity (e.g. crying, feeding or agitation)
Stertor (snoring)	Coarse noise generated in pharynx during sleep
Rattle	Coarse, irregular sound resulting from excessive secretions in upper airways
Grunting	Expiratory noise caused by partial closure of glottis during expiration to increase intra-alveolar pressure (positive end-expiratory pressure)

Table 2.6 Respiratory sounds audible without a stethoscope

> **Children occasionally exaggerate symptoms to avoid physical exercise.** In many cases, this is because they do not want to do sport or cannot perform to parental expectations.

Chest pain

Chest pain is uncommon in children. However it does occur, and is seen most often in late childhood and adolescence. Unlike in adults, in children it rarely has a cardiac cause and is often not the result of organic disease (**Table 2.7**).

Focused history

In addition to using the SOCRATES approach, make the following enquiries.

- Is the pain exacerbated by exertion, deep inspiration or coughing? Is it worse around mealtimes or at night?
- Are there any associated symptoms, such as light-headedness, tingling fingers, palpations, nausea, sweating or fainting?

Causes of chest pain	
System	Causes
Musculoskeletal	Costochondritis
	Intercostal muscle cramps (precordial catch syndrome)
	Rib fracture or slipping rib
Psychogenic	Family stresses
	Problems at school
Pulmonary: pleuritic chest pain	Pneumonia with or without effusion
	Empyema
	Pneumothorax
	Sickle cell disease (acute chest syndrome)
	Pleurodynia (coxsackievirus)
Gastrointestinal	Gastro-oesophageal reflux or peptic ulcer
	Oesophageal foreign body
	Cholecystitis or pancreatitis
	Acute viral hepatitis or subphrenic abscess
Cardiac: pericardial disease	Acute pericarditis
	Post-pericardiotomy syndrome
Cardiac: ischaemia	Kawasaki's disease
	Anomalous coronary arteries
	Tachyarrhythmias
	Familial hypercholesterolaemia
Other	Acute myocarditis
	Cardiomyopathy
	Aortic dissection
Neurogenic	Shingles
	Spinal cord or nerve root compression

Table 2.7 Causes of chest pain in children

- Is the pain worse on palpation of the chest wall?
- Is there a past history of underlying chronic disease that affects the chest, for example asthma, cystic fibrosis, cardiac disease, sickle cell disease or systemic lupus erythematosus?

Consider other, less common, causes of chest pain. Ask about:

- family history indicating cardiac problems, such as arrhythmias, cardiomyopathy, sudden death and Marfan's syndrome, or peptic ulcers (a positive family history increases the risk of a pathogenic cause)
- psychological factors, such as recent myocardial infarction in a relative, bereavement or problems at school (which suggests psychogenic chest pain)

> **Many young children lack the language skills to describe their symptoms accurately, or have difficulty localising them.** For example, toddlers with an exacerbation of asthma often describe 'tummy ache', and young children with supraventricular tachycardia describe 'chest pain'. In the context of other signs and symptoms, a wider list of possible causes is considered than that for an older child.

Vomiting

Vomiting is the involuntary forceful ejection of stomach contents through the mouth. Most cases are secondary to infective gastroenteritis and resolve spontaneously. However, there are several other, less common causes of vomiting that arise in the gastrointestinal system, and several are specific to children at particular ages (e.g. pyloric stenosis in babies).

Focused history

An appreciation of the duration of vomiting and consistency of the vomit helps determine the diagnosis and subsequent management.

Dehydration

Answers to questions about when the vomiting started, how frequently it occurs and the volume disgorged give clues to how dehydrated the child is likely to be. A longer history (>2 days) makes gastroenteritis less likely. A long history associated with weight loss suggests bulimia, particularly in a teenage girl.

Nature of the vomit

Green (bilious) vomit suggests malrotation or intestinal obstruction; both are surgical emergencies. Vomit that resembles coffee

grounds suggests upper gastrointestinal bleeding (haematemesis). Always consider nosebleeds as the source of the blood, or in breastfed babies, blood from a mother's cracked nipple.

Effortless vomiting in an infant suggests reflux or overfeeding. Projectile vomiting is associated with pyloric stenosis.

Timing

Early morning vomiting may indicate increased intracranial pressure, or pregnancy in teenage girls.

Diarrhoea

The presence of diarrhoea and illness in other family members make the diagnosis of gastroenteritis more likely.

Headache

Vomiting is associated with migraine and increased intracranial pressure.

Diarrhoea

Diarrhoea is the passage of more than three loose stools a day. The commonest cause is infective gastroenteritis. Other gastrointestinal causes include irritable bowel disease and coeliac disease; however, diarrhoea can be a symptom of disease in other systems, such as hyperthyroidism.

> **Clarify exactly what the child or their parent means by 'diarrhoea' at the start of the consultation.** Picture charts of different stool types help; what constitutes 'normal' stool is different for every individual.

Focused history

After clarifying that the diarrhoea is truly diarrhoea, determine the cause with further questions.

Onset and duration

Diarrhoea from birth suggests cows' milk protein allergy or intolerance. Consider inflammatory bowel disease in a child older than 10 years.

Diet

Diarrhoea after weaning is a feature of coeliac disease. In younger children, excessive intake of fruit, especially fruit juice, contributes to 'toddler diarrhoea'.

Frequency
Enquiries about the number of times a day the child opens their bowels help assess the impact of diarrhoea on the child's life. For example, if visits to the toilet are so frequent that the child is unable to attend school, their education will be negatively affected. Waking at night to open the bowels suggests significant diarrhoea.

Blood or mucus
These suggest infection or inflammation.

Infection
Transient lactase deficiency is common after gastroenteritis. It causes ongoing diarrhoea secondary to a lack of lactase in the small intestinal wall. The consequence is continued diarrhoea after the infective cause has resolved.

Undigested food
The presence of undigested food in the stool is typical of toddler's diarrhoea.

Poor growth or weight gain
Diarrhoea in the context of poor growth or weight gain is a feature of several chronic conditions, including Crohn's disease, cystic fibrosis and coeliac disease. Ask about other features associated with these diseases.

Abdominal pain

Abdominal pain encompasses any pain or discomfort in the abdomen. It is the result of many different pathologies, and may be gastrointestinal or genitourinary in origin, or secondary to infection. However, in many cases no cause is found, or there may a psychogenic cause.

A pain history is taken to narrow down the list of possible causes (use SOCRATES; see **Table 2.2** and page 54).

Focused history
Abdominal pain is a common presenting problem which is the result of mesenteric adenitis in many cases. The key is to exclude more serious causes of abdominal pain and their complications, e.g. appendicitis and peritonitis.

Location
Acute central abdominal pain is common in mesenteric adenitis; does the child have any symptoms of an upper respiratory tract infection, commonly associated with mesenteric adenitis?

Right iliac fossa pain suggests appendicitis. Loin pain is typical of pyelonephritis. Right upper quadrant pain suggests biliary pain; this is a finding in children with haemolytic anaemia who develop gallstones.

Associated features
Ask about associated features or symptoms, specifically the following.

- Is the child having diarrhoea or vomiting typical of gastroenteritis?
- Is the child constipated?
- Is there frequency or dysuria, indicating a possible urinary tract infection?
- Has the child lost weight?

Weight loss

This is a 'red flag' (a significant indicator of serious disease). It suggests a chronic disease such as inflammatory bowel disease.

Non-organic and psychosomatic pain

Be aware of non-organic pain in children. Ask about bullying. Children who are being bullied may complain of abdominal pain to avoid going to school. This results in a pattern of abdominal pain occurring in the mornings. Bullying can lead to psychosomatic abdominal pain: a real pain brought on by stress, with no other organic cause.

Fever

Fever is an increased core body temperature: > 37.5°C in children, although the exact level depends on the site where it is measured. It is especially common in children younger than 5 years. Most cases of fever are the result of a self-limiting viral infection, but these must be distinguished from the minority in which the cause is a serious bacterial infection (e.g. pneumonia or meningitis). Distinguishing between non-serious and serious cases is not always easy. However, a number of key features increase the likelihood of serious infection (see Table 17.9).

Focused history

History-taking in cases of fever is about identifying the focus of infection.

Associated symptoms

Cough, photophobia and neck stiffness suggest serious bacterial infection (see Table 17.9).

Hydration

Answers to the following questions give an idea of the child's general state of hydration and how unwell they are. Reduced fluid intake, decreased urine production and lethargy suggest significant dehydration and a more unwell child.

- Is the child still taking plenty of fluids and passing urine?
- How does their level of activity compare with how it is usually?

Rash

Different types of rash give clues to the underlying condition. For example, non-specific viral infection is associated with a maculopapular rash, whereas, meningococcal septicaemia is associated with with a non-blanching purpuric rash.

Travel history

A history of recent foreign travel suggests a tropical disease such as malaria.

Non-infective fever

Fever is not always secondary to infection; inflammatory conditions such as Kawasaki's disease and systemic onset juvenile idiopathic arthritis should also be considered. Answers to the following questions may increase the likelihood of a non-infective cause of fever.

- Has the fever persisted for 5 days or longer? (If so, consider Kawasaki's disease or systemic onset juvenile idiopathic arthritis)
- Is there conjunctivitis, a maculo–papular rash, lymphadenopathy or desquamation of the fingers? (If so, consider Kawasaki's disease)

- Is there any joint pain or swelling? (If so, consider systemic onset juvenile idiopathic arthritis and, rarely, rheumatic fever)

Collapse

Collapse is a sudden fall to the ground with loss of consciousness. Vasovagal syncope (or 'faint') is the most common cause. However, several more serious conditions are considered when assessing a child presenting with collapse (see Table 8.4).

Focused history

Answers to the questions relating to collapse help to differentiate between conditions causing collapse. None of the features described are individually characteristic of a certain diagnosis, but they help narrow down the list of possible causes and guide investigations.

Consciousness

Children may not understand what unconsciousness means. Therefore if a child has difficulty describing their experience, ask about the last thing they remember before the collapse. No recollection of what happened during the episode suggests that the child was completely unconcious (e.g. during a seizure). In contrast, the ability to recall events during the episode suggests that conciousness was not lost (e.g. in cases of pseudoseizure).

Patients with vasovagal syncope usually describe feeling light-headed, nauseous or sweaty just before a collapse. Patients with temporal lobe epilepsy describe an aura, i.e. an unusual subjective sensation such as a certain taste or smell, just before the onset of a seizure.

Palpitations

The presence of palpitations or tachycardia suggests a cardiac cause.

Witnesses

Stiffening or jerking movements in a patient who has collapsed do not necessarily indicate an epileptic seizure. Brief jerking movements of the limbs can occur during a simple faint. Ask witnesses the following questions.

- How long did the child take to recover?
- Were they sleepy after the episode?

- Did the child wet themselves or bite their tongue?

The answers will help differentiate between collapse with a cardiac cause and seizure. Children who have had a seizure tend to feel sleepy during the postictal period (the period immediately following an epileptic seizure) and take longer to return to their normal selves.

> Video of an episode of collapse, recorded on a mobile phone, is extremely helpful when determining the diagnosis. Witnesses to an episode provide vital information, but a video showing what happened provides valuable objective evidence.

Rash

A rash is a change in the appearance (colour or texture) of the skin. It is a very non-specific symptom. Rashes with a serious cause, for example meningococcal septicaemia or leukaemia, must be differentiated from those with a less serious cause.

Focused history

Ask the following questions.

- Where is the rash?
- When did it first appear?
- Could anything have triggered the rash?
- Has it changed in appearance?
- Has anyone else in contact with the child had it?

The appearance of a rash shortly after exposure to a potential allergen suggests an allergic reaction. Changes in the appearance of the rash, or others having had the rash, suggests an infective cause.

Drug history

Ask if any medications have been tried. Do any make the rash better or worse? Any creams that have helped may give a clue as to the diagnosis.

Nature of the rash

A non-blanching rash on the skin of an unwell, febrile child is a worrying sign; it raises the suspicion of meningococcal septicaemia. Petechial rash (characterised by tiny reddish or purplish spots caused by localised haemorrhage) in the context of weight loss, pallor, bleeding gums or easy bruising is likely to be a sign of leukaemia, whereas in a well child it probably represents immune thrombocytopenia.

A non-blanching rash in a well child is a presentation of Henoch–Schönlein purpura; do they have any other features of this condition? Rash is a feature of Kawasaki's disease; is there any other evidence to support this as the cause?

> The 'glass test' is an easy way for a parent to identify a non-blanching rash. A glass tumbler is placed over the rash and pressed down. If the rash does not disappear while pressure is applied, urgent medical advice must be sought.

Jaundice

Jaundice is the yellow (icteric) discoloration of the sclera, skin and mucous membranes caused by hyperbilirubinaemia (excess bilirubin in the blood). In children, the discoloration is generally apparent at a serum bilirubin concentration of 35–50 µmol/L; however, in neonates it may not be noticeable until bilirubin reaches a serum concentration of > 85 µm/L.

Hyperbilirubinaemia

This is the consequence of increased haemolysis (breakdown of red blood cells) or liver problems resulting in abnormal processing of bilirubin (see page 145).

Bilirubin in plasma is either unconjugated or conjugated (joined with glucuronic acid and therefore water-soluble).

- A high concentration of unconjugated bilirubin in the plasma results from increased production or altered metabolism of bilirubin, haemolysis, or reduced uptake and subsequent removal of bilirubin by the liver; the unconjugated bilirubin is either bound to albumin or free (unbound)
- Accumulation of conjugated bilirubin in the plasma occurs because of reduced excretion of bilirubin by hepatic parenchymal cells or obstruction in the biliary tract (see pages 144 and 205)

Jaundice resulting from excessive levels of unconjugated bilirubin is bright yellow or orange. Jaundice caused by excess conjugated bilirubin is greenish or muddy yellow (**Figure 2.3**).

Focused history

Detailed questioning in the context of the child's age will help narrow down the causes of jaundice.

Hepatic dysfunction

Jaundice may be the earliest and only sign of hepatic dysfunction (see page 218). Dark urine and pale stools suggest an obstructive lesion, for example biliary atresia.

Breastfeeding

Jaundice is commoner in breastfed babies. If a neonate is not feeding well, they can become dehydrated, leading to jaundice. Breastmilk jaundice usually resolves as the baby's hydration status improves.

Severe hyperbilirubinaemia results in lethargy and poor feeding, thereby exacerbating the jaundice. A serious condition called kernicterus can develop if a baby's jaundice is untreated (see page 143). Because breastfed babies are most at risk, their mothers should be supported in their efforts to establish successful breastfeeding.

Pruritus

In an older child, pruritis suggests cholestasis (decreased bile flow).

Blood type

Consider the possibility of haemolytic disease of the newborn in young babies with jaundice.

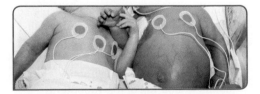

Figure 2.3 The baby on the right has jaundice caused by excess conjugated bilirubin, secondary to prolonged use of total parenteral nutrition; note the greenish tinge to the skin. The baby's non-jaundiced twin is on the left.

Family history

A family history of jaundice or jaundice with illness suggests a hereditary cause, for example Gilbert's syndrome, a genetic disorder in which people experience occasional, temporary episodes of jaundice.

Drug history

Consider any medications the child is receiving with the potential to cause hepatic dysfunction.

Limp

A limp is an abnormality of gait observed as an asymmetry when walking. It may arise as a consequence of pain anywhere in the lower leg, but it is usually caused by pain in the hip or knee. Although most cases are self-limiting (transient synovitis), be alert for serious underlying causes (septic arthritis) that require further treatment.

Focused history

A child's age narrows down the list of possible causes. When age is considered together with a good history, the diagnosis is usually apparent.

Onset

The timing of onset of a limp, i.e. acute or chronic, narrows down the possible causes (see Figure 9.1).

Trauma

Any history of trauma, either witnessed or unwitnessed, suggests an injury or strain to the bone or soft tissues.

Localisation

Ask about the location of the pain and any radiation. Bear in mind that young children may be unable to localise pain to a specific joint. If a specific joint seems to be affected, focus on this joint but remember that the underlying cause of the pain may be the joint above or below it.

Swelling

Joint swelling or tenderness, even if it has resolved, suggests an inflammatory or infectious cause.

Systemic symptoms

Symptoms such as fever, lethargy and abdominal pain suggest that the joint pain is secondary to a systemic condition.

Respiratory infection

In young children, a current or recent upper respiratory tract infection is consistent with transient synovitis.

Rash

Conditions associated with joint pain and a rash include systemic onset juvenile idiopathic arthritis and Henoch-Schönlein purpura.

> **Identification of child abuse requires the collection of information from multiple sources.** If a feature of a presentation raises the suspicion of child abuse, seek an explanation from the child as well as the parent or caregiver. Do not rely solely on the explanation provided by the accompanying adult.

> **There is evidence-based guidance on when to consider or suspect child abuse.** For example, guidance from the UK's National Institute for Health and Care Excellence says:
>
> - If abuse is considered a possible cause of the presentation, discuss your concerns with a more experienced colleague
> - If the level of concern is strong enough for abuse to be suspected, refer the child to children's social care

Child abuse

Always consider deliberate injury, especially in young children.

Lumps

A lump is a swelling palpable underneath the skin. The lump is commonly in the neck. However, lumps can appear anywhere in the body. A detailed history along with examination of the lump (see later in chapter) will often secure the diagnosis and therefore avoid uneccessary investigations.

> **Finding a lump can cause anxiety in parents who are worried about cancer.** In the majority of cases, the family can be reassured by the findings of a thorough history and examination.

Focused history

Ask when and where the lump appeared. A neck lump present at birth suggests a sternocleidomastoid tumour.

Growth and appearance

Answers to the following questions provide useful information.

- Has the lump grown? If so, how rapidly?
- Did anything precede the appearance of the lump, for example trauma?
- Is it tender?

Neck swellings that increase and decrease in size are probably the result of reactive lymphadenopathy in response to an upper respiratory tract infection or ear infection, both of which are common in children. Fat necrosis is a possibility in cases of preceding trauma at the site of the lump. A child with a tender neck lump usually has lymphadenitis. Red lumps suggest an infection.

Associated symptoms

Ask about:

- symptoms of thyroid disease, particularly if there is lump at the site of the thyroid gland (it could be a thyroid goitre)
- symptoms of inflammation and joint pain associated with arthritis (erythema nodosum is the presence of painful lumpy lesions on the shins, associated with autoimmune diseases)
- symptoms of cancer (e.g. weight loss or night sweats), because lumps could be enlarged lymph nodes (**Figure 2.7**), which may indicate leukaemia or other malignancies

> **A sternocleidomastoid tumour is not actually a tumour.** It is a benign lesion present from birth and usually accompanied by torticollis. The lesion is the result of fibrosis in the muscle and resolves with appropriate physiotherapy.

Faltering growth and weight loss

Faltering growth (previously known as failure to thrive) is a descriptive term and not a diagnosis in itself. It is defined as the falling

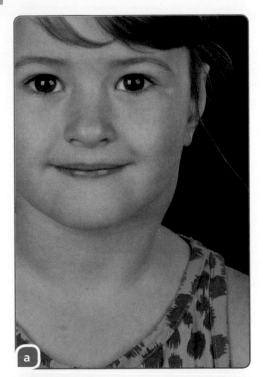

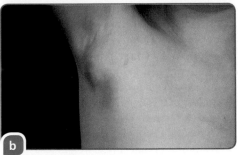

Figure 2.7 Visibly enlarged lymph nodes.

of weight measurements across two or more centile lines on a growth chart (see page 21), and warrants further evaluation of the child's nutrition and general health. It is most applicable to children under 2 years old.

See **Table 2.8** for causes of faltering growth. The cause of faltering growth is usually multifactorial. For example, an infant with congenital heart disease has an increased metabolic demand, which they may struggle to meet because of feeding difficulties secondary to breathlessness. Faltering growth is different from excessive weight loss in the newborn, which is attributed to feeding difficulties.

Focused history

In a child with faltering growth, explore whether they have inadequate intake or a condition that is causing increased demand on the body.

Birth history and birthweight

Consider the birth history and weight at birth alongside the subsequent growth chart. This helps determine the underlying reason for faltering growth. For example, an infant born to a mother with diabetes may have been abnormally large at birth and is now undergoing growth in a 'catch-down' pattern towards their genetic potential. Normal growth until weaning suggests coeliac disease.

Feeding

Ask about the volume of milk a baby takes at each feed, the type of milk (i.e. breast or formula; see page 38) and the frequency of feeds. The answers are used to assess whether a baby's intake is adequate to support growth.

Causes of faltering growth	
Cause	**Associated diagnoses**
Insufficient nutritional intake	Difficulties with breast and/or bottle feeding technique
	Neglect
	Poor suck or swallow (genetic or central nervous system conditions)
	Gastro-oesophageal reflux (feed refusal secondary to discomfort)
	Mechanical problem (e.g. cleft palate)
Inadequate nutrient absorption	Cow's milk protein intolerance
	Cystic fibrosis
	Coeliac disease
Increased intestinal loss of nutrients	Malabsorption
	Diarrhoea
	Vomiting
Increased metabolic demands	Congenital heart disease
	Hyperthyroidism
	Chronic or recurrent infection

Table 2.8 Causes of faltering growth in the first year of life

When there is no obvious cause for faltering growth, admitting the patient to hospital for a period of observation, e.g. a week, is helpful for obtaining evidence of how the child feeds and what the child eats.

Stool

Enquire about how often the child opens the bowels, and the consistency and colour of stools. This helps assess the adequacy of feeding in a newborn and identify malabsorption or liver problems at any age.

Passage of green stool continuing after the first few days of life suggests inadequate milk intake. Pale stool suggests obstructive jaundice. Frequent passage of loose stools suggests cow's milk protein allergy or intolerance.

Other symptoms

Ask specifically about signs and symptoms of possible pathological causes, such as gastro-oesophageal reflux, cow's milk protein allergy or intolerance and congenital heart disease. Features of genetic disease, jaundice and other conditions associated with faltering growth and weight loss are sought during the examination.

Common signs and how to examine a child

Starter questions

Answers to the following questions are on page 124.

4. Why are bottles of bubbles often found on paediatric wards?
5. When would you use a stethoscope to palpate the abdomen?

The aim of the examination is to detect signs that, together with the history, enable a list of possible causes to be identified. Providing the child cooperates, the paediatric examination includes assessment of all body systems, and entails plotting measurements on growth charts and recording basic observations (respiratory rate, heart rate, etc.). This is done to assess the overall well-being of the child rather than focus on the presenting problem alone.

Examination of the paediatric patient is an unpredictable experience. Older children and adolescents are generally cooperative. Difficulties tend to arise during examination of babies and toddlers; they may cry and resist examination by an unfamiliar person in an unfamiliar environment. If the child is upset and examination difficult, focus on the system causing the child's symptoms in an attempt to limit their distress.

> **Most young children take great delight in something like their new shoes or a cartoon character depicted on their T-shirt,** so saying how much you like them usually generates a smile. Negotiating cooperation with the offer of a sticker at the end of the examination is also helpful.

In adult medicine, examination follows a specific sequence, for example inspect, palpate, percuss and auscultate. However, this order is not necessarily followed in paedatrics.

To gather as much information as possible from a child who is not cooperating, it is necessary to be opportunistic. For example, you might look into the child's mouth when the child is screaming, or auscultate the chest at the start of the examintion, while the child is settled and not crying.

It is not unusual to be unable to place a hand or stethoscope on a child who is resisting examination. Fortunately, a wealth of information can be obtained by merely standing back and observing the child from a distance; observation is often the most informative part of the paediatric examination.

> **Never force a child to do anything they do not want to do.** It is helpful if they are made to feel at ease early on. Let them explore their environment, for example by simply letting them walk around the consultation room.

> **Differences in sensory processing can make elements of the examination particularly stressful for children with autism spectrum disorder.** They may have heightened sensitivity to stimuli that other children do not register. Simple measures can help them cope; for example, a child who is oversensitive to touch appreciates being warned which part of the body you wish to examine next.

General examination

Before starting the organ-specific examinations, a general examination is carried out. This consists of broadly observing the child and noting the following.

- Do they look well or unwell?
- Do they have any unusual facial features? (Dysmorphism may be a feature of a genetic disorder or an isolated finding)
- Are they interacting appropriately with others? (Lack of eye contact and difficulties in social interaction suggest autism spectrum disorder)
- Are they very quiet and drowsy? (This suggests a sick child)
- Are there any obvious abnormalities, such as limp?

This general examination takes place as soon as the child enters the consultation room, or even before, as they are coming from the waiting room. It helps provide clues as to what is wrong.

Also included in the general examination are assessment of growth and basic observations, i.e. measurements of respiratory rate, heart rate, blood pressure, temperature and oxygen saturation (the fraction of oxygen-saturated haemoglobin relative to total haemoglobin in the blood).

> Ideally, the child's body should be completely exposed to allow comprehensive examination. In practice, babies and toddlers are completely exposed but older children and adolescents are exposed only as necessary to carry out a thorough examination while minimising embarrassment.

Growth

All children have their weight and height measured on a regular basis by their health visitor to ensure they are thriving (growing adequately as expected).

The population-based spectrum of normal growth is represented by sex-specific standardised growth charts. Weight, height and head circumference measurements are plotted on these charts and used to identify children who are not growing as expected (a 'red flag'). Growth that is either too rapid or too slow prompts further investigation to determine why.

> The plotting and interpretation of measurements on a growth chart is a common examination question. Instructions are on the chart; find one and practise!

Measuring growth

Growth variables measured include height, weight and head circumference. Measurements are recorded in a standardised way using calibrated stadiometers and scales to avoid interexaminer variation and consequent spurious results.

Height

This is measured in children over the age of 2 years, with the examiner standing at the child's eye-level after the child has exhaled (**Figure 2.5**).

Length

Children younger than 2 years are unable to stand reliably, so their length is measured. This is a two-person task, because the child needs to be held still (**Figure 2.6**). Young children fidget, so it is difficult to obtain an accurate measurement. Therefore the mean of three measurements is recorded.

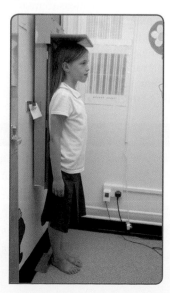

Figure 2.5 Measurement of height in a child.

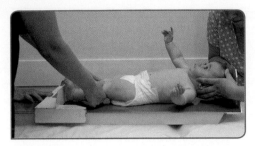

Figure 2.6 Measurement of an infant's length.

Weight

Calibrated scales are used to measure weight. Special scales are available to make it easier to weigh children who are in a wheelchair.

Head circumference

This is measured around the forehead (midway between the hairline and the eyebrows) and occiput, where the head circumference is greatest. The largest of three measurements is recorded.

> Specific growth charts are available for children with conditions with recognised differences in growth pattern, such as Down's syndrome and Turner's syndrome.

Interpreting growth charts

Growth measurements are plotted on a growth chart. At least two measurements taken at least 3 months apart are required to draw any conclusions regarding a child's growth; more measurements over a longer period give a more informative picture. One measurement cannot be interpreted, because it could be incorrect.

Patterns of concern

The following warrant prompt further observation or assessment:

- a fall across two centiles of height, weight or head circumference
- a fall across any centile if there are also abnormal findings on examination, such as dysmorphic features or signs of chronic disease

Investigation of short stature is discussed on page 332, and of faltering growth on page 63.

> The progress of puberty is assessed when evaluating growth, because precocious or delayed puberty is associated with certain abnormal growth patterns. The Tanner staging method is an objective, standardised way of carrying out the examination (see Figure 1.29).

Observations

Normal values for the basic observations recorded in paediatrics differ by age (**Table 2.9**). Observations are generally needed in the acute setting, in which they indicate how unwell the child is, for example by showing if the child is in shock. They are also used in the outpatient setting, for example measurements of blood pressure in a nephrology clinic, or oxygen saturation in a respiratory clinic.

An observation may be outside the normal range for various reasons, for example a chronic respiratory condition or an acute febrile illness. The crucial point is to identify when an abnormal observation warrants a comprehensive examination to identify the cause.

Normal observations			
Age	Heart rate (beats/min)	Respiratory rate (breaths/min)	Systolic blood pressure (mmHg)
Birth	110–170	25–60	60–100
6 months	105–165	25–55	65–115
1–5 years	85–150	20–40	70–120
6–11 years	70–135	16–35	80–130
12–18 years	60–120	14–26	95–140

Table 2.9 Normal observations in children

Heart rate and respiratory rate are increased if the child is distressed or crying. In these cases, repeating the measurements after the child has had time to relax or fall asleep will give true readings.

Carrying out observations

The following are commonly recorded observations:

- **heart rate**, measured by using a pulse oximeter, palpating a pulse or auscultating the heartbeat
- **respiratory rate**, measured by observing the child and counting the number of breaths they take every minute
- **oxygen saturation**, measured by pulse oximetry
- **temperature**, measured with a tympanic thermometer, except in premature neonates and babies up to a few months' old, in whom axillary temperature is measured (the ear canal is too small to allow a reliable tympanic reading to be obtained)
- **blood pressure**, measured by using a sphygmomanometer (automatic or manual) with a cuff that is appropriate for the size of the child; the bladder inside the cuff must cover > 80% of the circumference and at least two thirds the length of the upper arm (use of a cuff that is too small results in erroneously high readings)

Interpretation of observations

Observations are recorded so that abnormal clinical features can be detected and their causes determined. Paediatric observations are interpreted in the context of the child's age: for example, a heart rate of 150 beats/min is normal in a 3-week-old baby, but in a 15-year-old it is considered tachycardia. Causes of abnormal observations are shown in **Table 2.10**. Oxygen saturation should be > 95%, unless the child has a cyanotic congenital heart condition or chronic respiratory condition.

Respiratory examination

Respiratory illnesses are common in children. Many respiratory illnesses present

Abnormal observations	
Abnormal observation	Interpretation
Tachycardia	Early sign of shock, arrhythmia, fever
Oxygen saturation < 95%	Cardiac or respiratory disease
Tachypnoea	Early sign of shock or cardiac or respiratory disease
Hypotension	Late sign of shock

Table 2.10 Abnormal signs in standard observations

with similar signs, for example respiratory distress. Respiratory signs can also be a feature of non-respiratory illnesses such as heart failure. Different respiratory illnesses present with specific constellations of signs (**Table 2.11**). The respiratory examination is carried out with the aim of detecting respiratory signs that support or refute a specific diagnosis. Included within the respiratory examination is examination of the ears, nose and throat, which should be carried out on all febrile children as the commonest cause of fever is a upper respiratory tract infection.

Sequence

Inspection

The examination begins with inspection. Look at the patient from the end of the bed. Are they breathing comfortably or showing signs of respiratory distress? Respiratory distress is a warning that the child is unwell. Look for fingernail clubbing, which is associated with several respiratory conditions (see **Table 2.12**). Look at the child's skin for evidence of eczema, which is associated with asthma. Are there any central lines? These are placed in children with cystic fibrosis who need regular courses of IV antibiotics.

Palpation

Palpate the trachea; is it central? It deviates in cases of atelectasis (collapsed lung) and pneumothorax. Is chest expansion equal (**Figure 2.12**)? Unequal chest expansion implies lung pathology (see **Table 2.11**).

Respiratory disease: physical signs				
Condition	Chest shape or movement	Mediastinal shift	Percussion note	Breath sounds
Asthma or viral wheeze	Hyperinflated	None	Resonant	Wheeze on expiration
Consolidation	Decreased on side affected by pathology	None	Dull	Crepitations
Collapse	Decreased on side affected by pathology	To same side as affected by pathology	Dull	Decreased
Pleural effusion	Decreased	To opposite side of side affected by pathology	Stony dull	Absent, with or without bronchial sounds above fluid
Pneumothorax	Decreased	To opposite side of side affected by pathology	Hyper-resonant	Decreased
Bronchiolitis	Hyperinflated	None	Patients too young for percussion note to be determined	Crepitations and wheeze

Table 2.11 Physical signs of respiratory disease

Digital clubbing: causes	
System	Condition
Pulmonary	Cystic fibrosis
	Bronchiectasis
	Pulmonary abscess
	Empyema
	Interstitial fibrosis or pneumonitis
Cardiac	Cyanotic congenital heart disease
	Infectious endocarditis
Gastrointestinal	Ulcerative colitis
	Crohn's disease
Familial	No underlying pathology

Table 2.12 Causes of digital clubbing

> The trachea cannot be palpated in neonates and infants, because their necks are short and fat.

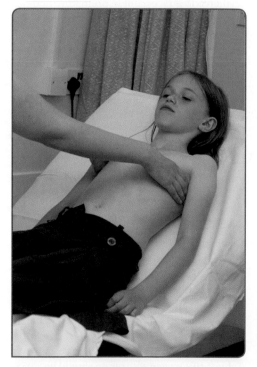

Figure 2.12 Assessment of chest expansion in an older child.

Percussion

Percuss both sides of the chest, anteriorly and posteriorly. Percussion does not tend to be carried out in babies, because the small size of the chest means that little useful information can be obtained using this technique.

The percussion note should be resonant. Sounds other than this point towards pathology located in the area where the sound is heard (see **Table 2.11**).

Auscultation

A stethoscope is used to listen, anteriorly and posteriorly, to both sides of the chest during the patient's inspiration and expiration. Normal breath sounds are vesicular in nature, i.e. the sounds are low pitched, and inspiration is longer and louder than expiration. Any other sounds suggest a disease process, for example localised crepitations (crackles) in cases of consolidation of the lung.

Examination of the ears nose and throat

An otoscope (**Figure 2.13**) is used to visualise the ear canal; look for signs of redness suggesting an otitis externa. Visualise the tympanic membrane: if it is red and bulging this also suggests an otitis media, if dull and retracted this suggests glue ear.

If a child is uncooperative there is a specific way of holding them to examine the throat (**Figure 2.14**), so a tongue depressor and light source can be used to visualise the tonsils. Red tonsils are commonly seen in viral upper respiratory tract infections. Enlarged, red tonsils with pus points are consistent with a diagnosis of tonsilitis and may require treatment with antibiotics.

The nose is examined with nasal speculum when there has been a foreign body inserted, e.g. a small toy, or in children with cystic fibrosis in whom polyps can be seen.

> **Abnormal breath sounds are occasionally heard without the use of a stethoscope,** for example wheeze.

Signs

Specific signs, when they appear together, can suggest the diagnosis; for example, reduced chest expansion and crepitations point towards a diagnosis of pneumonia. However, by far the commonest sign is the general 'respiratory distress'.

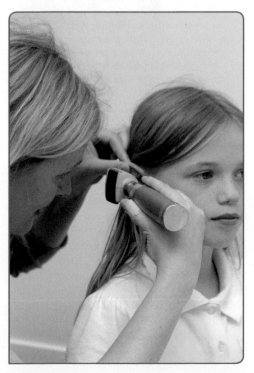

Figure 2.13 Using an otoscope to visualise the ear canal.

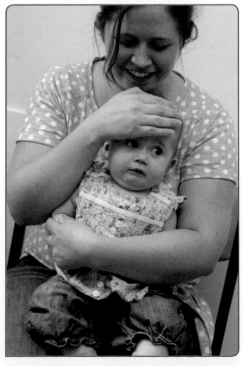

Figure 2.14 Holding an uncooperative child to enable the throat to be examined.

Respiratory distress

This is a general term for several clinical signs that sugggest that the body is working harder than normal to supply its tissues with oxygen:

- nasal flaring
- tracheal tug (an abnormal downward movement of the trachea)
- grunting
- intercostal and subcostal recession (**Figure 2.15**)
- use of accessory muscles (e.g. the sternocleidomastoid)
- head bobbing

Signs of respiratory distress do not always have a respiratory cause. For example, they are present in cases of sepsis and heart failure. A key skill is the ability to recognise these signs and consider them in the context of other information obtained during the examination to determine why the child is in respiratory distress.

Clubbing

Finger clubbing is an uncommon sign in paediatrics. Its presence suggests several possible diseases, not just respiratory in nature (**Table 2.12**).

Wheeze

This is a common sign detected during auscultation in the respiratory examination. The commonest reasons for its presence are asthma exacerbation and viral-induced wheeze. In babies, it is also heard in bronchiolitis and heart failure. The presence (or absence) of other signs must be determined to make the diagnosis. For example, the presence of crepitations and wheeze confirms bronchiolitis.

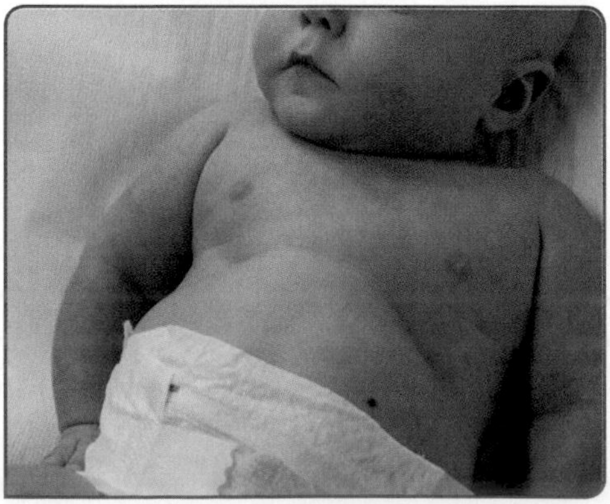

Crepitations

These are audible on inspiration and sound like crackles. They are most commonly heard in cases of consolidation of the lung (which characterises pneumonia) or bronchiolitis. The two conditions can be differentiated because there is no associated wheeze in pneumonia, whereas both crepitations and wheeze are heard in bronchiolitis. Occasionally, no clinical signs of pneumonia are present other than increased respiratory rate and cough, but consolidation will be apparent on a chest radiograph.

> **'Silent chest' is a sign of impending respiratory failure.** It is the absence of audible wheeze in a patient experiencing an acute exacerbation of asthma. As their condition deteriorates, increasing bronchoconstriction further restricts the movement of air into the chest, causing wheezing to decrease until eventually it can no longer be heard. Immediate management with bronchodilators is needed; if this fails intubation and ventilation are required.

Figure 2.15 Subcostal recession in an infant, indicating difficulty in breathing.

Cardiovascular examination

The cardiovascular examination is carried out to identify any abnormalities related to the heart or blood vessels. The commonest is a heart murmur, an unusual sound heard during a heartbeat. Heart murmurs are either abnormal murmurs associated with congenital heart disease or harmless 'innocent' murmurs produced by a structurally normal heart. In children, most murmurs are asymptomatic. Heart failure, which has many causes (see page 74), gives rise to many signs that are not specific to the cardiovascular examination, for example tachypnoea and wheeze.

Sequence

Inspection

Look at the patient from the end of the bed. Do they look cyanosed? Are there any signs of infective endocarditis, such as Osler's nodes? Do their features appear dysmorphic? Many syndromes are associated with structural congenital heart disease; for example, atrioventricular septal defect is frequently associated with Down's syndrome. Is a nasogastric tube being used? Heart failure is associated with poor growth, so the nasogastric tube may have been inserted for the delivery of additional high-calorie feed. Does the child have any scars suggesting previous cardiac surgery (**Figure 2.16**)?

Palpation

The rate, rhythm and volume of the peripheral pulses, including the femoral pulses, are assessed. Does the patient have tachycardia? Assess for radiofemoral delay (see page 75), which is present in coarctation of the aorta.

A hand is placed flat, with the palm down, over the precordium (the area to the left of the sternum) to detect precordial activity. The apex beat is palpated at the furthest lateral and inferior position. It is normally at the 4th or 5th intercostal space, in the mid-clavicular line; displacement to the left (laterally) suggests left ventricular hypertrophy.

Auscultation

Listen for the 1st and 2nd heart sounds and any heart murmurs. If a murmur is detected, the following features must be assessed to determine the cardiac lesion (if any) causing the murmur.

- **Location**: where the murmur is loudest
- **Intensity** (grade): systolic murmurs vary in intensity from grade 1, a faint murmur, to grade 6; murmurs of grade 4 and above are accompanied by an associated thrill (a palpable element)
- **Quality** (pitch): does the murmur sound harsh, soft or machinery-like?
- **Timing**: is it systolic, pansystolic or diastolic?
- **Radiation**: is the murmur heard elsewhere, for example the neck or back?
- **Variation with posture**: does the murmur change when the child is lying down or sitting up?

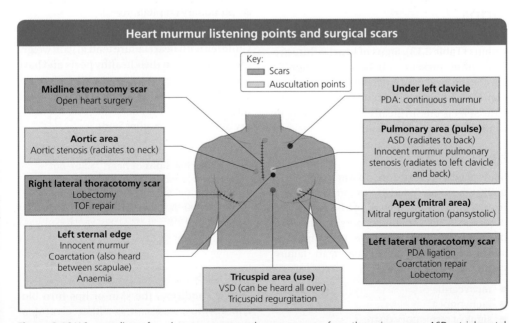

Heart murmur listening points and surgical scars

Key:
- Scars
- Auscultation points

Midline sternotomy scar
Open heart surgery

Aortic area
Aortic stenosis (radiates to neck)

Right lateral thoracotomy scar
Lobectomy
TOF repair

Left sternal edge
Innocent murmur
Coarctation (also heard between scapulae)
Anaemia

Under left clavicle
PDA: continuous murmur

Pulmonary area (pulse)
ASD (radiates to back)
Innocent murmur pulmonary stenosis (radiates to left clavicle and back)

Apex (mitral area)
Mitral regurgitation (pansystolic)

Left lateral thoracotomy scar
PDA ligation
Coarctation repair
Lobectomy

Tricuspid area (use)
VSD (can be heard all over)
Tricuspid regurgitation

Figure 2.16 Where to listen for a heart murmur, and common scars from thoracic surgery. ASD, atrial septal defect; LLSE, lower left sternal edge; PDA, patent ductus arteriosus; TOF, trachaeo-oesophageal fistula; ULSE, upper left sternal edge; VSD, ventricular septal defect.

Cardiac signs		
Sign	Elicited	Cardiac condition
Clubbing	On inspection	See Table 2.12
Central cyanosis	On inspection	Cyanotic congenital heart disease
Splinter haemorrhages and Osler's nodes	On inspection	Infective endocarditis
Tuberous or tendon xanthomata	On inspection	Familial hypercholesterolaemia
Thoracotomy or sternotomy scars (see Figure 2.14)	On inspection	Previous cardiac surgery
Radiofemoral delay	On palpation of pulses	Coarctation of the aorta
Weak pulses	On palpation of pulses	Shock, hypovolaemia, critical aortic stenosis
Bradycardia	On palpation of pulses	Heart block, normal variant
Tachycardia	On palpation of pulses	Anxiety, shock, pyrexia, supraventricular tachycardia
Sinus arrhythmia	On palpation of pulses	Normal variant
Displaced apex beat	On palpation of precordium	Ventricular hypertrophy, dextrocardia (the heart points towards the right side of the chest)
Increased apical activity	On palpation of precordium	Left ventricular volume or pressure overload
Heave at the lower left parasternal area	On palpation of precordium	Right ventricular hypertrophy
Thrill in the suprasternal notch or carotid arteries	On palpation of precordium	Aortic stenosis

Table 2.13 Cardiac signs seen in paediatrics

Signs

Many signs are associated with cardiac conditions (**Table 2.13**). Signs of heart failure are more often present in babies with a significant structural cardiac defect. They are less common in older children, because significant defects are surgically corrected early in a child's life to prevent heart failure.

Heart failure

Signs of heart failure develop when the heart's ability to pump blood is compromised; as a result, blood accumulates in the lungs and other parts of the body, causing them to become congested (see page 183). The constellation of signs indicating heart failure comprises:

- tachycardia
- tachypnoea
- signs of respiratory distress
- high-volume, bounding pulses
- hepatomegaly

- pumonary crepitations
- wheeze on auscultation

Children with heart failure tend to gain weight more slowly than their healthy peers and have increased energy requirement. Therefore the child is likely to be small for their age, and a nasogastric tube may be in place for the delivery of extra milk or other feeds.

> If a baby has signs of heart failure but the cardiovascular examination is otherwise normal, an extracardiac cause needs to be sought, for example aneurysm of the great cerebral vein (vein of Galen) in the head.

Cyanosis

In this condition, the skin or lips turn bluish. In most cases, it is either central or peripheral. The two need to be differentiated, because central cyanosis indicates cardiac or respiratory pathology and needs investigation, whereas peripheral cyanosis is a normal physiological response.

Central cyanosis associated with cyanotic congenital heart disease is clinically detectable when the level of deoxygenated haemoglobin in the bloodstream reaches 40 g/L. The discoloration is best observed in the mouth; look for a bluish tongue.

Peripheral cyanosis (acrocyanosis) is characterised by a bluish colour of the hands, the feet and the area around the mouth (circumoral cyanosis). The mucous membranes remain pink. It is a normal physiological response to vasoconstriction, for example the vasoconstriction that occurs when a person is cold.

> **In people with dark skin,** it may be easier to detect peripheral cyanotic discoloration in the lips and nails than on the hands.

Radiofemoral delay

The radial and femoral pulses are palpated simultaneously. Radiofemoral delay, a delay between the right radial pulse and the right femoral pulse, is a sign of coarctation of the aorta.

> **Sinus arrhythmia is a normal variant in which heart rate increases during inspiration and decreases during expiration.** This makes the pulse seem irregular unless the timing of inspiration and expiration are taken into account.

Heart sounds

There are two heart sounds: S_1 and S_2. S_2 is described as 'split', because the aortic component is heard before the pulmonary component. In children, S_2 is split more widely in inspiration than in expiration. The rapid heart rate of the newborn makes detection of the S_2 split difficult. Several congenital heart defects are associated with particular S_2 characteristics (**Table 2.14**).

Heart murmurs

The two broad groups of paediatric heart murmur are innocent, i.e. not associated with congenital heart defect, and pathological. In paediatric medicine, most heart murmurs are innocent. Most pathological murmurs are associated with a ventricular septal defect.

Innocent murmurs

These are sounds made by blood circulating normally around a structurally normal heart.

Congenital heart disease: S_2 heart sounds		
Defect	S_2 characteristics	Pathophysiology
Atrial septal defect	Widely split	Excessive filling of the right ventricle and delay in closure of the pulmonary valve
	Fixed split (the interval between aortic and pulmonary component does not vary with respiration)	The two atria function as a single unit, so respiration affects them equally
Aortic stenosis	Delayed and soft aortic S_2	In reversed splitting, the aortic 2nd heart sound follows the pulmonary component, because it takes longer for blood to be ejected from the left ventricle
	Reversed (paradoxical) splitting possible in severe cases	
Aortic atresia	Single S_2	Associated pulmonary hypertension causes early closure of the pulmonary valve
Pulmonary atresia		
Truncus arteriosus		
Transposition of the great arteries	The pulmonary component of S_2 is softer or inaudible	The pulmonary artery is located directly behind the aorta

Table 2.14 Features of S_2 heart sounds in congenital heart disease

The main types of innocent heart murmur are:

- Still's murmur, which is heard at the lower left sternal edge and can radiate upwards into the neck
- venous hum, heard below the clavicles; it is loudest when the child is sitting, and disappears when they lie down

A murmur is more likely to be innocent if:

- it is soft
- it is short
- there is no associated thrill
- there is no associated heave
- it is heard over a limited area
- it is mid-systolic (except venous hum)
- it has a musical, vibratory quality (low pitched)
- its intensity varies with posture
- no cardiac symptoms or other cardiac signs are present
- it is not heard over the back

Pathological murmurs

These are caused by turbulent blood flow through the heart, normally as a consequence of a structural or valvular problem. They are usually the only sign that a child has congenital heart disease (**Table 2.15**).

Features that suggest a pathological murmur include:

- an intensity of grade 3 or higher
- a harsh quality
- pansystolic timing
- being loudest at the upper left or upper right sternal border or the apex
- an abnormal S_2
- absent or diminished femoral pulses
- being audible over the back

Abdominal examination

The abdominal examination is carried out to identify any abnormalities related to the gastrointestinal and hepatic system. Signs detected in the abdominal examination can also suggest problems in other systems, for example splenomegaly is a symptom of hereditary spherocytosis, a haematological disorder.

Sequence

Inspection

From the end of the patient's bed, look for any obvious abnormalities. Is the child jaundiced? Do they appear to be in pain? This suggests acute abdomen (sudden, severe

Congenital heart disease: murmur location		
Type of defect	Timing of murmur	Location
Ventricular septal defect	Pansystolic	Loudest in 4th left intercostal space
		Radiates in all directions
Pulmonary stenosis	Ejection systolic	Loudest in pulmonary area
		Conducts to left posterior chest
Aortic stenosis	Ejection systolic	Loudest in the right upper sternum
		Conducts to both sides of the neck
		Suprasternal and carotid thrills
Atrial septal defect	Ejection systolic	Heard in the pulmonary area because of increased flow through the pulmonary valve
Coarctation of the aorta	Ejection systolic	Loudest over the back, between the scapulae
Persistent ductus arteriosus	Systolic, can extend into diastole	Loudest in the 2nd left intercostal space, lateral to the pulmonary area
		Radiates down to the apex
		Sounds like machinery

Table 2.15 Murmur location in congenital heart disease

abdominal pain requiring urgent assessment and treatment). Is a nasogastric tube in place? This shows that the patient is receiving extra nutrition, for example in cases of inflammatory bowel disease. The pumps used to administer feed through the nasogastric tube may also be present. Check the following to identify signs of gastrointestinal or liver problems (**Table 2.16**):

- hands
- eyes
- mouth
- chest
- abdomen; is a stoma present, showing that a bowel operation has been carried out (e.g. colectomy for ulcerative colitis), or a percutaneous endoscopic gastrostomy feeding tube, suggesting that the child has feeding difficulties (e.g. associated with cerebral palsy)?

Abdominal signs	
Sign	Associated disease or disorder
Clubbing	See Table 2.12
Leuconychia (white nails)	Hypoalbuminaemia
Koilonychia (spoon-shaped nails)	Iron deficiency anaemia
Palmar erythema, gynaecomastia, spider naevi	Liver disease
Asterixis (liver flap, a flapping tremor)	Hepatic encephalopathy
Jaundice	Hyperbilirubinaemia
Pale conjunctivae	Anaemia
Kayser-Fleischer rings	Hepatolenticular degeneration (Wilson's disease)
Mouth ulcers	Crohn's disease
Glossitis	Vitamin B12 deficiency
Angular cheilitis	Iron deficiency
Distended veins (caput medusae)	Portal hypertension
Faeces palpable in left iliac fossa	Constipation

Table 2.16 Signs detected in the abdominal examination

Inspect the external genitalia for hernias or scrotal swellings only if this is appropriate, i.e. when bilious vomiting is a possible sign of strangulated hernia.

> **Remember to check the child's flanks for hidden scars.** These suggest that they have undergone renal surgery.

Palpation

With the child lying flat on the bed, lightly palpate all areas of the abdomen to establish the location of greatest pain and any obvious masses. Repeat, but with deeper palpation.

> **Start palpating the abdomen away from the painful area.** Starting with the most painful area can upset the child early in the examination, making the rest of it more difficult.

Co-ordinate palpation for organomegaly (enlargement of the internal organs such as the liver, spleen or kidney) with the child taking deep breaths and the enlarged liver or spleen will hit your hand as you press it into the abdomen.

- To palpate for the liver, start from the right iliac fossa and move upwards to the right costal margin (**Figure 2.17a**)
- To palpate for the spleen, move from the right iliac fossa to the left costal margin (**Figure 2.17b**)

Ballot the kidneys (**Figure 2.18**). An enlarged kidney is palpable.

Percussion

Percuss over the abdomen, listening for any dullness. If organomegaly has been found on palpation, the lower borders of the spleen and liver are confirmed by percussing in the same direction in which palpation was carried out. Percussion over an enlarged liver or spleen produces a dull sound. A liver is enlarged if it can be palpated in a child over the age of 1 year. It is normal to feel 1–2 cm of liver in a younger child.

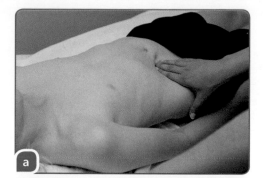

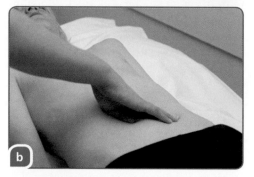

Figure 2.17 Palpation of the liver (a) and spleen (b).

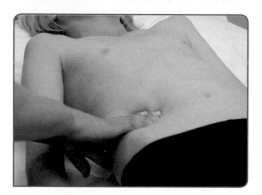

Figure 2.18 Balloting a kidney.

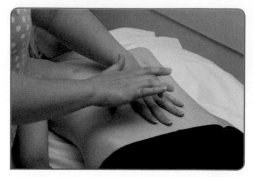

Figure 2.19 Percussing for ascites.

It can be difficult to differentiate the left kidney from the spleen. The following features help distinguish between the two organs.

■ It is not possible to palpate above a spleen

■ The spleen cannot be balloted

■ Percussion over a spleen is dull, but over a kidney it is resonant

■ A spleen has a palpable notch; a kidney does not

■ The spleen enlarges to the right iliac fossa, whereas the kidney enlarges down towards the left iliac fossa

Signs

Signs commonly detected in the abdominal examination are shown in **Table 2.16**. Pain on palpation of the abdomen occasionally represents a problem requiring surgery (e.g. appendicitis) but is most often secondary to mesenteric adenitis.

Abdominal distension

The five F's causing abdominal distension are:

■ **fat** – the child is overweight or obese
■ **fluid** – the distension represents ascites, a feature of nephrotic syndrome and liver disease
■ **faeces** – a severely constipated chid can present with abdominal distension
■ **flatus** – accumulation of wind secondary to bowel obstruction

Percuss for ascites by following a horizontal line from the umbilicus to the flank, bilaterally (**Figure 2.19**). If ascites is present, the percussion note becomes dull towards the flanks. This is confirmed by testing for shifting dullness. An enlarged bladder is identified by percussing from the pubic symphysis to the umbilicus.

Auscultation

The abdomen is auscultated for bowel sounds.

- **fetus** – a girl presenting with abdominal distension could be pregnant, even if sexual activity is denied

Organomegaly

This term means 'enlarged organ' and is generally applied to the liver or spleen. The liver usually becomes enlarged as a result of infection or a metabolic condition. The spleen is enlarged by haematological disorders or malignancy.

Ascites

This is the accumulation of free fluid in the abdominal cavity. It is found mostly frequently in children with a diagnosis of nephrotic syndrome, and is associated with liver failure.

Bowel sounds

Absence of bowel sounds suggests bowel obstruction, peritonitis, or if found after abdominal surgery, postoperative ileus.

Neurological examination

By considering the various signs detected during the examination, it is possible to determine whether a neurological problem affects the upper or lower motor neurones and to make a diagnosis.

A formal neurological examination is difficult in children under 6 years old, because they have difficulty understanding and complying with instructions. However, much information about a child's neurological system is gained via observation; for example, a preference for one hand under the age of 18 months suggests a hemiplegia, and an asymmetrical smile indicates a facial nerve palsy.

The developmental assessment (see page 93) overlaps to some extent with the neurological examination, because many neurological problems present as developmental problems. For example a neurological condition such as cerebral palsy causes delayed motor development.

> **Neurodevelopmental disorders are caused by disturbance of development of the central nervous system.** They manifest as developmental deficits, of varying severity, that often become apparent before a child starts school, when the achievement of expected milestones is delayed. Attention deficit hyperactivity disorder, autism spectrum disorder and intellectual disability are some of the most common neurodevelopmental disorders.

Sequence

Inspection

Stand back and watch the child in the waiting room or walking into the consultation room. Are they using both hands and upper limbs equally? This shows that there is no asymmetrical weakness. Do they have a tremor when placing bricks on top of one another? This indicates the possibility of a cerebellar problem. If the child is walking, is there any evidence of an abnormal gait (e.g. the toe striking the ground before the heel)?

> **Walking on tiptoes is a normal variant in children up to 3 years of age with an otherwise normal examination.** In other contexts, it indicates pathology such as cerebral palsy or dysplasia of the hip.

On closer inspection, is there evidence of muscle wasting or contractures? Are any café au lait spots present? These are associated with neurofibromatosis type 1. Does the child have adenoma sebaceum? This is a sign of tuberous sclerosis. Look behind the child's ear; is a ventriculoperitoneal shunt (a device is used to treat hydrocephalus) in place?

Look at the size and shape of the child's head. Macrocephaly is associated with neurofibromatosis.

Tone

In older children, tone is assessed in a similar way to in adults, by assessing resistance during passive movement of the limbs.

In infants, tone is assessed by:

- visual inspection of resting posture
- resistance to passive movement during handling
- observation of head lag on pulling the child to sit, and their general posture when held in ventral suspension (**Figure 2.20**)

Power

In older children, as in adults, power is tested by assessing strength of flexion and extension against resistance in all limbs. Instructions need to be demonstrated or adapted for younger children to aid their understanding. For example, 'Put your arms up like you're a chicken' is the request when testing abduction of the shoulders. Power in one side is compared with power in the other to identify whether one side of the body is relatively weak. A subtle upper motor neurone disorder is indicated by drifting of the hands when a child is holding their arms in front of them while their eyes are closed.

In babies, power is assessed by observation of spontaneous movements, noting any asymmetry. Further information is gained by assessing resistance while trying to restrict spontaneous movements.

Coordination

This is assessed to test for cerebellar dysfunction. In children who are able to follow instructions, it is tested by using the same techniques as for adults. For example, in the finger-to-nose test, ask the child to to fully extend one arm then move that side's index finger to touch their nose, while you look for tremor or past pointing. Demonstrate the movement first and make the test fun. The ability to make rapid finger or hand movements (**Figure 2.21**) and to draw can also be assessed.

In children who are unable to comply with coordination testing, difficulties with coordination are identified by watching them play (e.g. stacking bricks) or walk.

Reflexes

In older children, reflexes are tested by using a patella hammer. Children find it difficult to consciously relax, which makes reflexes difficult to elicit. If a child is unable to relax

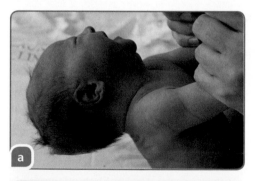

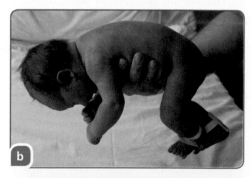

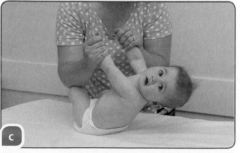

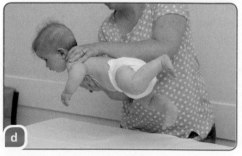

Figure 2.20 Assessment of tone in very young children. Head lag (a) and ventral suspension (b) in a newborn. Head lag (c) and ventral suspension (d) in an infant.

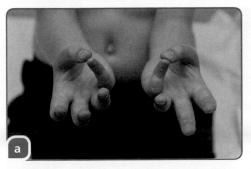
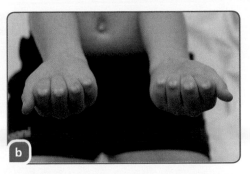

Figure 2.21 Assessment of cerebellar function, specifically coordination, in a toddler. The child is asked to make rapid movements of their fingers (a) and hands (b), and observed for evidence of dysdiadochokinesia (impaired ability to make rapidly alternating movements).

Primitive reflexes		
Reflex	Age of appearance	Age of disappearance
Palmar grasp	Present at birth	5–6 months
Plantar grasp	Present at birth	10–12 months
Stepping	Present at birth	2 months
Moro's	Present at birth	6 months
Tonic neck (arm extends when head turned to that side, other arm flexed like fencing posture)	Present at birth	2–3 months
Parachute (infant held in ventral suspension and brought rapidly towards ground. Infant holds out both arms to protect self)	8–9 months	Persists

Table 2.17 Ages of appearance and disappearance of primitive reflexes

by themselves, they need to be distracted so that the reflex can be obtained.

Neonates and infants are tested for the appropriate presence or inappropriate persistence of primitive reflexes (**Table 2.17**).

> **Up-going plantars (Babinski's sign) are normal in babies until the age of 12–24 months,** because their nervous system is not fully myelinated at this age. After this age, up-going plantars are a sign of upper motor neurone disorder.

Sensation

This cannot be reliably assessed in younger children, who have difficulty complying with the tests. However, in older children sensation is generally tested in the same way as it is for adults, e.g. using two-point discrimination test.

Cranial nerves

The cranial nerve examination is carried out differently in children of different ages (**Table 2.18**). In a neonate or infant, the whole examination is done by observation alone, because children this age are unable to follow instructions. In older children, cranial

Cranial nerve examination			
Cranial nerve	Function	Age < 6 years	Age > 6 years
I (olfactory)	Sense of smell	Not tested	Not tested routinely but substances familiar to the child (e.g. soap) can be used to test their sense of smell
II (optic)	Vision	Depends on developmental age Observe whether or not a baby fixes and follows an object in their visual field; do they reach for objects of various sizes? Use picture-matching cards for toddlers Check pupillary reflexes Fundoscopy, carried out by an ophthalmologist, if there are concerns about the fundus	Snellen chart or letter-matching cards Instruct the child to obscure one eye and to look straight at your nose, then assess their visual fields by wiggling a finger in each quadrant; repeat with the other eye obscured (**Figure 2.22**) Check pupillary reflexes Fundoscopy, carried out by an ophthalmologist, if there are concerns about the fundus
III (oculomotor), IV (trochlear) and VI (abducens)	Control of eye movements	With the baby's head held still, attract their attention with an object and monitor their eye movements as you move the object around	Ask the child to follow your finger with their eyes while keeping their head still (when examining a younger child, it may be necessary to hold their head or ask a parent to do so)
V (trigeminal)	Motor: muscles of mastication Sensory: facial sensation	Not formally tested	Feel for contraction of the masseter muscles when the child is asked to clench their jaw Check sensation (light touch) on the child's forehead, cheek and chin, on both sides of their face
VII (facial)	Control of muscles of facial expression	Observe for any asymmetry (e.g. of the nasolabial folds) Asymmetry may be apparent only when the baby is crying or smiling	'Smile and show me your teeth' 'Puff out your cheeks, like you're blowing up a balloon' 'Raise your eyebrows' 'Close your eyes as tight as you can'
VIII (vestibulocochlear)	Hearing and balance	Distraction test in babies aged 6 months	The whisper test is used to screen for hearing loss Rinne's test and Weber's test are used to lateralise and distinguish between conductive and sensorineural hearing loss Romberg's test is used to assess vestibular function
IX (glossopharyngeal) and X (vagus)	Swallowing, phonation, movement of palate	Listen for a hoarse voice or cry	'Open your mouth and say "Aah"' (watch for symmetrical movement of the soft palate and the uvula)
XI (accessory)	Movement of the sternocleidomastoid and trapezius muscles	Observe movements Look for torticollis	Ask the child to shrug their shoulders and turn their head to each side against resistance
XIII (hypoglossal)	Movement of the tongue	Observe movements of the tongue	'Stick out your tongue' (watch for any deviation from the midline)

Table 2.18 The cranial nerve examination in children

nerve function is tested in the same way as in adults.

> **When examining younger children, try to demonstrate what you want them to do rather than give verbal instructions.** Most children enjoy seeing the doctor poking out their tongue and puffing up their cheeks, and such actions encourage engagement in the examination they are undergoing.

Signs

Common neurological signs in paediatrics (**Table 2.19**) include:

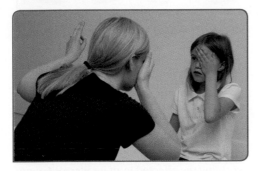

Figure 2.22 Gross assessment of visual fields in a school-age child.

- signs associated with upper motor neurone lesions, typically cerebral palsy
- skin lesions associated with neurocutaneous syndromes
- papilloedema, which is encountered in conditions associated with increased intracranial pressure

Abnormal gait is associated with many conditions (**Table 2.20**).

Increased tone and brisk reflexes

These are apparent in upper motor neurone disorders, most commonly cerebral palsy. Attention is paid to which limbs are affected, because this information is used when classifying the cerebral palsy (see page 257).

Abnormal gait and associated problems	
Type of gait	Possible cause
Spastic gait	Cerebral palsy
Ataxic (broad-based) gait	Cerebellar problem
Waddling gait	Muscular dystrophy
High-stepping gait	Peripheral neuropathy

Table 2.20 Types of abnormal gait in children, and associated problems

Neurological signs	
Sign	Cause
Unequal use of upper limbs	Weakness on one side
Tremor when stacking bricks	Cerebellar problem
Toe striking the heel before the ground when walking	Increased tone in abnormal leg(s); seen in hemiplegic or diplegic cerebral palsy
Muscle wasting	Neuromuscular condition or cerebral palsy
Multiple café-au-lait spots	Neurocutaneous condition (e.g. tuberous sclerosis)
Oversized head circumference	Neurofibromatosis, hydrocephalus, familial
Hand preference before 18–24 months	Neurological problem (e.g. cerebral palsy)
Increased tone	Upper motor neurone problem (e.g. cerebral palsy)
Reduced tone	Lower motor neurone problem or muscle disease (e.g. spinal muscular atrophy)
Papilloedema	Increased intracranial pressure
Little spontaneous movement, excessive head lag, child slipping through the hands of the person picking them up	Neuromuscular condition

Table 2.19 Signs detected in the neurological examination

Gower's sign

This is seen in children with neuromuscular problems, for example Duchenne's muscular dystrophy. It is demonstrated by asking the child to stand up from sitting on the floor. Proximal muscle weakness means the child will have difficulty rising, and will use their hands to push up from the floor and 'climb' up their legs.

Examination of a joint

Joint examinations are carried out if a child presents with joint pain or stops using a limb. The most frequently performed joint examination is the hip and knee examination, because limp is a common presentation. The hip and knee are the focus of the information in this section.

> The paediatric gait, arms, legs and spine examination, or 'pGALS', is a screening examination used on children presenting with musculoskeletal pain to identify specific areas of joint pain or immobility. These are then examined more closely.

Sequence

All joint examinations begin with the sequence 'look, feel and move'; this is followed by more specialist examinations applicable to the specific joint. Both joints are examined to enable comparison.

> Remember to examine the joint above and the joint below the one suspected of having the pathology, because pain can be referred from an adjacent joint.

Look

Each joint being examined needs to be adequately exposed. With the child standing, view the front, back and sides of the joint, looking for any muscle wasting, redness, swelling or scars, and comparing both sides.

Next, if the child is walking, observe their gait. Is their stance phase shortened? This antalgic gait indicates pain on weight bearing.

Genu valgum (knock knees; **Figure 2.23a**) is a normal variant in children aged 2–5 years.

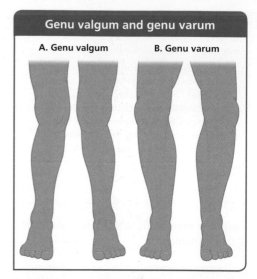

Genu valgum and genu varum

A. Genu valgum   B. Genu varum

Figure 2.23 Angular deformities of the lower limb. (a) Genu valgum (knock knees). (b) Genu varum (bow legs).

Genu varum (bow legs; **Figure 2.23b**) is a normal variant up to the age of 4 years.

Feel

With the patient lying down, assess the skin overlying the affected joint for warmth, comparing the temperature of this area of skin with the temperature of the skin over the normal joint. Increased temperature implies inflammation, for example in cases of juvenile idiopathic arthritis, or infection, for example in cellulitis or septic arthritis.

Next, feel the joint and perform measurements (**Table 2.21**) comparing both sides.

Move

The range of active and passive movement of the joint is assessed, and any restriction of normal movement noted (**Figure 2.24**). Restriction implies either a painful process preventing movement, for example septic arthritis, or a structural problem, for example slipped upper femoral epiphysis of the hip (page 283). Specific tests based on movement are carried out.

Thomas's test (hip)

When the natural lumbar curve is eliminated, a fixed flexion deformity of the hip is identified by failure of the knee to rest on the couch.

Specific examination of hip and knee		
Stage	Examination	Significance
Feel		
Hip	Over the greater trochanter	Pain implies bursitis
Knee	With the knee bent to 90°, palpate the joint line and patellar margin for tenderness	Tenderness indicates an inflammatory or infective disorder
	Feel for patellar tap by 'milking' fluid down from the suprapatellar bursa (**Figure 2.25**)	Bouncing of the patella is a sign of the presence of fluid, indicating an inflammatory or infective disorder
Measure		
Hip	True leg length (from the anterior superior iliac spine to the medial malleolus)	Discrepancy implies chronic disease reducing limb growth (the affected limb is shorter)
Knee	Around the quadriceps muscles and calf	Discrepancy suggests wasting from lack of use

Table 2.21 Specific examination of the hip and knee

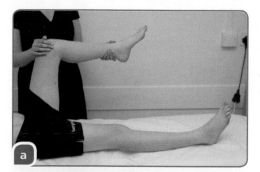

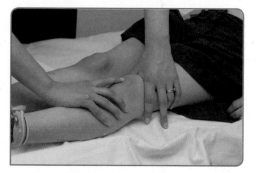

Figure 2.25 Patellar tap.

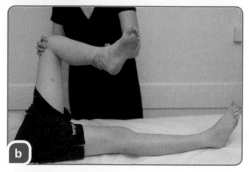

Figure 2.24 Examination of the hip. (a) Flexion. (b) Internal rotation.

Drawer test (knee)

Excessive anterior or posterior movement of the knee when manipulated at 90° implies rupture of the anterior or posterior cruciate ligament, respectively.

Examination of a lump

Lumps are examined to determine their nature. The child may have presented with a lump. Alternatively, the lump may have been detected during another examination, for example an abdominal examination, in which case it needs to be examined in more detail using a systematic approach.

Lumps are either filled with fluid (cystic) or solid. Neck lumps are commonly encountered in paediatrics. In the majority of cases they are reactive lymph nodes, but they can be the first presentation of cancer.

Sequence

Inspection

Define the position of the mass, and use a tape measure to determine its length and width. This information is particularly useful for neck lumps; it helps to narrow down the list of possible causes. For example, a lump in the midline cannot be a branchial cyst.

Palpation, percussion and auscultation

Palpate the mass – as gently as possible if the child experiences any pain – to define the following features (**Figure 2.26**).

- Shape
- Surface: is it smooth or irregular?
- Mobility: is the skin overlying the mass fixed to the mass? Is the mass mobile or fixed to deeper structures?
- Temperature
- Tenderness
- Consistency: is the mass very hard, like a stone? Rubbery? Spongy?
- Pulsatility
- Reducibility
- Transilluminability

The mass is then percussed and auscultated.

Signs

Features of different types of lump are shown in **Table 2.22**.

Neck lumps

There are many structures in the neck, so certain lumps are detected only in specific locations, for example thyroglossal cysts in the midline, and branchial cysts in the anterior triangle of the neck. Therefore the list of possible causes is narrowed down by a careful examination that pays particular attention to the location of the lump.

Hernia

Lumps in the groin are associated with hernias. These are seen most frequently in boys born prematurely, because the bowel is able to travel down the patent processus vaginalis. The lump is soft and reducible, and because it contains bowel, bowel sounds are heard when auscultating the mass. If the lump is hard, painful and non-reducible, it is an incarcerated hernia and requires urgent reduction to prevent bowel necrosis.

Examination of skin

A primary skin complaint requires thorough examination of the skin. Looking at the area of concern in detail, along with surrounding skin, is usually sufficient to make

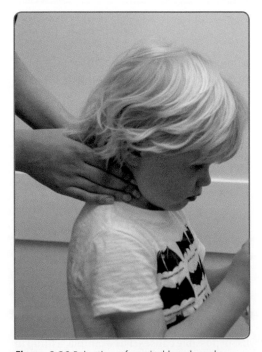

Figure 2.26 Palpation of cervical lymph nodes.

Lumps: interpretation of features	
Feature	Interpretation
Craggy, irregular surface	Malignancy (e.g. rhabdomyosarcoma)
Fixed mass (immobile)	Malignancy
Hot	Infection (e.g. abscess)
Tender	Infection
Hard (like stone)	Malignancy
Rubbery lymph node	Lymphoma
Spongy	Fluid-filled
Pulsatile	Vascular mass
Disappears when pushed in, reappears on coughing	Hernia
Mass glows red on transillumination	Fluid-filled
Dull on percussion	Fluid-filled
Resonant on percussion	Gas-filled
Bruits	Vascular mass
Bowel sounds	Mass contains bowel

Table 2.22 Features of lumps and their interpretation

a diagnosis. The skin is examined in examination of every system, for example for evidence of eczema in the respiratory examination. However, when the primary problem is a skin complaint, the dermatological examination is far more detailed and descriptive. The examination is based predominantly on inspection, and particular terms are used to describe the lesion.

Sequence

Inspection

Inspect the patient to identify the location of the lesion. Use a tape measure to determine its size, and note its shape, colour and other features (**Table 2.23**). Look at the surrounding skin; is it normal? Eczema herpeticum is a skin infection that occurs on eczematous skin.

> **Dermatological examinations should be carried out in a well-lit room so that the skin lesion can be seen clearly.** Use of a dermatoscope enables the lesion to be inspected in great detail. A tape measure is needed for accurate description of the lesion.

Inspect the skin over the rest of the body, including under the hair because skin conditions also present on the scalp. Pay particular attention to whether lesions are symmetrical (indicating flexural eczema), dermatomal (in cases of shingles) or only on exposed skin (suggesting contact dermatitis).

Palpation

Palpate the surface of the lesion. What is its texture? The lesions of plaque psoriasis are scaly. Note temperature and tenderness. Warm and tender lesions are likely to represent a skin infection.

Can any of the rash be scratched off? In psoriasis, flakes of skin can be scratched off.

Dermatological terms	
Morphological appearance	**Description**
Macule	Non-palpable flat area differing in colour from the surrounding skin
Papule	Palpable area of skin; diameter < 5 mm
Nodule	Palpable area of skin; diameter > 5 mm
Vesicle	Palpable fluid-filled lesion; diameter < 5 mm
Bulla	Palpable fluid-filled lesion; diameter > 5 mm
Pustule	Palpable pus-filled lesion; diameter < 5 mm
Plaque	Palpable raised area of scaly skin

Table 2.23 Definitions of terms used to describe skin lesions

In staphylococcal scaled skin syndrome, the skin can be rubbed off.

Complete the dermatological examination by palpating regional lymph nodes. These are likely to be enlarged in cases of infection (see **Figure 2.7**).

Signs

Pustules

These are a feature of many dermatological conditions. Localised pustules may represent impetigo, or if on the face and upper body, acne. Generalised pustules in a child with fever are likely to be caused by the chickenpox virus. Intensely itchy pustules are a sign of scabies infection.

Macules

These are a common feature of self-limiting viral illnesses. However, they are also seen in more serious diseases, such as measles.

Routine examination of the newborn

Starter questions

Answer to the following question is on page 124.

6. Why should a girl's dirty nappy be changed before a newborn examination?

The routine examination of the newborn takes place within 24 h of birth. It is done is to check that the neonate is healthy and to screen for congenital anomalies and potential disease. It is additional to the brief inspection of the baby carried out immediately after birth, usually by the attending midwife. The purpose of this first inspection is to determine if any emergency treatment is required.

The routine examination of the newborn is performed before the baby and mother are discharged to the care of a community midwife or health visitor. Prior to commencing the examination, information about the mother's health and peripartum period is gathered. The examination starts at the head and works down the body in a standard sequence to ensure nothing is missed.

Sequence

First, inspect mother's and baby's notes. Useful information to be gained includes:

- details of the pregnancy and birth
- results of antenatal screening tests
- maternal blood group
- antenatal scan results and birthweight
- whether the baby has received supplementary vitamin K (to prevent vitamin K deficiency bleeding; see page 45)

The examination is carried out when the baby is settled. It begins with visual inspection of the baby and observation of their spontaneous activity. Antigravity movements suggest normal power and tone. Paucity of movement is seen in neuromuscular problems. Before proceeding to handling that might disturb the baby, auscultate the chest and heart, and record the heart and respiratory rates.

Head and neck

Inspect head and neck for birth injuries and evidence of congenital anomalies (Table 2.24). Head circumference is measured and the result plotted on a growth chart, along with birthweight.

With the aid of a tongue depressor and torch, the hard and soft palate are visually inspected and palpated to look for a cleft. A small proportion of newborns have natal teeth, i.e. teeth which have erupted from the gum before birth. No intervention is required. However, because natal teeth have little root structure they can become loose and need

Head and neck signs in a newborn	
Sign	Condition indicated
Abnormal swelling	Birth injury (e.g. caput succedaneum or cephalhaematoma; **Figure 2.27**)
Absent fontanelle	Cranial synostosis
Head circumference on higher centile than weight	Asymmetrical intrauterine growth restriction, usually secondary to placental insufficiency
Asymmetrical facial movements	Facial nerve palsy resulting from traumatic forceps delivery
Absent red pupillary reflex or white pupillary reflex (leucocoria)	Congenital cataracts or retinoblastoma
Low-set ears	Possible genetic disorder (e.g. Down's syndrome or Turner's syndrome)

Table 2.24 Signs seen on examination of the head and neck of a newborn

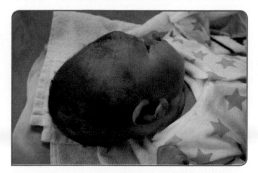

Figure 2.27 Caput succedaneum: swelling at the scalp.

removing by a maxillofacial surgeon to avoid aspiration.

An ophthalmoscope is used to check for bilaterally present red reflexes. All newborn babies undergo a hearing screen to identify congenital deafness. This takes place either before discharge from hospital or within the first few weeks of life.

> **Many cases of cleft palate are missed at the newborn examination.** Delayed detection can be avoided by using the appropriate technique. Submucous cleft palate, in which the cleft is covered by the lining of the roof of the mouth, is particularly easy to miss.

> The **red pupillary reflex** is often more of an orange or yellow colour in babies with dark skin.

Upper limb

Inspect the baby's arms and hands to look for any congenital defects or asymmetry. Observe their spontaneous movements, and check tone by moving the limb and assessing resistance. Floppy arms are a sign of a brachial plexus injury secondary to shoulder dystocia sustained during a difficult delivery.

> **Erb's palsy** is caused by damage to the upper part of the brachial plexus when the neck is stretched during the baby's passage through the birth canal. As a result, the arm is held in the 'waiter's tip' posture of shoulder adduction, elbow extension and wrist pronation. Most cases resolve spontaneously within a few weeks.

A single palmar crease, i.e. the presence of only one horizontal crease across the palm of the hand, can be normal but is more usually associated with Down's syndrome. Count the fingers, because some babies are born with extra or missing digits. This is usually an isolated finding but is occasionally accompanied by other congenital malformations as part of a syndrome.

> **Peripheral cyanosis, i.e. blue discoloration of the hands and feet secondary to vasoconstriction, is common in newborns.** However, it is not pathological and resolves spontaneously within a few hours.

Chest

This part of the examination comprises:

- assessment of the anterior and posterior chest walls for shape and symmetry
- measurement of respiratory rate (if not done prior to handling the baby)
- auscultation of the front and back of the chest for signs of respiratory distress, e.g. grunting or subcostal recession
- assessment of capillary refill time
- measurement of heart rate
- auscultation of heart sounds to check for murmurs

Oxygen saturation

A pulse oximetry probe is placed on the baby's right hand to measure preductal oxygen saturation, and on either one of their feet to measure postductal oxygen saturation. This is done to screen for cyanotic congenital heart disease, by identifying babies whose blood is insufficiently oxygenated. Further investigations are needed if there is a significant difference (> 5%) between the preductal and post-ductal measurements; this is an indication of congenital heart diseases or persistent pulmonary hypertension of the newborn. Normal oxygen saturation results do not exclude cyanotic congenital heart disease.

> The terms 'preductal' and 'post-ductal' describe the relation of parts of the aorta to the ductus arteriosus. Preductal oxygen saturation measurements reflect levels of oxygen in the blood leaving the branches of the aorta prior to the ductus arteriosus. Post-ductal oxygen saturation measurements reflect the levels in the blood after the ductus arteriosus.

> If the baby appears 'shut down' (with poor peripheral circulation) it is difficult to obtain accurate measurements from pulse oximetry. It is helpful if the baby is quiet: try asking the mother to hold or feed the baby, or let the baby suck your finger.

Abdomen

Inspect the abdomen for:

- distension or umbilical cord abnormalities
- normal cord insertion
- signs of infection in the umbilicus (redness and an offensive odour)

The abdomen is palpated to assess for organomegaly.

Groin

Run through the following checks.

- Palpate for the presence and quality of the femoral pulses; absent or weakly palpable femoral pulses are a sign of coarctation of the aorta
- Look for masses suggesting a hernia

- Check that the testes are palpable in the scrotum
- Assess for scrotal swelling
- Check the anal opening for atresia

> Some newborn girls have a clear or white vaginal discharge that is sometimes bloodstained. This is a consequence of the influence of hormones passed from mother to baby. It is not pathological.

Hip examination

The hip examination is a clinical screening test for developmental dysplasia of the hip. It combines comparison of leg length (using the Galeazzi's test) with instability testing using Ortolani's and Barlow's manoeuvres.

An audible and 'palpable' clunk elicited by Ortolani's manoeuvre shows that a hip is already dislocated (**Figure 2.28b**). For the

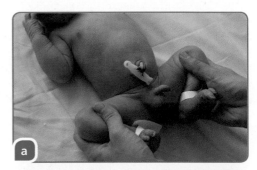
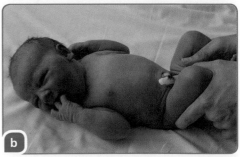

Figure 2.28 The neonatal hip examination.
(a) Ortolani's manoeuvre: both hips are gently abducted; a 'clunk of re-entry' is a positive result. Placement of a middle finger over the greater trochanter helps the examiner 'feel' the clunk.
(b) Barlow's manoeuvre: flexion and adduction of the hips, and backward pressure, with the aim of displacing the hip from the socket.

result of this test to be considered positive, the dislocation must also be reducible. If the dislocation is irreducible, the test result is negative and the leg is shorter on the affected side.

Barlow's manoeuvre determines whether a hip is dislocatable by putting the hip in the most unstable position and displacing it from the socket (**Figure 2.28a**). Abduction > 60° is normal. In bilateral developmental dysplasia of the hip, both hips have < 60° abduction.

Babies with an abnormal hip examination undergo an ultrasound scan at the age of < 4 months to look for developmental dysplasia of the hip.

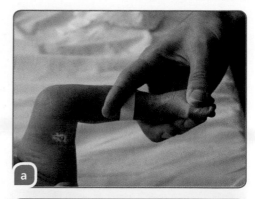

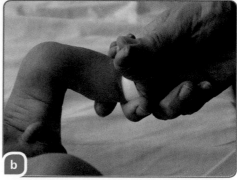

A useful mnemonic is:

- **Ortolani – O**ut to in (clunk of re-entry)
- **Barlow – dislocataB**le (provocative test)

Lower limbs and spine

Examine the legs for:

Figure 2.29 The normal full range of ankle movements in a neonate.

- malformations or limb disproportion, indicating skeletal dysplasia
- abnormal movements and swelling suggesting a fracture secondary to birth injury
- asymmetry of the skin fold creases, which indicates developmental dysplasia of the hip
- any limitation of the full range of movement in the feet and ankles (**Figure 2.29**)
- talipes (club foot)
- an abnormal number of toes on either or both feet

The baby is then turned over and the spine inspected for any dimples or tufts of hair. These are possible signs of spina bifida occulta.

Primitive reflexes

Bring the examination of the newborn ends to a close checking the primitive reflexes.

- Moro's reflex is tested by observing the movement of the arms as the baby falls backwards (**Figure 2.30**)
- Stroking the cheek and putting a finger in the neonate's mouth stimulates the rooting and sucking reflexes, respectively
- Palmar and plantar grasp reflexes are tested by placing a finger in the palm of the baby's hand or the inner sole of one of their feet; the baby's fingers or toes should grasp it
- Stepping reflex is tested by standing baby upright with their feet on a solid surface. The baby will lift its feet as if stepping

The absence of primitive reflexes suggests a neurological problem. For example, babies with a brachial plexus injury have an asymmetrical Moro's reflex.

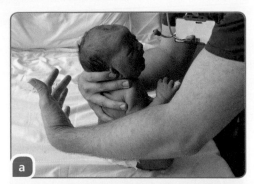

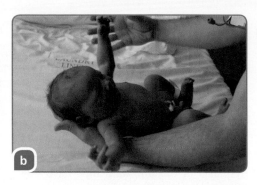

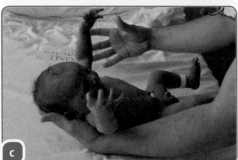

Figure 2.30 The primitive Moro's reflex. (a) The baby is allowed to suddenly fall backwards. (b) The arms open out fully and symmetrically. (c) The arms then move back inwards.

Developmental assessment

Starter questions

Answers to the following questions are on page 124.

7. What has arms and legs coming out of its face?

The developmental assessment takes many forms: from informal reviews of developmental milestones when a child presents with an acute illness, to formal examinations in which progress in each of the four developmental domains (see page 94) is scored using a standardised scoring system such as the Griffith or Bayley scales. If a child's development falls outside expected norms, a thorough paediatric assessment is warranted to establish if this is the result of pathology.

Standardised scoring systems are useful for monitoring developmental progress over time, but are time consuming (requiring 2–3 h). When initial concerns are raised by parents or nurseries, use short screening tests such as the Schedule of Growing Skills II or DENVER II are used by GPs or health visitors to identify children requiring referral for further assessment.

Developmental history

The developmental history provides information about the child's development to date: whether it is normal for age, whether any concerns have been raised by the parents or others involved in the child's life, and finally whether there are any risk factors that increase the likelihood of developmental problems. It includes information on:

- the pregnancy and birth (e.g. whether the child was born prematurely or needed resuscitation at birth)
- the child's general health (including details of any major illnesses, medication use, etc.)
- concerns regarding the child's growth or nutrition (the growth chart is reviewed)

- the attainment of common developmental milestones to date
- family members (including details of developmental delay and any hereditary conditions)
- parental concerns
- concerns raised by staff at the child's nursery or school

Developmental examination

A developmental examination can be carried out in any child-friendly setting with a few basic items (toys, bricks, crayons etc.). The developmental milestones and the ages at which they are expected to be achieved are shown in **Table 2.25**.

For each domain, begin with a few tasks that the child should be able to perform at their age. If they are successful, proceed to progressively more advanced tasks until they are unsuccessful. If they are unable to perform the initial task, work backwards until a task is found that they can perform.

> **Tailor the examination to the age of the child.** For example, assessments of a baby's progress in the domains of fine motor skills and communication and language are carried out before assessment of their gross motor skills, because the latter entails a greater level of physical interaction, which might upset the baby.

Inspection

The examination begins as soon as the child is seen, usually in the waiting room.

Developmental milestones				
Age	Gross motor skills	Fine motor skills*	Communication and language†	Social skills
6 weeks	Head lag on pull to sit; holds head in line on ventral suspension	Fixes and follows, initially through 45°, then 90°; closed hands	Quietens in response to sound	Smiles at parent's face
3 months	No head lag on pull to sit; raises head to 90° when prone	Fixes and follows through 180°; hands open; beginning to bring hands to midline	Turns head to sound, and coos in response	Social smiling (realises that smiling makes another person smile in response)
5–6 months	Rolls front to back; sits with support	Voluntary grasp of objects; brings objects to mouth; transfers objects from hand to hand	Turns in response to name; babbles	Holds bottle when feeding; looks for removed objects (understands object permanence)
8–10 months	Sits unsupported; starts to crawl; pulls to stand	Pokes at objects with finger; progresses from palmer to pincer grasp	Babbles using two-syllables; shouts	Waves bye-bye; finger feeds
12 months	Cruises between objects; stands	Bangs bricks together; throws objects	Says 'mama' and 'dada'; understands simple sentences	Claps hands; displays stranger awareness
15 months	Walks stably	Uses pincer grip for small objects	Jabbers; repeats words; understands words for some objects	Points and pulls; drinks from a cup
18 months	Carries toys while walking; runs unstably	Scribbles; turns 2 or 3 pages of a book at a time; builds a tower of 2 or 3 cubes (Figure 2.32a)	Points to named body parts and common objects (e.g. door); follows one-step requests	Holds a cup in both hands; feeds self
2 years	Runs stably	Turns pages of a book singly; copies a line	Says 2-word sentences; has 50-word vocabulary	Plays alone; eats with a fork and spoon
2.5–3 years	Climbs stairs one at a time; kicks a ball	Builds a tower of 6–8 cubes; draws a person with arms and legs emerging from the head (Figure 2.32b); copies a circle	Says 3- or 4-word sentences; follows 2-step requests	Begins toilet training; puts on shoes and underwear
3.5–4 years	Pedals a tricycle; jumps well; hops	Builds a tower of 9 or 10 cubes; draws a person with arms and legs emerging from the body (Figure 2.32c); copies a square	Asks lots of 'why' questions; counts to 10; uses past tense	Eats with a knife and fork; uses toilets unaided
5 years	Stands on one foot; comes down the stairs one at a time	Copies a triangle; writes own name; does up buttons	Counts to 20	Chooses own friends; role plays

*Includes visual development.

†Includes hearing.

Table 2.25 Milestones in the four developmental domains

- Assess their general level of activity and interest in their surroundings
- Observe their interaction with their parents and any other children in the waiting room
- Assess their general state of health
- Look for any dysmorphic features

The child's attention span can be gauged while they are sitting at a table during assessment of their fine motor, communication and language, and social skills tested.

> **The developmental examination does not always give a true picture of the child's abilities.** They may be tired or simply not in the mood to cooperate on the day. If this is the case focus on one domain or bring the child back for another attempt in the future.

Gross motor skills

This part of the examination is carried out to assess the child's ability to make and coordinate large movements, for example with their arms, legs and whole body. In babies, it can be done in one sequence (**Figure 2.31**). For older children, instruct them to perform different activities e.g. hopping, jumping or climbing stairs. Testing for the presence or absence of primitive reflexes is left until the end of the examination, because it may distress babies.

> **Try to make the assessment of gross motor skills fun for toddlers; be prepared to join in.** It can be carried out at the start of the examination if the child is active, or at the end if they are happy sitting at the table.

Fine motor skills

The child's ability to make and coordinate small movements of the hands and fingers is assessed; these fine motor skills are required when manipulating small objects and performing more intricate tasks. Simple objects such as cubes (**Figure 2.32a**) or a pen and paper (**Figure 2.32b** and **c**) are used to assess fine motor skills in a toddler. Older children

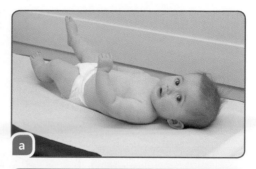
a

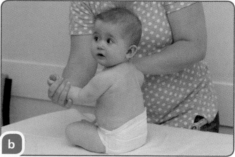
b

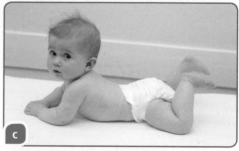
c

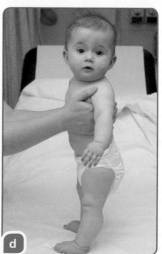
d

Figure 2.31 Assessment of gross motor skills in an infant. (a) Observe the baby to assess their tone and spontaneous movements. (b) Assess sitting posture. Can the child sit independently? Is their back rounded or straight and upright? (c) Place them prone on the bed. Do they lift their head or shoulders off the bed? (d) Hold the baby standing. Are their legs able to bear weight? Can they stand independently and take a few steps?

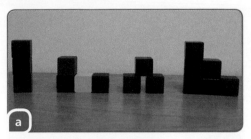

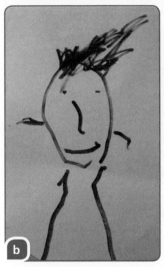

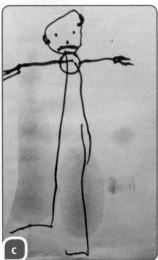

Figure 2.32 Development of fine motor skills. (a) Cubes placed to create a tower, train, bridge and steps as the child develops. (b) When asked to draw a person, a child aged 3 years typically produces an image of a figure with limbs emerging from the head. (c) A child aged 4 years draws a figure with limbs emerging from the body, and with hands and feet.

are asked to draw more complex pictures, e.g. a house, or to tie their shoelaces.

Visual development

Vision is also assessed, because the ability to perform tasks requiring fine motor skills depends on adequate vision. This part of the examination is carried out by observing if the baby can identify and pick up progressively smaller objects (see **Table 2.25**). Note any hand preference, or any asymmetry, which may indicate cerebral palsy.

Picture cards are used to assess vision in children aged 18 months to 3 years; they are given the name of an object and asked to point to the card depicting it. Letter-matching cards are used from the age of 3 years. A standard Snellen or LogMAR chart is used to assess the vision of children old enough to read letters.

Remember to look for the presence of a squint. In addition, check the red pupillary reflex as part of the assessment of vision. Absent red reflex suggests a cataract.

A referral to an ophthalmologist is made if more detailed assessment of visual acuity is required or fundoscopy needs to be carried out to investigate any abnormalities of the eye.

Communication and language

Skills in communication and language, both expressive and receptive, are assessed. Adequate hearing is necessary for the acquisition of these skills, unless another mode of communication, such as sign language, is taught.

Ask the parents of an infant about the sounds they make at home. For older children, simply having a conversation with them will give a good idea of language skills. General conversation with the child during the developmental examination is used to assess hearing.

When assessing language, identify whether any delay is in receptive language (the child's ability to understand what others are saying), expressive language (the child's ability to use words) or both. A question can be reformulated to assess receptive language alone or both receptive and expressive language. For example:

- in response to 'Show me your nose', a child with adequate receptive language will understand the instruction and point to their nose
- in response to 'What is this [the examiner points to the child's nose]?', a child with adequate receptive and expressive language will understand the question and reply 'My nose'

Difficulties with communication and language have many causes. Depending on the nature of the language delay, the child may be referred to the speech and language therapy team, the audiology department (for a formal hearing test) or the communication clinic.

> **For children growing up in homes in which more than one language is used,** referral to a speech and language therapist is appropriate only if they are experiencing difficulties understanding and using the family's primary language. It is normal for multilingual children to use a mixture of languages. This mixing decreases over time until they become proficient in the individual languages.

Ask the parent how the child communicates their needs and wishes at home. Do they point? Use words? Cry? Do they ask questions?

> All children have a **formal hearing test,** using headphones, when they start school.

Social skills

This part of the examination assesses the child's progress in developing the social skills needed to interact appropriately with others and to carry out daily activities, including self-care.

Look for features that suggest autism spectrum disorder, such as reduced eye contact or repetitive play. Ask the parents if their child has mastered skills such as feeding themselves (and using cutlery), helping with dressing or using the toilet, to determine whether they have achieved the expected milestones.

A referral to the communication clinic is made if formal assessment of a child's social skills is needed.

> **Remember to wave bye-bye at the end of the examination.** Babies start to wave back from 1 year of age, and this milestone is easy to elicit if you have established a rapport with the baby.

Investigations

Starter questions

Answers to the following questions are on page 124.

8. How many ways are there to collect a urine sample?
9. Why might you want to trigger a seizure in a child?

Investigations are carried out to confirm or refute differential diagnoses. The commonest are blood tests, urine tests and imaging studies (e.g. radiography and ultrasound). Children, especially younger children, can find it difficult to undergo investigations; invasive tests are particularly distressing. For this reason, no investigation is considered 'routine' in paediatrics. Investigations are carried out only if the information obtained will determine management.

Blood tests

In children, the commonest indications for blood tests are abdominal pain and suspected infection; however, tests are not required in all cases and should be used to support a clinical diagnosis rather than replace clinical judgement. The range of normal values depends on the age of the child, so it must be checked to ensure that results are interpreted correctly.

Obtaining blood samples

The procedure for obtaining blood samples from a young child differs markedly from that used when taking samples from an older child or adult. A play therapist prepares the child by explaining the procedure in an age-appropriate way. An assistant helps to position the limb and restrict its movement when the samples are taken, while the play therapist and parents use distraction techniques to keep the child calm.

The use of topical anaesthetic cream and distraction techniques (or reassurance in an older child) can eliminate the distress associated with venepuncture or cannulation; however, the cream must be applied an hour before the procedure. Topical refrigerant anaesthetic (cold spray) is less effective but acts instantly; it is therefore particularly useful when blood tests are required in an outpatient setting. Sucrose solution can reduce the distress of venepuncture in young babies, by providing a pleasant distraction from any pain. Allowing a baby to breastfeed has a similar effect.

Generally, a butterfly needle and syringe are used to withdraw blood. In neonates, a lancet is used to obtain capillary blood from the heel (a heel prick blood sample).

Full blood count

A full blood count is carried out to assess the levels of red blood cells, white blood cells and platelets in a whole blood sample. Common reasons for requesting a full blood count are:

- to check for anaemia, indicated by a low red blood cell count
- to check for evidence of infection, generally indicated by a high (but occasionally low) white blood cell count, typically with a predominance of neutrophils in bacterial infections and lymphocytes in viral infections
- to check for thrombocytopenia, indicated by a low platelet count

Simultaneous low levels of red blood cells, white blood cells and platelets indicate bone marrow failure, the most common causes of which are leukaemia and infection with viruses such as parvovirus B19 and Epstein–Barr virus.

Blood film

A blood film, also known as a blood smear, is obtained when information about the numbers or appearance of the blood cells is required. It is particularly useful to confirm haemolysis or detect blast cells in cases of suspected leukaemia.

A small drop of blood is placed on a slide and spread thinly across its surface. The blood sample is stained and viewed under the microscope to look for abnormalities.

Clinical chemistry

Clinical chemistry covers a wide range of tests carried out on blood and various other bodily fluids. The fluids most commonly tested are:

■ serum, i.e. the liquid component of blood that has been allowed to clot
■ plasma, i.e. the liquid component of blood that has been prevented from clotting

In contrast, a sample of whole blood is used in a full blood count.

Urea and electrolytes

Tests to measure urea and electrolytes are also referred to as kidney function tests. In paediatrics, they are mainly used to check for dehydration. There are four components: sodium, potassium, urea and creatinine.

Sodium

Hypernatremia (a high level of sodium) usually indicates dehydration. However, in rare cases it is the result of excessive intake of salt, for example in cases of fictitious or induced illness.

Hyponatremia (a low level of sodium) develops when there is:

■ an excess of water in the body, for example in cases of excess IV fluid replacement or syndrome of inappropriate antidiuretic hormone secretion
■ excessive sodium loss via the kidneys or gastrointestinal tract

Potassium

Excessively high or low potassium causes abnormalities in the cardiac rhythm.

Hypokalaemia (low potassium) is most commonly encountered in patients with excessive gastrointestinal losses (e.g. vomiting or diarrhoea) or with the shift to the extracellular space and osmmotic diuresis in diabetic ketoacidosis.

True hyperkalaemia (high potassium) is uncommon. However, a high level of potassium is a common result that represents a complication of haemolysis during sampling.

Urea and creatinine

These are waste products produced during protein and muscle metabolism. A high level indicates poor kidney function or dehydration. Typically, urea is the first to be increased in acute renal impairment or dehydration, followed by an increase in creatinine. A high creatinine concentration accompanied by a relatively normal urea concentration indicates chronic renal impairment.

Liver function tests

These tests are done to assess the health and function of the liver. Coagulation tests are also useful in the assessment of liver function, because many clotting factors are synthesised in the liver. The prothrombin time becomes prolonged when liver function is poor.

Albumin

This is one of the main proteins produced by the liver, and a good indicator of liver function. A high level indicates dehydration. Low levels are seen in cases of malnutrition, liver disease and nephrotic syndrome.

Alanine transaminase (ALT) and aspartate aminotransferase (AST)

These enzymes are normally present within the liver cells. Increased levels usually indicate hepatocellular damage, but AST is also increased in cases of cardiac or skeletal muscle damage.

Alkaline phosphatase (ALP)

This enzyme is present in bile ducts and bone. Increased ALP indicates a problem with the biliary tree or a bone disorder. Differentiate between the two by looking at the γ-glutamyl transferase concentration, which is increased in liver disease but not bone disease.

Bilirubin

This is a by-product of haem breakdown. Increased levels lead to jaundice (see page 144).

C-reactive protein

This is a non-specific measure of inflammation. Increased levels indicate the presence of infection or inflammation, but do not identify which parts of the body are affected.

C-reactive protein is measured in children with a suspected infection, to try to differentiate between a bacterial infection and a viral infection. Generally,

- a large increase in C-reactive protein suggests bacterial infection
- a small increase in C-reactive protein, or no increase, is more usual in viral infections

The test has poor sensitivity and specificity, so the result is always interpreted in conjunction with the clinical picture and the results of other investigations. It is useful in the diagnosis and monitoring of inflammatory conditions such as juvenile idiopathic arthritis and inflammatory bowel disease.

Blood gases

Measurement of blood gases provides information on oxygenation, ventilation (gas exchange and removal of carbon dioxide) and the body's acid–base balance. Blood gases are mainly requested in paediatric medicine as part of the general assessment and treatment of a seriously ill child, for example a child with diabetic ketoacidosis or sepsis. Rarely, it is indicated in the management of paediatric respiratory disorders such as asthma and bronchiolitis.

In adults, blood gases are measured using arterial blood. In contrast, in children capillary blood gases (or venous blood gases taken during cannulation) are measured. The blood is taken from the heel of a baby or via finger pricking in an older child. In pediatrics, arterial blood gases are rarely measured outside the intensive care setting.

Coagulation tests

Coagulation tests are requested when a child presents with an unusual pattern of bleeding or bruising, or has suspected hepatic dysfunction.

- Prothrombin time is a measure of the extrinsic pathway of the clotting cascade
- Activated partial thromboplastin time is a measure of the intrinsic pathway of the clotting cascade
- Fibrinogen, a protein essential for the formation of blood clots, is measured; its levels are decreased in liver disease and disseminated intravascular coagulation

Microbiology

Microbiological tests are used to identify the pathogen causing an illness and to inform the choice of antibiotic and the duration of treatment.

The first stage of analysis is microscopy and Gram stain to determine if any organisms are visible. The sample is then cultured, and the sensitivity of any organisms cultured to various antibiotics is assessed.

Urine tests

The most common indication for urine testing in paediatrics is suspected urinary tract infection (see page 229). Urine is also analysed to aid diagnosis of various other conditions:

- Urine is tested for the presence of ketones and glycosuria (glucose in the urine) in cases of suspected diabetic ketoacidosis
- Toxicological tests are carried out to detect the presence of drugs in cases of accidental or deliberate ingestion
- Urine organic acids is a test for the acidic products of carbohydrate, fat and protein metabolism; it is used in the diagnosis of inborn errors of metabolism

Obtaining urine samples

Analysis of a midstream clean-catch urine sample is the gold standard for diagnosis of urinary tract infection. However, a midstream sample is difficult to collect in young children, especially those who are not toilet trained; a clean-catch sample is the next preferred option. The commonest method for obtaining a clean-catch sample is for the child to sit with their nappy off, on top of a sterile bowl on a parent's lap.

Alternatives to obtaining a clean-catch sample are collection using special adhesive sterile bags applied to the cleaned perineum, and sterile pads in the nappy. However, samples obtained this way are often contaminated with skin commensals and are suitable only for tests unrelated to infection. For urgent samples, especially in infants, a catheter can be used or suprapubic aspiration carried out.

Dipstick urinalysis

This is a simple bedside investigation to detect the presence of protein, glucose, ketones, blood, nitrites and white blood cells. The dipstick has patches that change colour when they come into contact with urine containing these entities. The colours are then compared against a scale on the packet and the results recorded.

Dipstick analysis for nitrites is unreliable in children under 3 years of age. Microscopy is required in all cases of suspected urinary tract infection.

Microbiology

Urine samples are commonly sent for microbiological analysis. White blood cell count is determined to assess the likelihood of infection.

Imaging

Imaging studies are non-invasive investigations in which radiation (in radiography and CT), magnetic fields and radiowaves (in MRI) and soundwaves (in ultrasound) are used to visualise the internal parts of the body. Compared with adults, children are more sensitive to radiation and thus for a child the cancer risk associated with high or repeated radiation doses is heightened. No specific level of exposure is considered safe, so radiography and CT are carried out only when the benefit from the information gained outweighs the risk from radiation exposure.

An advantage of MRI and ultrasound is that there is no exposure to radiation. However, the patient must remain still for the duration of an MRI scan, and children find this difficult.

Radiography

In plain radiography, X radiation is used to create a single two-dimensional image of an area of the body. The most commonly radiographs requested in paediatrics are:

- chest radiographs, for the identification of pneumonia or pneumothorax
- radiographs of individual limbs, to identify any fractures

Because of the risks associated with radiation exposure, radiographs are ordered only in cases in which the information gained is necessary to guide management; they are not ordered routinely. For example, it is not necessary to obtain a chest radiograph to confirm a case of community-acquired pneumonia, a condition diagnosed clinically and for which the treatment is antibiotics, regardless of any radiographic findings.

Chest radiographs

In paediatrics, chest radiographs are most commonly obtained to assess the lung fields, usually in children with fever of unknown origin or respiratory signs and symptoms without a clear cause. Key features looked for on a radiograph are collapse, consolidation and pneumothorax. Chest radiographs also provide information about the heart. The size or appearance of the heart on a chest radiograph may raise the suspicion of congenital heart disease, or a chest radiograph may be ordered to look for signs of heart failure in a child with known congenital heart disease.

In older children, chest radiographs are obtained in a posteroanterior direction while the child is in deep inspiration. This is achieved by asking them to 'Take a deep breath and hold...' Young children and babies are unable to hold their breath in response to this request; in these cases, the radiographer tries to time the exposure with the child's spontaneous inspiration. Because of the practical difficulties of obtaining a chest radiograph in babies, the image is taken anteroposteriorly, with the baby placed on their back on top of the radiographic plate.

In infants, the cardiothoracic ratio can be as high as 0.65. This is because of their wide superior mediastinum, the result of the prominent thymic shadow that is present in the first few months of life before involuting. In older children, the cardiothoracic ratio is 0.5, similar to that in adults.

> **Take care when interpreting heart size on an anteroposterior film.** The heart may look artificially big, as a result of the direction in which the X-rays travel when the image is obtained.

Abdominal radiographs

These are infrequently obtained in paediatric practice, because of the high level of radiation required to obtain an image. Abdominal radiography is mainly requested to identify free air in the abdomen in cases of suspected bowel perforation, or to identify dilatated loops of bowel, signifying obstruction. The child should sit upright so that any free air accumulates under the diaphragm. Babies are unable to sit upright for this investigation. Therefore, in a neonate with suspected bowel perforation, the radiograph is obtained with the child in the left lateral decubitus position, allowing any free air to collect around the liver.

Skeletal survey

A skeletal survey is a series of plain radiographs of all the bones in the body. It is used as part of the investigation of suspected non-accidental injury in babies and young children, to identify both new and healing fractures.

Computerised tomography scan

In CT scanning, radiation is used to obtain cross-sectional images ('slices') of structures in any part of the body. Sequential images can be combined to produce a three-dimensional image. The most commonly scanned area of the body in paediatrics is the head. CT scans are also used by respiratory physicians to identify congenital lung anomalies such as cystic lesions, which may not be apparent on a chest radiograph. CT also shows localised areas of bronchiectasis and tumours. The radiation dose in CT scanning is very high, therefore in children other imaging modalities are used wherever possible and appropriate.

Magnetic resonance imaging

In MRI, a strong magnetic field and radiowaves are used to produce detailed images of the structures within the body, especially the soft tissues. No radiation is used, so it is safe to use in paediatrics. However, claustrophobia is common, and children find it difficult to remain still while the scan is obtained. Sedation may help older children cope with the procedure. Young children may require general anaesthesia to ensure that they remain in one position.

In paediatrics, MRI is most commonly used to obtain images of the brain, for example in children with developmental delay, focal seizures or onset of seizures at a very young age. MRI images are obtained of almost any other area of the body for various indications, for example in cases of suspected osteomyelitis.

CT versus MRI: benefits and indications

Both CT and MRI have specific advantages and disadvantages (**Table 2.26**). The choice of investigation depends on the situation.

- CT is better in an acute situation (e.g. in cases of trauma) or when a diagnosis is urgently required (e.g. when there is suspicion of a mass with increased intracranial pressure, or cerebral abscess)
- MRI is better for detailed examination of the brain

Ultrasound

In ultrasonography, high-frequency soundwaves are used to create images of internal structures. It is non-invasive and safe, because it does not require the use of radiation. It is

Comparison of CT and MRI		
	CT	MRI
Advantages	Fast and readily available	No exposure to ionising radiation
	Good for identifying acute haemorrhage, infarction, hydrocephalus, abscess, intracranial calcification	Provides high-resolution, anatomically detailed images with excellent soft tissue contrast
		Good for early identification of infarction and infection (e.g. encephalitis)
Disadvantages	Significant ionising radiation exposure	Noisy, and induces claustrophobia
	Poor resolution in posterior and temporal fossae	Examination takes > 30 min (sedation or general anaesthetic required in children unable to lie still throughout the procedure)

Table 2.26 Advantages and disadvantages of CT and MRI

also usually well tolerated. In paediatrics, ultrasound images of the abdomen and hip are most commonly requested. Cranial ultrasound is routinely used on neonatal units to screen for intraventricular haemorrhages.

Abdominal ultrasound

Ultrasound views of the abdomen are used in investigations of abdominal pain, particularly appendicitis and intussusception. They are also used to assess for abnormalities of the renal tract.

Cranial ultrasound

This is mainly used in neonatology, but it can be used to assess any baby with an open fontanelle. Standard views are obtained through the anterior fontanelle. Compared with CT or MRI, the advantages of cranial ultrasound in imaging of the brain are:

- It is non-invasive
- It does not expose the child to radiation
- It can be carried out at the bedside, usually by neonatal doctors rather than radiologists

Common indications include identification of intraventricular haemorrhage or post-haemorrhagic ventricular dilatation in premature babies, and identification of ischaemic changes in hypoxic ischaemic encephalopathy.

Hip ultrasound

This scan is obtained in assessments of a child with limp. The aim is to identify fluid inside the joint capsule. If fluid is detected, it

is not possible to differentiate between septic arthritis and transient synovitis based on the ultrasound image: aspiration of the joint fluid is necessary to make the diagnosis.

Hip ultrasound is also the investigation of choice for young babies with suspected developmental dysplasia of the hip.

Contrast studies

Studies using contrast agents, usually barium, are used to visualise the upper gastrointestinal tract (i.e. the oesophagus, stomach and proximal part of the small intestine) or the large bowel. Barium studies are carried out to identify strictures or blockages of the bowel, or malrotation. Gastro-oesophageal reflux is also identified.

An upper gastrointestinal barium study requires the child to drink a solution containing barium. In a lower gastrointestinal study, a barium enema is given. A series of radiographs are then obtained, in which the outline of the gastrointestinal tract is made apparent by the radiopaque barium.

> **To make it more palatable to children, the contrast agent can be added to a fruit-flavoured drink.** Alternatively, it can be delivered via nasogastric tube.

Micturating cystourethrogram

Micturating cystourethrography is a radiological investigation carried out to identify reflux in the urinary tract during urination. Contrast is introduced via a urinary catheter inserted into the bladder. A series of radiographs of the renal system are then obtained to identify any abnormality in urinary flow as the child passes the contrast-containing urine.

Radioisotope scans

Radioisotope scans provide information on the structure and function of the kidneys. The radioisotope is injected into the bloodstream, and cameras are used to detect the uptake of radioactivity by the kidney. Lack of perfusion of radioisotope through the kidney, or localised areas of the kidney, indicates scarring. If there is an obstruction in the renal system, it takes longer for the radioisotope to be excreted. Other information obtained includes the difference in filtration function between the two kidneys (fractional excretion).

> **Wash your hands thoroughly after carrying out a radioisotope scan,** particularly after helping a child use the toilet or changing their nappy. It can take days before all the radioisotope is excreted.

Three types of radioisotope scan are available.

- Mercaptoacetyltriglycine (MAG3) scans provide information on both the substance of the kidneys and excretion from the kidneys, and is usually used instead of the two separate scans below
- Diethylenetriaminepenta-acetic acid (DTPA) scans provide information on obstruction of the ureters, for example obstruction of the pelviureteric or vesicoureteric junction
- Dimercaptosuccinic acid (DMSA) scans provide more detail on renal scarring than MAG3 scans

> A mnemonic for the uses of radioisotope scans is:
>
> - **DTPA** shows the **P**eeing of the kidney
> - **DMSA** shows the **S**ubstance of the kidney

Respiratory tests

Respiratory tests are carried out to identify problems with breathing and determine their cause. They most commonly used tests measure lung volumes, evaluate the efficiency of gas exchange and identify problems with the airway. Baseline measurements are commonly recorded and lung function monitored over time. Lung function testing is rarely used in children under 5 years old because it is difficult for them to perform the test adequately.

Lung function tests

Lung function tests are carried out to measure airflow resistance, lung volumes and gas exchange, and thereby assess how well the lungs are working. A child's height is the strongest predictor of lung function, so standardised charts are available that show expected measurements by height. However, comparison of the most recent measurements with previous measurements for the same child are more useful for monitoring lung function and assessing response to treatment. Although spirometry gives a more complete picture of lung function, peak expiratory flow rate (PEFR) is much easier to carry out and is usually the first-line lung function test in children.

Lung function tests are helpful for:

- making a diagnosis, for example asthma is diagnosed if use of a bronchodilator reverses exercise-induced decreases in PEFR
- monitoring chronic disease, for example cystic fibrosis, asthma or neuromuscular disease
- assessing the risk of general anaesthesia or air travel in children with severe chronic lung disease or thoracic abnormalities (e.g. scoliosis)

Peak expiratory flow rate

This is easily measured with a portable peak flow meter. The test is used to identify asthma, which is characterised by reversible airflow limitation with diurnal variation. To measure PEFR, the child takes a deep breath in, places their lips around the mouthpiece of the peak flow meter and blows out as hard and as fast as possible. The accuracy of the reading is increased if the child is encouraged to take a good deep breath in and a good breath out. Peak flow meters can be used at home to monitor PEFR.

Spirometry

This is carried out to measure flow rates and dynamic lung volumes during forced inspiration and expiration through a mouthpiece. It produces a flow–volume loop, which can distinguish between the following conditions:

- obstructive small airways disease
- restrictive lung disease

> **Spirometry and PEFR measurements are unreliable in children under 5 years of age because they have difficulty understanding and complying with the test.** Furthermore, for a young child who uses an inhaler, the test can be confusing because they require forceful expiration rather than the inspiration the child has been taught for good inhaler technique.

Spirometry also measures forced vital capacity (FVC) and forced expiratory volume in 1 s (FEV_1). Typical patterns occur in different airways:

- Normal values for $FEV_1/FVC\%$ are > 80%
- FVC is reduced in restrictive lung disease
- FEV_1 is reduced in obstructive small airways disease

A measurement repeated 10 min after a bronchodilator is given (reversibility testing) that shows a > 10% increase in FEV_1 indicates reversible airways disease (e.g. asthma). A decrease in FEV_1 with exercise, usually on a treadmill, also suggests asthma. As with measurement of PEFR, the child needs to take a deep breath in, but in spirometry the subsequent blow out needs to be sustained for as long as possible – until they 'run out of breath'.

> **Visual incentives** seen by the child on the spirometer screen, such as cartoon characters blowing up a balloon, and encouragement from medical staff and parents during the test, are vital to get the child to blow as hard and as long as possible so that meaningful results are achieved.

Exercise tests

Children over the age of 5 years can usually manage these tests, which are usually done using a treadmill. The tests are useful to show exercise-induced bronchoconstriction in asthma. The child exercises for 6 min, and their heart rate and lung function before exercise and at 2, 5 and 10 min after exercise are measured. If FEV_1 or PEFR decreases, a bronchodilator is given and lung function retested 2 min later. In children with asthma, lung function improves in response to the bronchodilator (bronchodilator reversibility).

Pulse oximetry before and immediately after exercise can also be measured. Oxygen desaturation with exercise occurs in cases of interstitial lung disease, which is unusual in children.

Sleep studies

Sleep studies are used to assess for obstructive and central apnoea, hypoventilation and hypoxaemia during sleep. They range from simple overnight pulse oximetry, usually carried out at home, to full polysomnography, which is carried out only at specialist centres.

Pulse oximetry

In pulse oximetry, two diodes emitting light at different wavelengths (red and infrared) and a photodetector unit are used to measure the oxygen saturation of circulating haemoglobin and the heart rate (pulse). The diodes are contained in a device that is attached to a thumb or toe by either adhesive tape or a clip. A decrease in oxygen saturation associated with an increase in heart rate suggests obstructive apnoea. This is usually a consequence of tonsillar hypertrophy in children (see page 172). However, a normal trace does not exclude obstructive sleep apnoea. A decrease in oxygen saturation with a large decrease in heart rate suggests that the pulse oximetry probe has lost adequate contact with the skin; the result is either a movement artefact or the device has fallen off.

Polysomnography

This is the measurement of several physiological variables during sleep. It is used in investigations of obstructive sleep apnoea, hypoventilation associated with neuromuscular weakness and hypoventilation resulting from abnormal respiratory control (central causes). The data recorded vary with each centre and the purpose of the study, but may include:

- sleep stage
- movements of the chest or abdomen
- electromyography of the diaphragm
- arterial oxygen saturation
- heart rate
- end-tidal carbon dioxide
- eye movements

Polysomnography is a much more complex investigation than pulse oximetry and is therefore carried out only in specialist centres and for patients with specific conditions (e.g. narcolepsy). However, it provides much more data and is more accurate than pulse oximetry.

Cough swabs and sputum cultures

The presence of a pathogenic organism in secretions from the lung confirms an infection, and the sensitivity or resistance of the organism to different antibiotics is used to guide treatment. However, children find it difficult to expel sputum, and any sputum coughed up is usually swallowed. Therefore oropharyngeal cough swabs are usually collected from children with conditions such as cystic fibrosis. The child is encouraged to cough while a small dry swab on a stick is placed at the back of their throat. Alternatively, sputum is induced by the use of nebulised hypertonic saline (3–7%), which irritates the lung, eliciting a cough and expectorated sputum, which is collected. The presence of *Aspergillus* on a cough swab contributes to a diagnosis of allergic bronchopulmonary aspergillosis, which is confirmed by the presence of *Aspergillus* immunoglobulin (Ig) E and IgG in serum.

Sweat test

The gold standard test for cystic fibrosis is the sweat test. Sweat is stimulated by pilocarpine iontophoresis at the skin surface and analysed for chloride content. Children with cystic fibrosis have sweat with a high chloride concentration (> 60 mmol/L).

Mantoux test

This test, also known as the tuberculin sensitivity test, is carried out in cases of suspected tuberculosis. Tuberculin is injected intradermally (**Figure 2.33**). The response to tuberculin is a delayed hypersensitivity reaction, so it is measured 48 h after the injection. A positive result indicates tuberculosis infection. The result is positive if the diameter of the resulting induration (the palpable raised, hardened area) is > 5 mm in a child who has not had bacillus Calmette–Guérin (BCG) vaccination, or > 15 mm in a child who has.

Electroencephalography

In electroencephalography (EEG), several electrodes are glued to the scalp to record the electrical activity of the brain. It is a painless

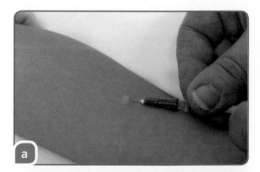

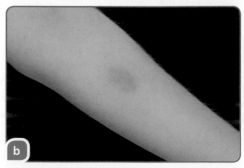

Figure 2.33 The Mantoux test. (a) Injection of tuberculin. The intradermal nature of the test results in a 'bleb' under the epidermis. (b) A positive result, with induration as well as redness.

investigation that usually takes about half an hour. It is carried out to support a clinical suspicion of seizures and to help characterise the type of epilepsy.

A standard EEG is done while the patient is awake. Likely triggers, such as hyperventilation and exposure to flashing lights, are used to trigger seizure activity. In cases where the standard EEG is normal but there is high clinical suspicion of epilepsy additional information is obtained from a repeat EEG carried out while the child is sleep or after a period of sleep deprivation; it may show changes not seen on the EEG obtained when the child was awake.

Cerebral function monitoring

This is a continuous but more basic type of EEG used in neonates at risk of hypoxic ischaemic encephalopathy (**Figure 2.34**). Three thin electrodes are inserted subdermally on the baby's scalp; they continuously record background electrical activity in the brain and any seizures (including subclinical seizures). The voltage of the background activity indicates whether the brain is functioning normally or the child has encephalopathy. Monitoring is carried out at the bedside, usually for at least 6 h and up to 3 days, primarily in babies undergoing therapeutic cooling. If seizures are detected on the CFM anti seizure medications are commenced.

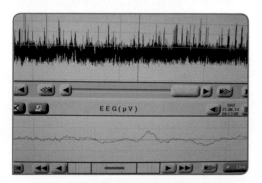

Figure 2.34 The cerebral function monitor, showing electrical activity in the brain over time.

Cardiac tests

In children, cardiac tests are done to assess the structure and function of the heart. In paediatric cardiology, the main concerns are the diagnosis and monitoring of congenital heart disease; acquired cardiac conditions (see page 190) are less common in children.

Electrocardiography

Electrocardiography (ECG) is used to record the electrical activity of the heart. It is a useful investigation for detecting problems with cardiac rhythm and ventricle size. It is also used to monitor the development or progress of known complications, such as pulmonary hypertension in cases of lung pathology.

Certain ECG appearances are characteristic of specific types of congenital heart disease (**Table 2.27**). However, these are more easily diagnosed by echocardiography.

Age-specific variables

Correct interpretation of a child's ECG requires knowledge of their age. A normal

Congenital heart disease: ECG appearances	
ECG appearance	Congenital defect
Right ventricular hypertrophy	Pulmonary hypertension (any cause)
	Severe pulmonary stenosis
	Tetralogy of Fallot
	Transposition of the great arteries
Left ventricular hypertrophy	Aortic stenosis
	Coarctation of the aorta
	Mitral regurgitation
	Obstructive cardiomyopathy
Biventricular hypertrophy	Ventricular septal defect
Right atrial hypertrophy	Tricuspid stenosis
Right bundle branch block	Atrial septal defect
	Complex defects

Table 2.27 ECG appearances in congenital heart disease

ECG for a neonate and during the first couple of years of life differs from that for an older child or adult, because in younger children, relative hypertrophy of the right ventricle is normal. Therefore in children a lead is usually placed on the right side of the chest (the V4R lead) to evaluate right ventricular hypertrophy, rather than the usual position of the V4 lead in adults, on the left side of the chest.

There is variation in the age at which the apparent right ventricular hypertrophy in children disappears. However, all features of right ventricular hypertrophy (other than the inverted T wave in V1–V2) should have disappeared by the age of 2 years; persistence of these features indicates an underlying abnormality. By the age of 10 years, the inverted T wave in V1–V2 has resolved and the ECG should be the same as that in an adult.

To diagnose underlying cardiac problems from ECG results, the age and heart rate of the child needs to be considered because:

■ ECG voltage criteria for the diagnosis of pathological ventricular hypertrophy differ according to the child's age
■ age and heart rate nomograms are used to assess the PR interval; a long PR interval is seen in first-degree heart block
■ The QT interval also varies with heart rate, so the corrected QT interval (QTc) is used for children, in whom the normal value is < 0.45 s
■ T-wave inversion is a finding in myocarditis and pericarditis or left ventricular hypertrophy or strain, but inverted T wave in V1–V2 is normal in children up to the age of 10 years

Echocardiography

An echocardiogram is an ultrasound image of the heart. It provides a two-dimensional cross-sectional view showing the anatomy of the heart and any structural defects. Dynamic views are used to assess the size and behaviour of the heart chambers and valves. Doppler and colour flow mapping assist by showing flow and pressure gradients across valves and any defects (holes), thereby enabling assessment of the severity of any valve incompetence or narrowing and the haemodynamic significance of any defect.

Allergy tests

Allergies are classified into IgE-mediated and non–IgE-mediated allergies (see page 289).

■ In IgE-mediated allergies, the immune system produces excessive amounts of IgE antibody specific to a certain allergen
■ In non–IgE-mediated allergies, the immune system response does not include IgE production; the mechanisms of these allergies are poorly understood

Symptoms of an IgE-mediated allergy occur rapidly soon after exposure to the allergen. This is not usually the case with non–IgE-mediated allergies, in which symptoms tend to appear much later. Therefore the type of allergy test carried out depends on whether an immediate or a delayed reaction is being investigated.

Skin prick tests

Skin prick tests are used to confirm suspected IgE-mediated (i.e. immediate-type) allergies. A drop of a standardised allergen test extract is placed on the volar aspect of the forearm. A lancet is pressed through the drop of allergen extract and into the skin causing a light scratch. A positive control (histamine) is applied to detect suppression of reactivity such as that caused by antihistamines. The diluent used to preserve the allergen extracts is used as a negative control.

After 30 min, the largest diameter of the raised wheal (not the larger red flare) at the point of application of each allergen is measured. A result larger than that of the positive control, when there is no reaction to the negative control, is positive (**Figure 2.35**).

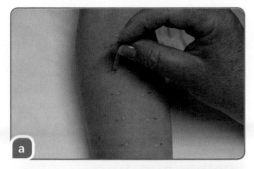

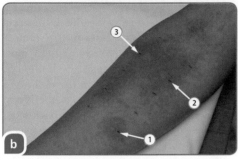

Figure 2.35 Allergy testing. (a) The skin prick test. (b) The results after 30 min: ①, the positive control; ② and ③, positive reactions, in this case to peanuts and Brazil nuts. The wheal diameter, not the red flare, is measured to assess the reaction.

Skin prick tests are interpreted alongside the clinical history, because 15% of people with a positive result on skin prick testing do not develop symptoms on exposure to the relevant allergen. However, the tests have a high negative predictive value, i.e. if the result for a certain allergen is negative, it is highly unlikely that the child is allergic to that allergen. The response to skin prick tests is suppressed by antihistamines, H_2 receptor antagonists and topical (but not oral) steroids, so the use of these medications is suspended for a minimum of 48 hours before the test is performed.

Serum-specific IgE is measured if skin tests cannot be carried out (e.g. in patients with severe eczema) or when the skin prick test, together with the clinical history, give equivocal results. However, a blood test is required for measurement of serum-specific IgE, and it is less sensitive than skin prick tests for the identification of inhaled allergens.

Food challenge

A food challenge is the introduction of a food to which a patient may be allergic, first by placing on the lip and then by eating. It is required for the diagnosis of delayed non–IgE-mediated reaction to a food, because there are no skin prick tests or blood tests for these conditions.

A food challenge is offered when:

■ there is an unclear history of food allergies
■ the results of blood tests and skin tests for allergy to a specific food are inconclusive
■ the child is suspected to have outgrown a food allergy

Because of the risk of anaphylactic shock (see page 403), food challenges are carried out only in specialist centres with facilities for full resuscitation.

Invasive tests

More invasive tests are occasionally required to diagnose or assess the severity of certain conditions. In children, most invasive tests require the use of general anaesthesia or heavy sedation so that the child remains still during the procedure, and so their discomfort and distress minimised. Therefore invasive tests are carried out only if the potential information cannot be obtained by other means (e.g. MRI).

Treatment may be carried out at the same time as an invasive test. For example, cardiovascular conditions are simultaneously diagnosed and treated when an 'umbrella' device is used to close cardiac defects during cardiac catheterisation.

Bronchoscopy

Bronchoscopy is the use of an endoscope to visualise the larynx and inside of the airways for diagnostic and therapeutic purposes. It is used to exclude abnormal airway anatomy or malacia. It is also used during lavage to obtain samples for analysis (presence of certain cell types indicates persistent low-grade inflammation).

A rigid bronchoscope is a hollow metal tube down which instruments and optics are passed into the major airways. This type of bronchoscope is required for the removal of an inhaled foreign body. It also provides good views of the larynx.

A flexible bronchoscope is a fibre-optic instrument that reaches the smaller, more distal airways. It can be used to evaluate stridor but is more useful for investigation of unexplained chronic cough or wheeze, suspected airway malformations or compression, atelectasis and recurrent pneumonia (in the same lung area), because of the access to the distal airways and upper lobes.

Cardiac catheterisation

Cardiac catheterisation is used to assess heart structure and function in children with congenital or acquired cardiac disease. The child is sedated and a local anaesthetic used to numb the area at which the catheter (a thin, flexible tube) will be inserted. The catheter is inserted into a large blood vessel (usually a vein, but occasionally an artery), usually in the groin. Under radiographic guidance, the catheter is placed in different areas of the heart, enabling:

- measurement of blood pressures in different heart chambers and blood vessels
- evaluation of the oxygen content of the blood in each heart chamber
- injection of dye in angiography, the results of which provide precise anatomical information in cases of structural congenital heart disease

Cardiac catheterisation is also used to treat conditions, for example when an umbrella occlusion device, introduced via the catheter, is used to close a patent ductus arteriosus or atrial septal defect, or balloon dilatation is used to treat valve stenosis (see page 183).

Endoscopy

An endoscope is a flexible camera used to visualise internal parts of the body, such as:

- the oesophagus, stomach and duodenum (in upper gastrointestinal endoscopy)
- the lower gastrointestinal tract, typically the large colon (in sigmoidoscopy or colonoscopy)

This investigation is carried out while the child is under heavy sedation or general anaesthesia. It is used in investigations of Crohn's disease and ulcerative colitis, to visualise the bowel wall and aid the collection of samples for biopsy if indicated by the detection of abnormalities (see page 214). Complications are unusual but include bleeding and gastrointestinal perforation.

Lumbar puncture

In this investigation, a needle is inserted between the bony processes of the spine to obtain a sample of cerebrospinal fluid, most commonly for the diagnosis of meningitis. In babies, an assistant holds the child in a curled position, and topical anaesthetic and sucrose are given to comfort them. In older children, sedation or general anaesthesia is usually required.

The cerebrospinal fluid is examined under a microscope to look for bacteria and white blood cells; it is then cultured. Levels of protein and glucose are also measured (see Table 8.3 for interpretation).

> **The duration of antibiotic treatment in confirmed cases of meningitis** is determined by the type of organism cultured from the cerebrospinal fluid samples.

Contraindications for lumbar puncture include signs of increased intracranial pressure or coagulopathy.

Biopsy

Biopsy is the examination, under a microscope, of a sample of body tissue. The term is also often used to refer to sample itself and the act of obtaining the sample. Biopsy can help to diagnose a specific condition and to assess its severity (e.g. the degree of inflammation) or determine its grade (e.g. the aggressiveness of a cancer).

Biopsy is helpful in cases of:
- inflammation; samples of the bowel wall, the liver (in hepatitis) or the kidney (in nephritis) are obtained

- infection; samples of the lymph nodes are obtained (e.g. in tuberculosis)
- various skin conditions
- cancer; samples of bone marrow (in leukaemia) or solid organs are obtained

Skin biopsy

This is carried out to diagnose skin lesions (e.g. blistering lesions) and rare genetic and metabolic conditions that cannot be confirmed by blood tests or other investigations. The most common technique is to use an instrument called a punch tool to obtain a small cylinder of skin tissue. The specimen is analysed under a microscope or used to culture fibroblasts for genetic testing.

Bone marrow biopsy

This is done to obtain bone marrow for pathological analysis, particularly if leukaemia is suspected. Samples are usually taken from the posterior iliac crest by aspiration or use of a trephine needle. The investigation is carried out while the child is under general anaesthesia.

Bedside tests

Bedside tests (also known as point-of-care testing) are medical diagnostic tests carried out at the time and place of patient care. They are convenient and provide quicker results, thereby enabling clinical management decisions to be made immediately. Bedside tests in paediatrics include blood glucose testing, measurement of blood gases and electrolytes, dipstick urinalysis and pulse oximetry.

Pulse oximetry

Pulse oximetry is a non-invasive method of assessing oxygenation. Although very useful, artefacts or inaccurate results are obtained if there is movement or inadequate contact with the patient's skin. Erroneously low readings are obtained in cases of poor perfusion. Conversely, the results are falsely reassuring in patients with anaemia or whose blood contains methaemoglobin (in the blood disorder methaemoglobinaemia) or carboxyhaemoglobin (in cases of carbon monoxide poisoning).

Hyperoxia test

The hyperoxia test is carried out, usually in a newborn baby, to determine whether the cause of cyanosis is a respiratory disorder or cyanotic congenital heart disease.

- Most children with cyanotic congenital heart disease have low oxygen levels with low or normal levels of carbon dioxide
- High carbon dioxide levels strongly suggest lung disease

The test is sometimes called the nitrogen washout test.

A preductal (right radial) arterial blood gas measurement is obtained after the baby has been breathing 100% oxygen for 15 min. An oxygen level > 33 kPa excludes congenital heart disease; a level < 20 kPa strongly suggests it.

In practice, the results of pulse oximetry rather than arterial gases are usually used to guide treatment; the aim is to achieve 100% oxygen saturation. Occasionally, a child with non-cyanotic congenital heart disease with heart failure has cyanosis if frank pulmonary oedema is present, but unlike in cases of cyanotic congenital heart disease, the cyanosis improves with administration of oxygen.

Management options

Starter questions

Answer to the following question is on page 124.

10. When would you suspect an adolescent with a chronic condition is not taking their medication?

The acute treatment and long-term management of medical conditions in children comprise medication, therapy and supportive care. These are provided by medical and nursing staff, specialist nurses and allied health professionals (e.g. health visitors, physiotherapists and dieticians; see Chapter 17). Ideally, the child receives treatment at home, with the aim of avoiding unnecessary disruption to their lives (daily routines, school attendance, leisure activities, etc.).

Compared with adults, the average length of stay for an acute admission to hospital is short for children (24 h), because ongoing management is usually provided by parents or carers. A child with a chronic condition is likely to require medication over months or years, so its effects on their growth and development, including puberty, needs to be considered.

Adherence to treatment

As with adults, adherence to treatment is variable. Children usually depend on their parents to bring them to appointments, administer medication and carry out certain treatments. Therefore the condition needs to be explained to parents, and the need to administer medication as instructed or carry out other treatments emphasised.

Treatment options and the benefits of medication or other treatments must be explained to the child in terms they understand. The degree of a child's involvement in decision making depends on their age and level of understanding.

Consent

The principles of consent are the same in paediatrics as they are in adult medicine: the patient must be given enough information about the benefits and risks of a treatment, along with any other options (e.g. withholding the treatment), to enable them to make an informed decision, which may include granting their consent to undergo a specific treatment. All patients over 16 years of age are presumed to have the capacity to make this decision unless there is evidence to the contrary.

In younger children, the decision is made by the parents, or those with parental responsibility, on behalf of the child and acting in the child's best interests. From about the age of 12 years, children may be capable of making their own decisions regarding medical treatment. A child's competence to consent to or refuse treatment is based on an assessment of whether they understand the information provided and are sufficiently mature to use this understanding to reach a decision. It is termed Gillick competence in the UK, Australia, New Zealand and a number of other countries (see Table 17.10). Assessment of competence is specific to each individual circumstance; however, certain criteria apply in all situations (see page 436).

In many countries, the Fraser guidelines are followed when deciding whether it is appropriate to provide contraceptive advice to a girl younger than 16 years without informing her parents. These originated in the UK and have been adopted in other countries, such as Australia and Canada.

Basic and advanced resuscitation in children

Resuscitation is the act of reviving a patient who has lost consciousness as a result of a life-threatening illness or injury, who is usually not breathing or breathing ineffectively (respiratory arrest) and who may also have diminished or no cardiac output (cardiorespiratory arrest). Unlike in adults, most instances of cardiorespiratory arrest in children are not caused by primary cardiac problems but are secondary to other causes, mostly respiratory insufficiency. Resuscitation of a child follows the 'ABC' sequence:

1. Airway
2. Breathing
3. Circulation

Resuscitation is classified as 'basic' or 'advanced'. Basic life support is the initial treatment to support breathing and circulation, either until the child responds or until they can be given full medical care. Basic life support, often called 'mouth to mouth' or 'cardiac massage', can be given outside the hospital; it can be provided by bystanders or by paramedics or medical personnel using basic equipment (e.g. bag and mask to administer oxygen).

Advanced paediatric resuscitation is carried out in accordance with Advanced Paediatric Life Support, a set of protocols and practical skills that extend basic life support to further support an open airway (via intubation) and ensure adequate ventilation and circulation (e.g. with administration of IV fluids, inotropes or other cardiac drugs, or defibrillation).

> **Cardiorespiratory arrest generally has poor outcomes in children.** A seriously ill child is assessed systematically, because directed interventions at the compensated or decompensated stages of the illness or injury prevent progression to cardiorespiratory arrest.

The parents' presence in the resuscitation room is supported. They can then see that everything possible is being done to help their child. Bereaved parents who were present when their child was being resuscitated report less anxiety and depression several months after the death.

Basic life support

Treatment of the seriously ill child follows a structured ABC approach, with interventions made at each step as abnormalities are identified, and the next step of the assessment not started until the preceding abnormality has been treated and corrected. The basic life support algorithm is outlined here.

Airway
Open the airway by tilting the head and lifting the chin. The best position differs between infants and older children, because of the comparatively large occiput and small neck in the former. An infant's head is placed in a 'neutral' position, and an older child's head in a 'sniffing' position (with the head tilted further back) (**Figure 2.36**). Adjuncts such as oropharyngeal or nasopharyngeal airways are helpful for maintaining the airway.

Breathing
Look, listen and feel for any breaths. If there is no respiratory effort, five 'rescue breaths' are given, either mouth to mouth or with a bag and mask and oxygen supply, if available (**Figure 2.37**). In infants, the face mask (or rescuer's mouth) should cover the mouth and nose. For older children, it should cover only the mouth, with the nostrils occluded by the rescuer's finger and thumb. Check that the chest is seen to rise and fall.

Circulation
Check for a central pulse. If there is no pulse, or the pulse rate is < 60 beats/min with poor perfusion, chest compressions are started at a rate of 100–120 compressions/min in a ratio of 15 compressions to 2 breaths. Chest compressions are carried out on the lower third of the sternum and depress the sternum by at least one third of the depth of the chest;

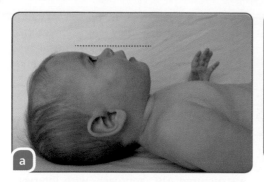
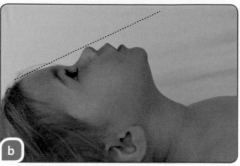

Figure 2.36 Optimal head positions to open the airway. (a) The head of an infant is placed in a 'neutral' position. (b) An older child's head is placed in a 'sniffing' position.

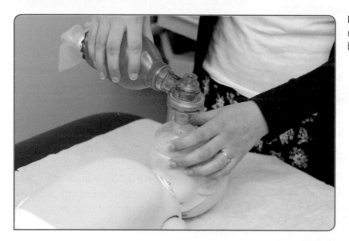

Figure 2.37 Position of bag and mask for administering rescue breaths to an infant.

the pressure is released completely after each compression. In infants, use two fingers or encircle the chest with both hands. In older children, use one or both hands.

Advanced paediatric resuscitation

This follows the principles of Advanced Paediatric Life Support. Advanced management of cardiorespiratory arrest in children varies depending on the type of heart activity recorded by ECG (**Figure 2.38**). Cardiac arrest in children is usually asystole preceded by progressive bradycardia. This is a non-shockable rhythm, as is pulseless electrical activity. Both asystole and pulseless electrical activity are treated by providing effective ventilation and performing chest compressions, in addition to addressing reversible causes such as

hypovolaemia. Ventricular fibrillation and pulseless ventricular tachycardia can both be treated with DC shocks, but they are uncommon in paediatrics.

In an emergency, the child's weight is estimated instead of being measured to guide determination of appropriate drug dosages, volumes for the administration of fluids and sizes of equipment such as endotracheal tubes. Recognised weight formulae are available for this and are readily accessible in treatment areas for seriously ill children.

Medication

Medication is given either as a short course (in cases of acute illness) or over a long period

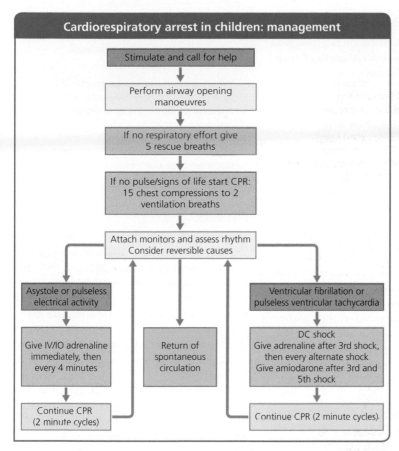

Figure 2.38 The algorithm for advanced management of cardiorespiratory arrest in children. CPR, cardiopulmonary resuscitation; DC, direct current; IO, intraosseous.

(in chronic conditions). Most medications used in adults are also used in children, but some are contraindicated or have to be used with caution, for example:

- **Aspirin** is contraindicated in children younger than 15 years, because of the risk of Reye's syndrome
- **Tetracyclines** cause discoloration and pitting of tooth enamel if given to children younger the 8 years
- **Codeine** causes respiratory depression in children

Drug absorption, distribution, metabolism and elimination (pharmacodynamics) vary by age. Therefore doses and dosing intervals differ between children of different ages, from preterm babies to adolescents, and between children and adults. The appropriate dose also depends on the indication for the drug and the route of administration.

Accordingly, for paediatric prescribing a paediatric formulary is required, for example the *British National Formulary for Children*.

> **When prescribing for children, calculation of dosages is based on both age and weight** (rather than weight alone, as in adults). The dose for a child is not proportional to that for an adult; for example, an 8 kg child would not be given a tenth of the appropriate dose for an 80 kg adult.

A child who has a chronic condition such as epilepsy needs a plan formulated in partnership between themselves, their parents, their school and a healthcare professional, to cover aspects such as recommendations on the administration of prescribed medicines in school. In the UK this is called the 'individual healthcare plan'.

Medication adherence

Poor adherence to medication is a common problem limiting the effectiveness of treatment. Contributing factors include:

- difficulty in taking the medication (e.g. inability to swallow tablets, poor inhaler technique)
- unpleasant taste
- difficult timings (e.g. not fitting around the school day)
- perceived lack of efficacy by the child or their parents
- real or perceived adverse effects

Adolescents with chronic illnesses such as diabetes or epilepsy often omit to take their medication because they do not want to be different from their peers; they do not always admit to this. Some children also use refusal to adhere to treatment to assert their authority and gain some control over their lives. These problems are best resolved through an honest, non-judgemental discussion, and negotiation if necessary.

A home visit by a nurse specialist often identifies underlying social problems reducing medication adherence in children with a chronic condition, for example a chaotic home environment or the family's lack of understanding of the condition.

Routes of administration

Most paediatric medicines are given orally as a liquid or tablets. A dose of liquid medicine is measured with an oral syringe or a measuring spoon. A medicine may be mixed with small quantities of food or drink, particularly if its taste needs to be masked. However, certain medicines should not be mixed with food, and some capsules or granules should not be dissolved in a drink.

Intravenous administration is chosen if a medicine cannot be given orally, for example if the child is vomiting. The subcutaneous route is used for insulin. Intramuscular injections are avoided unless only single doses are required and IV cannulation would be more problematic; however, some drugs and vaccines are only administered intramuscularly.

Rectal and buccal treatments may be used for seizures and are useful because the drug can be administered at home or school.

> When prescribing topical treatments for skin conditions, the 'fingertip dose' is a useful guide to the amount of cream required. This is the amount of cream squeezed out to the length of the distal phalanx of the child and is enough to cover an area the size of the child's outstretched hand.

Inhalers

These enable rapid delivery to the lungs of low doses of drugs in cases of asthma and cystic fibrosis (see pages 160 and 163. The delivery of drugs in this way to the inner surface of the lungs can be considered a form of topical treatment. To ensure adequate delivery of the inhaled drug, it is vital that the child is taught correct inhaler technique, and that their technique is checked on at least an annual basis.

Several types of inhaler are available. The choice depends on the child's age, the medication to be given and the child's preference. The most commonly used type is a metered dose inhaler. This is used with a spacer and mask by children under 4 years or a spacer and mouthpiece by children under 12 years (**Figure 2.39**), because children find it difficult to push down on the inhaler at the same time as they breathe in; use of the spacer or mask allows the child to breathe normally while using the inhaler. Smaller devices ideal for use by teenagers at school are dry powder and breath-actuated inhalers. Nebulisers are used to administer certain antibiotics in cystic fibrosis and some cases of severe acute asthma exacerbation (see page 406).

Drug licensing

Because of the practical difficulties and ethical issues associated with drug trials in paediatric populations, pharmaceutical companies often choose not to include the use of a drug in children when applying for licences. Therefore in children many medications are used 'off-licence' or 'off-label'. This

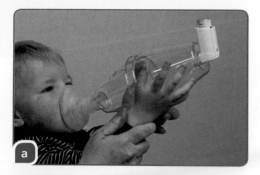

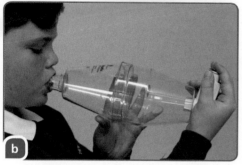

Figure 2.39 Use of a large-volume spacer with a mask (a) and a mouthpiece (b) for administration of asthma medication.

common practice is accepted providing that it is in accordance with the consensus of a respected body of professional opinion.

Analgesics

Pain management in children follows a two-step approach depending on the level of pain:

- simple non-opioid drugs such as paracetamol (acetaminophen) and ibuprofen and other non-steroidal anti-inflammatory drugs (NSAIDs) for mild pain
- opioid analgesics (usually a titrated dose of morphine) for moderate to severe pain

Other forms of pain management are used in specific situations. For example, sucrose is given to a neonate and topical anaesthetic cream is applied to the skin of an older child for distraction from pain and pain relief during venepuncture. Inhaled nitrous oxide ('gas and air') is effective in an acute situation for procedures such as manipulating an injured limb.

> Aspirin is never used for analgesia in children, because of the risk of precipitating Reye's syndrome, which is characterised by acute non-inflammatory encephalopathy and fatty degeneration of the liver. However, it is used for its antiplatelet properties in the management of Kawasaki's disease.

Paracetamol

This is a mild analgesic compound that also has antipyretic properties. It has no anti-inflammatory activity. It is commonly used in children and is available over the counter.

Mode of action

Paracetamol's mode of action is unclear. It is considered a weak inhibitor of prostaglandin synthesis, but it also has central effects, with activation of descending serotonergic pathways.

Indications

Paracetamol is used for pain, including post-operative pain, and for pyrexia with discomfort. It is given orally, rectally or by IV infusion.

Contraindications

Paracetamol is used with caution in children with liver disease or chronic malnutrition. In all children, the cumulative dose over the previous 24 h needs to be assessed before each dose is given (the limit varies with age).

Adverse effects

Paracetamol causes liver failure in overdose, which may be accidental in young children or deliberate in older ones. The toxicity is dose-related. Overdoses of paracetamol are treated with N-acetylcysteine.

> Dosages of paracetamol and ibuprofen are based on the child's age rather than their weight. This avoids confusion for parents administering it at home after the child has been discharged from hospital.

Ibuprofen

This is an NSAID. It is used as an analgesic and antipyretic, and given orally or intravenously. Other NSAIDs include diclofenac, indometacin and naproxen.

Mode of action

Ibuprofen, like other NSAIDs, decreases the activity of the enzyme cyclo-oxygenase, thereby inhibiting production of prostaglandins.

Indications

Ibuprofen is for mild to moderate pain, pain and inflammation associated with soft tissue injuries, and pyrexia with discomfort. It is used in cases of juvenile idiopathic arthritis (see page 278) for the pain and inflammation, and in patent ductus arteriosus (see page 181) where it acts at a cellular level to initiate closure in the neonatal period.

Contraindications

Ibuprofen is used with caution in children with asthma, because of the risk of bronchospasm. It is contraindicated in children with active gastrointestinal bleeding or a history of peptic ulcer.

Adverse effects

Compared with other NSAIDs, ibuprofen has fewer adverse effects, with lower incidences. The main adverse effect is gastric irritation.

Morphine

Being an opioid, morphine is an effective analgesic. To avoid the potentially serious complication of respiratory depression, the dose is titrated so that the dose used is the lowest necessary to control the pain. Morphine is given orally, subcutaneously or intravenously depending on the clinical setting. A slow-release oral preparation is available for palliative care.

Mode of action

Morphine decreases the feeling of pain via its direct action on the central nervous system. It binds to opioid receptors, thereby mimicking the effects of the endogenous endorphins that normally activate these receptors. Morphine also acts on receptors in the myenteric plexus in the intestinal tract; this reduces gut motility, resulting in the adverse effect of constipation.

Indications

Morphine is used for the relief of severe pain. Gradually tapering doses are administered to babies with neonatal opioid withdrawal (neonatal abstinence syndrome) caused by maternal drug use.

Contraindications

These include an acute abdomen and heart failure secondary to chronic lung disease.

Adverse effects

In addition to respiratory depression and constipation, the adverse effects of morphine include hypotension, drowsiness and nausea. Morphine has a high potential for addiction and abuse. If the dose is reduced after long-term use, withdrawal symptoms are likely to be experienced.

Corticosteroids

Corticosteroid drugs, also called steroids and glucocorticosteroids, are synthetic analogues of the corticosteroid hormones produced by the body (in the adrenal cortex). Corticosteroids have an anti-inflammatory effect, but they also suppress the immune system. They are used in the treatment of many inflammatory conditions, including asthma, allergic reactions, inflammatory bowel disease (ulcerative colitis and Crohn's disease) and immune conditions (e.g. nephrotic syndrome and arthritis). They are also used to reduce swelling in brain tumours, and as replacement therapy in adrenal insufficiency (congenital adrenal hyperplasia and Addison's disease).

Drugs in this group

There are various types of steroid, with different potencies and available in different preparations. The following are commonly used:

■ oral prednisolone for acute asthma and chronic inflammatory conditions such as juvenile idiopathic arthritis
■ inhaled steroids, such as beclometasone as a preventer medication in the

management of asthma or nebulised budesonide for croup
- oral dexamethasone for croup
- IV hydrocortisone when oral therapy is inadequate, for example in acute severe asthma, in anaphylactic shock and in patients on long-term steroid therapy who are acutely unwell
- topical steroids (e.g. hydrocortisone), to treat various skin conditions, including eczema

Mode of action

Corticosteroids combine with glucocorticoid receptors in the cytoplasm of cells. The corticosteroid–glucocorticoid receptor complexes translocate to the nucleus, where they bind to specific areas of DNA, thereby activating or suppressing the synthesis of various proteins. These proteins include enzymes that regulate vital cellular activities over a wide range of metabolic functions, including all aspects of inflammation.

Contraindications

There are few absolute contraindications to the use of steroids. However, they are used with caution in children with diabetes mellitus or hypertension because they increase blood sugar levels, affecting diabetic control and causing hypertension.

Adverse effects

Steroid treatment is effective, but long-term treatment has many potential adverse effects, including:

- weight gain (resulting from increased appetite)
- mood swings and sleeping difficulties
- bone thinning
- easy bruising
- moon facies
- cataracts

Growth is carefully monitored, because steroid use can cause growth to be stunted, and the patient's adult height will be shorter than would have been expected. Therefore the lowest effective dose is used.

Suppression of endogenous adrenal steroid hormones is also a major concern. Patients should avoid close contact with anyone who has had an infection (e.g. chickenpox). Children on long-term steroid therapy (or their parents) carry a 'steroid treatment card' to explain what must be done if they become unwell, and to provide information for health care providers in an emergency.

Antibiotics

Antibiotics are used for the treatment and prevention (prophylaxis) of bacterial infections. They are classified as bactericidal or bacteriostatic.

- Bactericidal antibiotics kill bacteria
- Bacteriostatic antibiotics inhibit infection by preventing bacteria from dividing

Antibiotics are ineffective against viral illnesses such as the common cold. Narrow-spectrum antibacterial antibiotics are used to target specific types of bacteria, such as Gram-negative bacteria (e.g. coliforms) or Gram-positive bacteria (e.g. streptococci). Broad-spectrum antibiotics are used against a wide range of bacteria, including both Gram-positive and Gram-negative organisms.

Oral antibiotics are usually effective. However, IV antibiotics are used:

- in more serious or deep-seated infections
- when the oral route is not tolerated
- when there is no oral preparation of the appropriate antibiotic

Indications

When a bacterial infection is suspected, empiric therapy is started either with a narrow spectrum antibiotic based on the most likely organism to cause the infection in question (**Table 2.28**) or with a broad-spectrum antibiotic, such as the third generation cephalosporins, when the child is acutely unwell, with sepsis or meningitis, pending laboratory culture results. When the responsible microorganism has been identified, definitive narrow-spectrum antibiotic therapy should be started to reduce the risk of resistance emerging.

Drugs in this group

The most useful way to classify antibiotics is in relation to the class of organisms they are used to target (**Table 2.29**). However, there is

Antibiotic therapy			
Type of infection	Condition	Antibiotics	Most common causative organisms
Upper respiratory tract infection	Tonsillitis	Penicillin V (oral) Benzylpenicillin (IV) In penicillin allergy: ■ azithromycin (oral) ■ erythromycin (IV)	*Streptococcus pyogenes* (group A β-haemolytic streptococcus)
	Acute otitis media	Amoxicillin (oral) Co-amoxiclav (IV) In penicillin allergy: ■ azithromycin (oral) ■ cefotaxime or ceftriaxone* (IV)	*Streptococcus pneumoniae* *Haemophilus influenzae*
Lower respiratory tract infection	Community-acquired pneumonia	Amoxicillin (IV or oral) Penicillin allergy or mycoplasma suspected: ■ azithromycin (oral) ■ cefuroxime (IV)	*Streptococcus pneumoniae* *Mycoplasma pneumoniae*

*10% of patients with a penicillin allergy have an allergy to cephalosporins.

Table 2.28 Empirical antibiotic therapy for children

Antibiotic classification by target organisms	
Target organisms	Antibiotics
Gram-positive bacteria (e.g. *Staphylococcus aureus, Streptococcus* spp.	Penicillins: benzylpenicillin (IV), penicillin V (oral), amoxicillin, ampicillin, flucloxacillin
	Cephalosporins: first-generation (cephalexin), second-generation (cefuroxime)
	Macrolides: erythromycin, azithromycin
Gram-negative bacteria (e.g. *Haemophilus influenzae, Escherichia coli, Klebsiella* spp., *Enterobacter* spp.)	Trimethoprim
	Aminoglycosides (gentamicin)
	Third-generation cephalosporins (cefixime, cefotaxime, ceftazidime)
Anaerobic bacteria (e.g. *Clostridium* spp.)	Metronidazole
Mycoplasma spp.	Erythromycin
	Newer macrolides: azithromycin, clarithromycin

Table 2.29 Target organisms and appropriate antibiotics

some crossover, for example with the cephalosporins; first-generation cephalosporins are active predominantly against Gram-positive bacteria, and successive generations have increased activity against Gram-negative bacteria (but often with reduced activity against Gram-positive organisms).

Contraindications

Any history of allergy should be sought before prescribing any antibiotic, especially penicillins. However, true allergy must be differentiated from common adverse effects of antibiotics (e.g. loose stools) or a previous rash caused by the illness, not the medication. Amoxicillin is not prescribed if glandular fever is suspected, because it leads to a rash; this is not an allergic reaction.

Many antibiotics are excreted from the kidneys, therefore to reduce toxicity the dose is decreased in patients with renal failure. This is especially necessary when certain antibiotics are used, for example gentamicin, which can cause hearing loss in patients with impaired renal function. Levels of antibiotic in the blood may need to be measured before each dose.

Adverse effects

Most antibiotics are well tolerated. Adverse effects result from the pharmacological or toxicological properties of the antibiotic, or allergic reactions to it. Diarrhoea, resulting from disruption of the intestinal flora, and nausea are common.

> The therapeutic index is the maximum tolerated dose divided by the minimum effective dose. Some antibiotics, such as the penicillins, are very safe and therefore have a very high therapeutic index. Others, such as gentamicin, have a low maximum tolerated dose and therefore a low therapeutic index.

Supplemental oxygen

Oxygen makes up 21% of air. However, for medical purposes, up to 100% oxygen can be delivered. It is regarded as a drug and is recorded on medication charts when prescribed.

Indications

Supplemental oxygen is given when a child breathing in air is unable to keep blood oxygen saturation (Spo_2) at a level sufficient to maintain adequate oxygenation of body tissue, including the vital organs. Low Spo_2 characterises hypoxia, which is the consequence of either a respiratory condition or poor lung perfusion.

Supplemental oxygen is used in:

- acute situations, such as an exacerbation of asthma or septic shock
- chronic conditions, such as chronic lung disease of prematurity

Pulse oximetry is used to monitor Spo_2 in these situations. Supplemental oxygen can also be given to reduce the work of breathing in respiratory conditions, because the greater than normal amount of oxygen inhaled per breath means that less effort is required for the body to obtain sufficient oxygen for its needs.

Mode of action

Supplemental oxygen is delivered into the lungs either via a mask in a child who is breathing spontaneously or via mechanical ventilation. Oxygen diffuses across the alveolar membranes, enters the bloodstream and binds to haemoglobin in red blood cells. The oxygen is then transported, bound to the red blood cells, along the pulmonary veins into the heart and then around the body.

Dosage

The target Spo_2 depends on the underlying condition. Spo_2 is normally at least 97%, so this is the target in most conditions. However, in bronchiolitis $Spo_2 > 93\%$ is acceptable (see page 166).

> Chronic respiratory obstruction and insufficiency are uncommon in children, so 100% oxygen can generally be given to acutely unwell children without concern about oxygen-induced hypoventilation or carbon dioxide retention.

Once a child's condition has stabilised, the lowest concentration of oxygen required to maintain good levels of Spo_2 is used. This is because 100% oxygen causes free radical damage to the lungs, with associated ongoing inflammation. Preterm babies receiving supplemental oxygen are closely monitored to check for the development of any complications, especially retinopathy of prematurity (see page 140).

Methods of administration

Oxygen, at up to 100%, is usually delivered at a low flow rate (up to 5 L/min) via nasal prongs or a simple face mask. It can also be delivered via high-flow systems and ventilation. Generally, humidification is required when flow rates > 2 L/min are used, because:

- cold, dry air increases the loss of heat and fluid, thereby worsening bronchoconstriction
- high flow rates dry out the mucous membranes, causing airway damage and thickening of secretions, which are then difficult to clear in cases of airway obstruction

Ventilatory support

Mechanical ventilation is a type of artificial ventilation in which the actions of a machine assist or replace spontaneous breathing. In paediatrics, the usual type of mechanical ventilation is positive pressure ventilation, in which air or oxygen is pushed into the trachea, unlike the negative pressure process of spontaneous breathing. There are two types: invasive ventilation and non-invasive ventilation. The choice between the two depends on the amount of spontaneous breathing the child is doing.

- In **invasive ventilation**, a tube is placed in the trachea to provide full support from the ventilator; this type of ventilation is indicated in cases of respiratory failure or exhaustion and failed non-invasive ventilation (if a child is breathing spontaneously, the action of the ventilator synchronises with their breaths)
- In **non-invasive ventilation**, a face mask or nasal prongs are applied, and usually continuous positive airway pressure is used to maintain positive end expiratory pressure and thereby keep the airways open at the end of expiration; the patient must be making spontaneous respiratory effort and have good respiratory drive

Both types of ventilation can be used at the home of a patient with a chronic condition. For long-term invasive ventilation, tracheostomy is required

Indications

Mechanical ventilation is indicated for poor spontaneous ventilation and ineffective gas exchange at the alveolus (respiratory failure). Indications for mechanical ventilation in paediatrics, other than general anaesthesia, are acute or chronic conditions including:

- prematurity (respiratory distress syndrome)
- respiratory arrest
- acute life-threatening severe asthma
- bronchiolitis
- hypotension (e.g. in sepsis and shock)
- protection of the airway in an unconscious patient
- neuromuscular problems

> **In respiratory failure, oxygen supplementation alone may improve oxygenation.** However, it will not assist with ventilation and the removal of carbon dioxide.

Complications

Mechanical ventilation carries a risk of potential complications. These include pneumothorax, airway injury, alveolar damage, ventilator-associated pneumonia and subglottic stenosis (in preterm babies).

Fluid management

The body needs to maintain a balance between fluid intake and fluid output, which includes the fluid naturally lost from the skin and respiratory system. Infants and young children have a higher fluid requirement because of the higher water content of their bodies, higher ratio of surface area to body mass, higher respiratory and metabolic rate, and immature renal function.

In addition to maintenance fluids, dehydrated children require additional fluid to correct the deficit. This is usually provided as 0.9% saline (sodium chloride in water) with 5% dextrose, administered intravenously over 24–48 h. However, fluid management differs depending on the underlying condition; for example, no dextrose is given initially in cases of diabetic ketoacidosis (see page 410). Also, boluses of 0.9% saline are used for initial resuscitation.

The following formula is used to calculate maintenance fluid requirements in children:

- 100 mL/kg for the first 10 kg, plus
- 50 mL/kg for the second 10 kg, plus
- 20 mL/kg for the next 60 kg

This gives the total amount required in 24 h (divide by 24 for an hourly volume).

Nutrition

Good nutrition is essential for maintenance of general health and to aid recovery from illness. A few days of poor nutritional intake during an acute illness in a usually healthy child is of little concern; however, children with chronically insufficient intake of nutrients require caloric supplementation or feeding via a different route (e.g. via nasogastric tube).

Children who are overweight or obese are identified, and they and their parents receive support to help the child follow a healthy diet and increase their levels of physical activity (see page 215). Children with certain medical conditions, such as cystic fibrosis (see page 163) or cows' milk protein allergy (see page 293), require special diets; they receive help from a dietician.

Supplementary feeding

Infants with congenital heart disease who struggle to feed because of breathlessness, children with anorexia after chemotherapy, and children with neurodevelopmental problems or swallowing difficulties all require supplementary feeding to ensure that they receive adequate nutrition. Occasionally these 'supplementary' feeds are the child's sole source of nutrition. Adequate supplementary feeding may be achieved with a continuous overnight feed, enabling a child to maintain an appetite for oral food intake during the day.

Tube feeding

Feeding via nasogastric tube or percutaneous endoscopic gastrostomy feeding tube (**Figure 2.40**) enables feed to be delivered directly into the stomach in children whose oral food uptake is insufficient.

- A nasogastric tube passes through the nose and into the stomach via the oropharynx and oesophagus; nasogastric tube feeding is used when temporary supplementary feeding is required
- A percutaneous endoscopic gastrostomy feeding tube is inserted, under endoscopic guidance, directly into the stomach via an

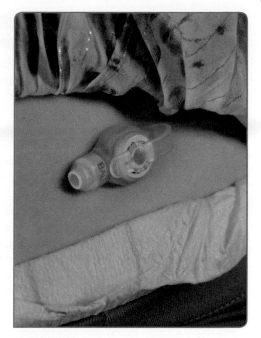

Figure 2.40 A percutaneous endoscopic gastrostomy (PEG) tube inserted on the left side of the abdomen to assist feeding in a child with severe cerebral palsy.

incision in the abdominal wall; it provides long-term nutritional support

Parenteral (IV) nutrition

This is a last resort for children for whom enteral (into the stomach) feeding is not possible. It is most commonly used for premature babies in the first few days of life, while milk feeds are being established, and in babies with necrotising enterocolitis, who are designated nil by mouth for a prolonged period.

In older children, parental nutrition is used in cases of intestinal failure (e.g. resulting from short bowel syndrome, or after abdominal surgery) or hypercatabolic states (e.g. in cases of severe burns). Complications of parental nutrition include central line infection and cholestatic liver disease.

Answers to starter questions

1. If the child is adopted, the mother may have no knowledge of their antenatal or family history. When seeing adopted children, there is often a lack of information regarding the pregnancy and birth history. Often the parents know significant details, but this is not always the case.

2. Mobile phone recordings are helpful when taking a history for an episode of collapse or seizure, or the character of a cough. Encourage parents to film episodes if it is safe to do so; watching the footage can provide useful information that helps make a diagnosis.

3. Medics and non-medics often use the word 'bilious' differently. Non-medics often use it to mean vomiting fluid, for example the yellow or clear fluid vomited when there is no food left in the stomach after prolonged vomiting. The medical term bilious vomiting is the vomiting of 'cabbage water' green bile due to obstruction of the bowel downstream from the entry of the bile duct into the bowel.

4. Bubbles are a useful distraction therapy when conducting painful procedures on children, such as venepuncture. Using them makes the procedure less traumatic for the patient and parents, and makes it easier to perform for the doctor.

5. Some children presenting with abdominal pain do not have a genuine problem, but are using it as an excuse not to go to school, for example. When you actively palpate the abdomen the child may complain of pain. If while auscultating the abdomen you press the stethoscope into the abdomen, rather than your fingers, children with no genuine pain do not complain because they do not realise what you are doing.

6. Female infants may have an anal atresia, but still pass meconium (early stool) because of a vaginal fistula. Cleaning the perineum (or asking a parent to do this) ensures an atresia is not missed during the examination.

7. A person drawn by a 3-year-old! A child's first attempts at drawing a person follow a predictable order, starting with large scribbles that gradually become more orderly. They begin to draw things which are familiar to them: circles become heads with features, arms and legs are initially just lines coming out of the head. Gradually the drawings become more accurate with more features in the correct place.

8. There are many ways to collect a urine sample; the gold standard is a clean catch where the child urinates into a sterile container. However, this is hard for young children who are not yet potty-trained. Catheterisation is used when the sample is needed urgently, for example a septic child who needs antibiotics. Bags and pads are also used to collect urine, but these samples are prone to contamination from organisms around the perineum.

9. It is very helpful to witness a seizure because eyewitness descriptions are often difficult to interpret and because it will give information about what triggers the seizures (e.g. photostimulation). It is also helpful to capture a seizure when having an EEG: the neurophysiologist looks for corresponding brainwave changes at the time of the seizure that can help classify epilepsy.

10. Frequent admissions with severe exacerbations of their chronic condition, e.g. wheeze, diabetic ketoacidosis, would suggest a child is not taking their medication. Teenagers with chronic conditions often go through a phase of rebellion and they should be educated on the importance of taking medications.

Chapter 3
Neonatology and perinatal medicine

Starter questions

Answers to the following questions are on page 154.

1. Why are preterm infants' arterial oxygen saturations kept below 95%, rather than at 100%?
2. Why is jaundice in a baby less than 24-hours-old an emergency?
3. Why are pregnant women advised to avoid gardening?
4. Why are some term infants actively cooled after resuscitation?

Introduction

Neonatology is the care of neonates (newborn babies), whether they are born at term or preterm (i.e. premature). A term neonate is a baby born after 37 weeks of gestation. A preterm neonate is one born at 23–37 weeks of gestation. Babies born before 23 weeks are usually not resuscitated because they are unlikely to survive.

Perinatal medicine is the care of the fetus or baby in the perinatal period. Definitions of this period vary, but it is generally considered as being from 22 weeks' gestation to 1 week after birth.

Preterm neonates face a unique set of health problems. They are cared for in neonatal units by nurses and physicians specialising in the treatment of premature babies and the management of complications of prematurity.

Case 1 Yellow newborn baby

Presentation

Jade is a term neonate (39 weeks' gestation) and her mother's first child. She was born by spontaneous vaginal delivery. Jade's newborn examination at 18 h was normal. On day 3, 56 hours after Jade's birth, the midwives notice that she appears jaundiced, i.e. her skin appears yellow. The paediatric junior physician is asked to review her.

Initial interpretation

Jaundice that first presents on day 3 is probably physiological jaundice, i.e. due to the normal increased breakdown of red blood cells in the first days after birth and a reduced ability of the liver to cope with the resulting increase in haem in the blood (see page 145). The most common pathological causes, such as haemolysis, present within 24 h of birth. However, if the baby is unwell and lethargic, infection (a cause of jaundice) needs to be excluded. Insufficient feeding, which particularly occurs in primigravida breast feeding mothers, leads to dehydration and worsening jaundice.

Further history

Jade's birthweight was 3.2 kg, which is on the 50th centile. She has been breastfeeding regularly, every 2 h, and has passed urine and meconium (the first stools), which are dark in colour. There have been no periods of lethargy.

Examination

Jade is jaundiced, but she is alert and well perfused, with a normal fontanelle and skin turgor. At birth she had a caput (swelling of the scalp), but this is resolving and only residual bruising is now visible. Her weight on day 3 is 3.1 kg.

Interpretation of findings

Because she is alert and the examination findings are normal, Jade does not appear to have an infection. At 3%, the weight loss is normal, with breast-fed neonates losing up to 10% of their birth weight (up to 5% for formula-fed neonates), in the first 5–7 days of life. This suggests good breastfeeding, as does the production of urine, so dehydration is unlikely to be the cause of the jaundice.

Investigations

The degree of jaundice cannot be determined by visual assessment alone. It requires measurement of circulating bilirubin, the compound that causes jaundice. A transcutaneous bilirubinometer reading is made and is plotted on a treatment threshold graph appropriate for Jade's gestational age at birth and chronological age (age since birth). It is found to be at the threshold for instituting phototherapy. Therefore Jade's serum bilirubin concentration needs to be measured to confirm the high reading.

Diagnosis

The diagnosis is physiological jaundice, because there are no features associated with jaundice of pathological cause. The bruising resulting from the caput is likely to have exacerbated the condition because the extravascular blood in the bruise is broken down into bilirubin, which then circulates in the blood.

Jade is undressed and placed in an incubator under a phototherapy light box to reduce the level of bilirubin in her blood, and breastfeeding is continued. Monitoring of serum bilirubin taken 24 and 36 hours later shows a gradual decrease and the phototherapy is stopped. Jade is discharged from hospital on day 5; her bilirubin levels have stayed within normal limits.

Case 2 Newborn with difficulty breathing

Presentation

Sam is born at 27 weeks' gestation. Before delivery, his parents receive counselling from the neonatal team so they are aware of the problems Sam is likely to experience because of his prematurity. Sam has poor respiratory effort at birth; his breathing is irregular, he is grunting and there is marked subcostal and sternal recession.

Initial interpretation

The most likely cause of Sam's breathing difficulty is neonatal respiratory distress syndrome, caused by surfactant deficiency resulting from his prematurity. Infection can lead to a similar presentation so is always considered.

Further history

Sam's mother's amniotic membranes ruptured 36 h before the start of labour. She received a full course (2 doses) of antenatal steroids more than 24 h before delivery. She has had no signs of infection, for example increased body temperature, since her membranes ruptured nor was there a positive culture result on testing of a sample obtained by high vaginal swab, carried out due to the prolonged rupture of membranes.

Examination

Sam has irregular breathing, with a respiratory rate of 20 breaths/min (normal >40 breaths/min). He is showing signs of respiratory distress with grunting and

Management of a preterm birth

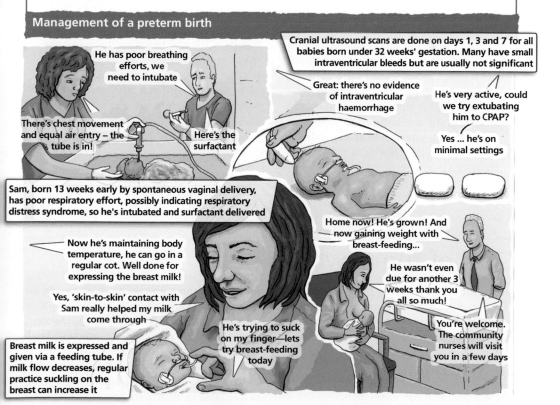

He has poor breathing efforts, we need to intubate

Cranial ultrasound scans are done on days 1, 3 and 7 for all babies born under 32 weeks' gestation. Many have small intraventricular bleeds but are usually not significant

Great: there's no evidence of intraventricular haemorrhage

He's very active, could we try extubating him to CPAP?

There's chest movement and equal air entry – the tube is in!

Here's the surfactant

Yes ... he's on minimal settings

Sam, born 13 weeks early by spontaneous vaginal delivery, has poor respiratory effort, possibly indicating respiratory distress syndrome, so he's intubated and surfactant delivered

Home now! He's grown! And now gaining weight with breast-feeding...

Now he's maintaining body temperature, he can go in a regular cot. Well done for expressing the breast milk!

He wasn't even due for another 3 weeks thank you all so much!

Yes, 'skin-to-skin' contact with Sam really helped my milk come through

He's trying to suck on my finger—lets try breast-feeding today

You're welcome. The community nurses will visit you in a few days

Breast milk is expressed and given via a feeding tube. If milk flow decreases, regular practice suckling on the breast can increase it

Case 2 *continued*

deep subcostal and sternal recession. His heart rate is 80 bpm (normal >120 bpm), and he is blue and floppy.

Interpretation of findings

Sam is not a well baby. Being blue and floppy demonstrates oxygen deprivation. Because of his extreme prematurity (gestational age at birth, ≤28 weeks) and the signs of respiratory distress, respiratory distress syndrome is likely. The amniotic membranes act as a barrier to infection so the prolonged rupture of membranes (rupture occurring > 24 h before delivery) put Sam at risk of infection.

Investigations

Sam is intubated and given surfactant via an endotracheal tube. He is transferred to the neonatal unit, where he receives mechanical ventilation via a ventilator. Antibiotics are started because of the possibility of infection. A chest radiograph at 4 h of age shows features of respiratory distress syndrome: the lung fields have a ground glass appearance and an air bronchogram, a column of air representing bronchi made visible by the atelectasis of surrounding alveoli, is present (see **Figure 3.4**).

During the first 12 h of admission to the neonatal unit, Sam is difficult to ventilate and high pressure is needed to inflate his lungs. His oxygen requirement increases to a maximum of 45% oxygen. He is given a second dose of surfactant at 12 h, after which the pressure required for ventilation decreases.

> If a baby's condition is stable, a chest radiograph is usually delayed until 4 h of age to maximise the time for reabsorption of lung fluid. The presence of fluid would make it difficult to interpret the appearance of the lung fields on a chest radiograph obtained before 4 h.

Diagnosis

Sam has respiratory distress syndrome. Because of his extreme prematurity, this remained a risk despite the administration of antenatal steroids. Blood test results (CRP and blood culture) and the chest radiograph show no sign of infection, so antibiotics are discontinued after 36 h. Sam is ventilated for 6 days in total before being extubated and switched to non-invasive ventilation via continuous positive airway pressure (CPAP).

Care of the newborn baby

Treatment of the newborn baby depends on whether they were born at or before term. Different skills and staff are needed at the birth of a preterm baby compared with a term baby.

Term neonates

In the developed world, the vast majority of births are straightforward. In a healthy term pregnancy, the baby can be delivered by an experienced midwife in a birthing unit or outside hospital, for example at the mother's home, without the need for medical staff. However, if there are maternal or obstetric complications (see page 148) the birth needs to take place in a unit where an obstetrician is available to ensure that mother and baby are well during and after delivery.

Once the baby is born, the time is noted. If the baby is crying it is immediately dried then placed on the mother's bare chest and covered with a warm towel. This skin-to-skin contact comforts the baby and stimulates the mother's milk supply. If skin-to-skin contact is not possible, the baby is wrapped in a towel for warmth.

At 1 min, 5 min and 10 min, the baby's breathing, pulse rate, reflex irritability (grimace), colour and muscle tone are assessed to calculate the Apgar score. A low score, e.g. ≤ 6 at 1 min, alerts staff that the baby is unwell and that resuscitation is needed (**Table 3.1**).

A high Apgar score, e.g. ≥ 9 at 5 minutes, indicates that the baby has transitioned well from the interuterine environment to the extra-uterine environment (see page 17). However, some babies do not adapt immediately and require resuscitation; this is usually needed in situations in which there has been evidence of fetal distress (e.g. fetal bradycardia).

If the baby does not breathe instantly and their heart rate is low (i.e. < 100 bpm), they are helped to breathe by the administration of artificial breaths through a bag valve mask. This helps to inflate the lungs, by pushing out the amniotic fluid and oxygenate the baby; oxygenation helps increase the heart rate. If this intervention fails to help, the baby requires more advanced resuscitation, including chest compressions and the use of resuscitation drugs, adrenaline (epinephrine) and sodium bicarbonate (**Figure 3.1**).

Preterm neonates

The preterm baby must be delivered in a hospital where appropriate obstetric and neonatal teams are present. When the baby is delivered, their condition is stabilised and they are transferred to the neonatal unit as swiftly as possible so that intensive care can begin without delay.

During stabilisation, the baby is at risk of becoming cold, so they must be placed under a radiant heater.

- If their gestational age at birth is > 28 weeks, they are dried and wrapped in a warm towel
- If they are younger than 28 weeks' gestation, their trunk and limbs are placed in a plastic bag loosely sealed around the neck, without being dried, to minimise the loss of heat and fluids

Fetal distress is identified by an increase or significant decrease in fetal heart rate or lack of variability on cardiotocography, an acidotic fetal blood sample, or meconium-stained liquor.

An Apgar assessment must be carried out. A preterm baby with a good heart rate (≥ 100 bpm) and respiratory drive usually still requires low-level respiratory support (facial oxygen or CPAP) before being

Apgar score criteria					
Score	Respiration	Pulse rate (bpm)	Reflex irritability (response to stimulation)	Colour of trunk	Muscle tone
0	Absent	Absent	None	White	Flaccid
1	Gasping	< 100	Grimace	Blue	Some flexion
2	Regular	> 100	Cry	Pink	Normal, with spontaneous movement

Table 3.1 The Apgar score criteria. Apgar stands for **A**ppearance, **P**ulse, **G**rimace, **A**ctivity, and **R**espiration. It is used to assess and record the condition of a newborn baby, to determine whether they require any assistance

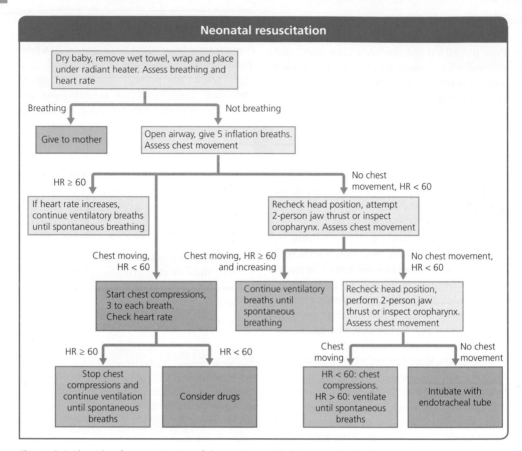

Figure 3.1 Algorithm for resuscitation of the newborn. HR, heart rate (in bpm).

transferred to the neonatal unit. A baby with poor respiratory effort or signs of significant respiratory distress, which is usually experienced by extremely preterm babies with a gestational age at birth ≤ 26 weeks, requires intubation, ventilation and the administration of surfactant (see page 133) before transfer.

Problems of prematurity

Compared with babies born at term, preterm babies are more vulnerable to particular health problems, so they fall under the care of specialist neonatologists. Preterm babies are categorised by birthweight (**Table 3.2**) or gestational age at birth (**Table 3.3**); the lower the birthweight or gestational age at birth, the greater the risk of problems associated with prematurity, as well the mortality and morbidity. Problems of prematurity can be short term and resolve with prompt recognition and treatment, or they can result in long-term morbidity.

About 8% of babies are born preterm in the developed world. Multiple births are responsible for 30% of very low birthweight infants.

Hypothermia

All preterm babies are at risk of hypothermia, defined as a body temperature of < 36°C. This

Prematurity: classification by birthweight	
Classification	Definition
Low birthweight	< 2500 g
Very low birthweight	< 1500 g
Extremely low birthweight	< 1000 g

Table 3.2 Classification of prematurity by birthweight

Prematurity: classification by gestational age		
Classification	Gestational age (weeks)	Percentage of births
Late preterm	34–37	6.5% all births
Moderately preterm	32–34	75% of all preterm births
Very preterm	< 32	2% all births
Extremely preterm	< 28	25% of all preterm births

Table 3.3 Classification of prematurity by gestational age at birth

is because they have thin skin, a large body surface area from which heat can be lost and limited stores of subcutaneous fat for insulation. A baby born at 26 weeks' gestation has about 3% body fat, increasing to about 8% at 30 weeks' gestation and 10–15% at term.

Preterm babies become hypothermic unless careful attention is paid to keeping them warm. Methods to avoid hypothermia include nursing the baby in a heated, humidified incubator and placing a hat on their head to prevent heat loss. As gestational age increases, the baby can be dressed in clothes. Hypothermia is associated with increased mortality in babies born before term.

Infection

Preterm babies are at increased risk of infection, including septicaemia, pneumonia and skin infections. This is because they have less passive immunity (from antibodies crossing the placenta) from the mother, because maternal immunoglobulin does not cross the placenta until about 30 weeks. In addition, their immature immune systems are unable to mount a strong immune response to infectious agents.

The skin of preterm neonates is thin and fragile and therefore prone to breakdown and vulnerable to infection. To treat other problems associated with prematurity, they may also have many invasive devices in situ, including endotracheal tubes and central lines. The use of these devices make it easier for infectious agents to enter the body.

Infection in preterm neonates is treated promptly with intravenous antibiotics. Antibodies against the specific infective organism are used rather than broad-spectrum antibiotics, because use of the latter increases the risk of antibiotic resistance. Staff caring for the babies must pay strict attention to hand hygiene, and invasive lines are inserted using aseptic (sterile) technique and removed promptly when no longer needed. Most preterm babies require several courses of antibiotics, which makes them susceptible to fungal overgrowth and infection, so prophylactic antifungal agents are given in some neonatal units to babies <28 weeks' gestation or <1kg at birth, twice weekly for the first four weeks of life.

Feeding difficulties

Preterm babies have a fragile gut and are therefore vulnerable to a serious bowel condition called necrotising enterocolitis (see page 138). In addition, babies do not have an efficient suck and swallow reflex until about 34 weeks' gestation. Because of these two problems, preterm neonates < 34 weeks receive intravenous nutrition (total parenteral nutrition) at the same time that milk is gradually introduced via a nasogastric tube into the stomach. The rate of increase of the enteral feeds depends on the gestational age and weight of the baby, but it is usually several days before full enteral feeds are established. Expressed breast milk is preferred to formula milk, because it contains antibodies and has better nutritional content. Furthermore, the use of formula milk is associated with a greater risk of necrotising enterocolitis.

Once the baby has an established suck reflex, they can feed from the breast or bottle. This may be difficult at first, because the baby's low energy reserves mean that they tire easily, but most preterm babies are able to establish breast or bottle feeding by the time their corrected gestational age reaches 36 weeks.

Mortality and morbidity

Preterm babies, particularly the extremely preterm, are at greater risk of mortality and morbidity than babies born at term. Many factors influence survival.

- The likelihood of survival increases with gestational age at birth (**Figure 3.2**) and birthweight
- Ethnicity: for example in developed countries preterm African-Caribbean babies have a higher rate of survival than Caucasian babies
- Preterm girls are more likely to survive than preterm boys

Preterm babies are more likely than term babies to be readmitted to hospital, especially in the first year after discharge, and usually with respiratory or feeding problems. Long-term neurodevelopmental impairments include physical disability (physical, visual or hearing), learning difficulties and behavioural problems. The likelihood of neurodevelopmental disability decreases with increasing gestational age at birth (**Figure 3.3**).

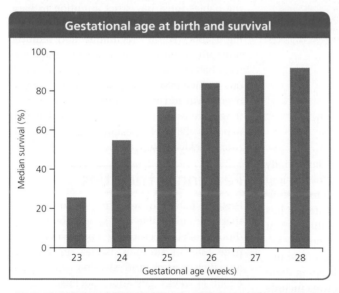

Figure 3.2 Median percentage survival of preterm babies in developed countries by gestational age at birth.

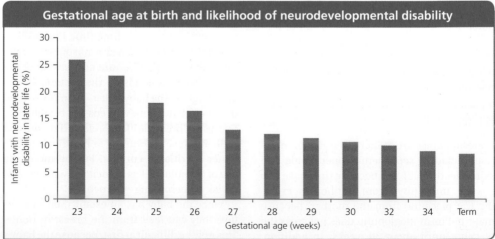

Figure 3.3 Percentage of premature babies who go on to have neurodevelopmental disability in later life, by gestational age at birth

In an average school class, three or four children will have been born preterm.

In anticipation of the long-term problems that a child born preterm may experience, regular outpatient follow up is arranged during the first year of life to monitor their development and growth, and arrange appropriate interventions if necessary.

Respiratory conditions associated with prematurity

Respiratory problems are common in preterm babies. This is because the lungs of a preterm baby are immature and lack a compound called surfactant. The two commonest respiratory problems encountered in the preterm neonate are respiratory distress syndrome and chronic lung disease.

Respiratory distress syndrome

Respiratory distress syndrome (also known as hyaline membrane disease) is caused by a lack of surfactant in the lungs, causing widespread alveolar collapse (atelectasis). The more preterm the baby is born, the more likely they are to have respiratory distress syndrome.

Epidemiology

Respiratory distress syndrome is common in babies born before 28 weeks' gestation. It occurs in 30% of babies born at 31 weeks' gestation and occasionally in term infants, especially if the mother has diabetes mellitus.

Aetiology

Impaired surfactant synthesis and secretion leads to stiff lungs (decreased compliance); there is therefore increased effort to breathe and diffuse atelectasis. Damage to the endothelial and epithelial cells of the distal airways results in a fibrinous hyaline membrane lining the alveoli soon after birth. The epithelium begins to heal within a few days and endogenous surfactant synthesis begins.

Clinical features

The condition is characterised by signs of respiratory distress at delivery or within 4 hours of birth:

- tachypnoea (rapid breathing, >60 breaths/minute)
- expiratory grunting
- recession (intercostal, sternal and subcostal)
- cyanosis (low oxygen saturation, <93% in air)

Other causes of respiratory distress should also be considered (**Table 3.4**).

Diagnostic approach

Diagnosis is clinical and confirmed by a chest radiograph, which shows lung fields with a diffuse granular or 'ground glass' appearance with an air bronchogram, (larger airways outlined). The heart border is obscured with severe disease (**Figure 3.4**).

Management

Management of respiratory distress syndrome includes giving steroids to the mother during the antenatal period when there is a threat of preterm delivery, to mature the baby's lungs and thereby reduce the severity of the condition. If the baby has signs of respiratory distress syndrome after birth severe enough to require mechanical ventilation, they are given exogenous surfactant via an endotracheal tube as soon as possible. Most require two doses 6–12 hours apart. Oxygen is given to maintain adequate saturation.

Respiratory distress in neonates: causes	
Cause	Underlying aetiology
Congenital pneumonia	Associated with group B streptococcal infection
Respiratory distress syndrome*	Lack of surfactant
Transient tachypnoea of the newborn**	Delay in clearance of amniotic fluid in the lungs
Pneumothorax	Alveolar rupture
Persistent pulmonary hypertension of the newborn	Incomplete fetal circulation adaptations at birth (see page 17)
Meconium aspiration syndrome**	Meconium causes: ■ Blockage in airways ■ Chemical pneumonitis ■ Persistent pulmonary hypertension ■ Secondary infection
Congenital lung anomalies	Congenital diaphragmatic hernia Tracheo-oesphageal fistula
Pulmonary hypoplasia	Reduced lung volume during fetal development (due to reduced amniotic fluid or reduced space in thorax)
Upper airways obstruction	Choanal atresia
Non-respiratory causes	Perinatal asphyxia (lack of neurological drive)
	Congenital heart disease
	Severe anaemia

*Mainly preterm infants.
**Mainly term infants.

Table 3.4 Causes of respiratory distress in neonates

- If the respiratory distress syndrome is severe, the baby requires oxygen via mechanical ventilation to ensure adequate lung expansion and gas exchange
- If the condition is mild, i.e. the baby is not working too hard to breathe and needs only minimal oxygen to maintain saturation >91%, mechanical ventilation is unnecessary and oxygen via nasal cannula or CPAP may alone be sufficient

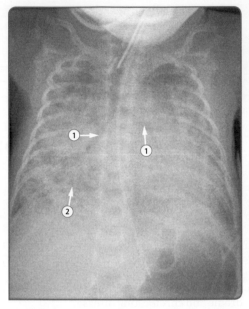

Figure 3.4 Chest radiograph with typical appearance in respiratory distress syndrome. ①, Air bronchogram, air-filled bronchi appearing dark against the atelectatic alveoli which appear light grey/white; ②, fine granular 'ground glass', appearance of the lung fields due to the atelectatic alveoli and interstitial fluid.

Complications of mechanical ventilation include pneumothorax, pulmonary haemorrhage and chronic lung disease.

Prognosis

The prognosis is good, with most babies recovering from respiratory distress syndrome.

Chronic lung disease

Chronic lung disease, also known as bronchopulmonary dysplasia, is a late respiratory complication that occurs in babies with a very low birthweight. It is diagnosed when a neonate still requires supplementary oxygen to maintain an oxygen saturation >95% at a gestational age of > 36 weeks (with a chronological age of > 4 weeks).

Epidemiology and aetiology

Chronic lung disease is uncommon in infants with a birth weight >1250 g or born at more than 30 weeks' gestation. About 25% of low-birthweight infants (<1500 g) are diagnosed with bronchopulmonary dysplasia. The cause of chronic lung disease is lung tissue inflammation, which is secondary to many factors including respiratory distress syndrome and prolonged mechanical ventilation (volume and pressure trauma), oxygen toxicity and infection (**Figure 3.5**).

Clinical features

Clinical features include:

- the need for supplemental oxygen, usually via nasal cannula, to maintain oxygen saturation >95%
- subcostal recession
- fine crackles on inspiration, audible with a stethoscope

Diagnostic approach

Chronic lung disease is diagnosed when a neonate continues to require supplemental oxygen after 36 weeks' gestational age (and at least 4 weeks' chronological age). A chest radiograph is not routinely carried out, but if obtained may show areas of hyperinflation (air trapping), under-inflation (collapse), fibrosis or cysts.

Management

The aim of management of chronic lung disease is prevention of its occurrence through considerate treatment of respiratory distress syndrome. If the baby needs ventilation to overcome respiratory distress syndrome, it should be as gentle as possible, using the lowest volumes and oxygen concentration, to allow adequate gas exchange with minimal lung trauma and secondary inflammation.

Good nutrition is vital to optimise lung growth and repair, and thereby reduce the likelihood of chronic lung disease. Neonates with chronic lung disease need extra calories, because they use a large amount of energy during breathing, and this slows their growth.

A baby with chronic lung disease who requires oxygen but is otherwise well, for example one who has reached a corrected gestation of term and is feeding well orally and gaining weight, need not stay in hospital and can be discharged with equipment for the delivery of home oxygen therapy.

Prognosis

Nearly all babies survive after discharge and cease supplemental oxygen by 1 year corrected age. Chronic lung disease makes babies vulnerable to chest infections in the first year, particularly bronchiolitis, so parents must be aware of its signs and symptoms and seek prompt medical advice if they become concerned.

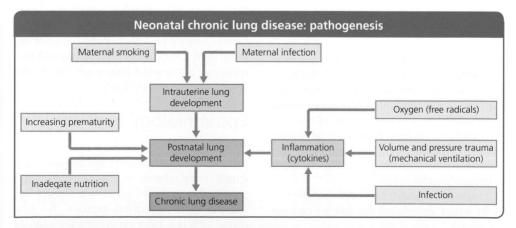

Figure 3.5 Pathogenesis of neonatal chronic lung disease.

> Children who had chronic lung disease are likely to have emphysema-like symptoms in mid- to late-adulthood. If they also smoke cigarettes regularly this can present much earlier.

Monthly injections of palivizumab, a monoclonal antibody against respiratory syncytial virus infection, are given to babies who are on home oxygen therapy during their first winter to reduce the risk of respiratory syncytial virus bronchiolitis.

Neurological problems associated with prematurity

Two main neurological problems are encountered in the premature baby: apnoea of prematurity and intraventricular haemorrhage. As with most problems in neonatal medicine, the aim is to prevent its occurrence. However, this may not always be possible, despite prompt stabilisation and good neonatal care.

> Apnoea is thought to contribute to sudden infant death syndrome (SIDS), sometimes known as 'cot death'. The parents of babies considered to be at high risk, for example those with a family history of SIDS, are given apnoea monitors to use at home. An alarm sounds if the baby stops breathing, thereby alerting the parents.

Apnoea of prematurity

All premature babies born at < 28 weeks' gestation will have apnoea, which is defined as a pause of breathing of > 20 s. Apnoea in the premature baby has many causes:

- immature respiratory drive
- gastro-oesophageal reflux
- infection
- seizures
- hypoxia

It is most commonly secondary to immature respiratory drive. The frequency of apnoea increases with decreasing gestational age at birth.

A preterm baby who has apnoeas occuring frequently in succession requires mechanical ventilation. The ventilator supports the baby to breathe until they are mature enough to breathe by themselves; the age of maturity varies between babies. All preterm babies are given caffeine mediation daily, with the aim of stimulating the respiratory centre of the brain to initiate breaths.

Prognosis is good. Most apnoeas resolve by 34 weeks' gestational age and the caffeine is stopped.

Intraventricular haemorrhage and periventricular leukomalacia

Intraventricular haemorrhage and periventricular leukomalacia are acquired lesions of the central nervous system that affect preterm infants and cause long-term disability. Intraventricular haemorrhage is defined as a haemorrhage into the brain ventricles. Periventricular leukomalacia follows ischaemic brain injury and occurs at the watershed area (border) of the arterial distribution, at the white matter adjacent to the lateral ventricles of the brain.

Epidemiology and aetiology

Intraventricular haemorrhage occurs when small blood vessels in the subependymal germinal matrix (the vascular structure lining the brain ventricles) rupture. The germinal matrix is most prominent between 24 and 34 weeks of gestation but is almost completely regressed by term, which is why term neonates do not tend to have intraventricular haemorrhages. Intraventricular haemorrhages occur in about 20% of babies born at < 32 weeks' gestation.

There are multiple causes for intraventricular haemorrhages, the main one being prematurity itself, with associated loss of cerebral autoregulation and significant fluctuations in cerebral blood flow and pressure. Other risk factors are:

- hypertension
- hypotension
- high levels of carbon dioxide in the blood
- low levels of oxygen in the blood

Periventricular leukomalacia results from ischaemic injury to oligodendrocytes in the developing brain and cytokine-induced damage from a maternal (chorioamnionitis) or neonatal infection. It has similar risk factors to intraventricular haemorrhage, although it is associated with infections (cytokine effect) and low (rather than high) carbon dioxide levels in the blood.

Clinical features

Intraventricular haemorrhages and periventricular leukomalacia are usually asymptomatic and only detected when a cranial US scan is carried out. Sudden deterioration in the baby's clinical state, for example with prolonged apnoea, bradycardia or a large, rapid decrease in haemoglobin levels, may indicate an intraventricular haemorrhage.

Diagnostic approach

Intraventricular haemorrhages are diagnosed by a cranial US scan. Babies born at < 32 weeks' gestation have at least three scans in the first week of life, when the germinal matrix is most likely to bleed, to identify a silent intraventricular haemorrhage. They are graded according to severity, from grade 1 (least severe) to grade 4 (most severe) (Table 3.5). Periventricular leukomalacia is noticed at birth if due to ischaemia or an infection in utero. All preterm babies have a routine cranial US scan at 28 days and 36

Intraventricular haemorrhage: grading	
Grade	Cranial ultrasound finding
1	Haemorrhage limited to germinal matrix
2	Haemorrhage into ventricle, no ventricular dilatation
3	Haemorrhage into ventricle, ventricular dilatation evident
4	Haemorrhage into brain parenchyma

Table 3.5 Grading of the severity of intraventricular haemorrhage

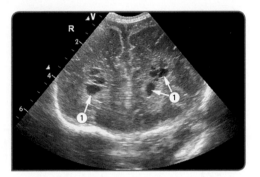

Figure 3.6 Cranial US scan in the coronal plane through the frontal lobes, showing periventricular leukomalacia. The echodensities ① are cysts involving the brain parenchyma.

weeks corrected age that shows periventricular echodensities (cysts) if periventricular leukomalacia is present (Figure 3.6). An MRI scan is performed at term corrected age if periventricular leukomalacia is seen on the ultrasound scan to confirm the extent of the injury.

Management

There is no treatment for intraventricular haemorrhage or periventricular leukomalacia. Therefore the aim is to prevent its occurrence by reducing the risk factors, for example hypoxia. If an intraventricular haemorrhage is identified, its progression is monitored by carrying out weekly cranial US scans during the baby's stay in hospital.

Larger intraventricular haemorrhages are associated with ventricular dilatation (hydrocephalus, Figure 3.7), because blood in the

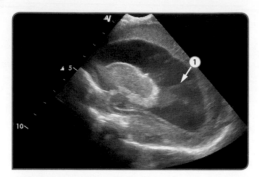

Figure 3.7 Cranial ultrasound scan in the parasagittal plane showing dilation of the ventricle (hydrocephalus) ①.

ventricles prevents drainage of cerebrospinal fluid. Hydrocephalus frequently resolves spontaneously. However, if it causes head circumference to increase, the cerebrospinal fluid must be drained. This requires either repeated lumbar punctures or insertion of a shunt (see page 250).

Prognosis

The likelihood of survival and long-term outcome depend on the severity of the haemorrhage or periventricular leukomalacia and whether it is unilateral or bilateral.

■ Grade 1 and 2 intraventricular haemorrhage have good outcomes, with only a minority of children experiencing mild cognitive impairment
■ Unilateral grade 3 or 4 intraventricular haemorrhage can cause hemiplegia (paralysis on one side of the body)
■ Extensive bilateral lesions can lead to quadriplegic cerebral palsy, visual impairments and intellectual disability

Gastrointestinal problems associated with prematurity

Feeding difficulties (see page 206) are common in preterm babies. A preterm neonate's suck reflex is immature, and the small size of their stomach makes it difficult for them to tolerate feeds, resulting in vomiting. Gastro-oesophageal reflux is also frequently encountered in the neonatal unit. However, the gastrointestinal problems associated with prematurity usually resolve as the baby gets nearer to term.

Necrotising enterocolitis

Necrotising enterocolitis is a serious acute inflammatory bowel condition that occurs in the 2nd or 3rd week of life in premature babies. It is the most common gastrointestinal emergency in neonates and is associated with high morbidity and mortality.

Epidemiology and aetiology

In necrotising enterocolitis, there is necrosis of the bowel, i.e. bowel tissue dies as a result of lack of blood flow. The exact cause of the condition is unknown, but it is associated with prematurity, hypoxia, infection and artificial milk formula feeds. It occurs more frequently in preterm babies, affecting 2–5% of those with very low birthweight, but it can affect babies born at any gestation.

Clinical features

The classic presentation of necrotising enterocolitis is the triad of:

■ bile-stained (green) aspirates from the stomach
■ abdominal distension (**Figure 3.8a**), with or without discoloration
■ bloody stools

The condition can also present with non-specific signs, for example the baby may be quiet or in shock, with tachycardia or hypotension. The stages of necrotising enterocolitis are shown in **Table 3.6**.

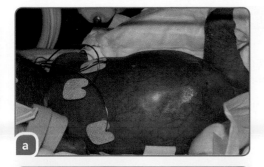

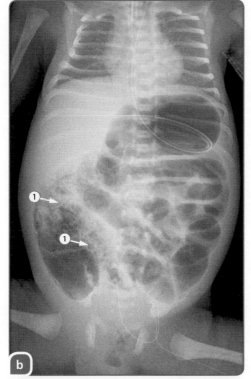

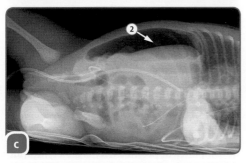

Diagnostic approach

Diagnosis is based on the clinical features of necrotising enterocolitis, because no single test is confirmatory. However, an abdominal radiograph can support the diagnosis because the bowel is usually dilated (**Figure 3.8b**). In children with severe symptoms, the abdominal radiograph shows gas in the bowel wall (pneumatosis intestinalis). This finding is pathognomonic for necrotising enterocolitis; the gas is from gas-producing microorganisms. Also in severe cases, the gut necrosis may lead to bowel perforation, in which case the radiograph shows free air in the abdomen (**Figure 3.8c**).

Management

The aim is to prevent necrotising enterocolitis by introducing feeds gradually, preferably using breast milk, which compared with formula milk is much gentler on the gut.

Babies with necrotising enterocolitis are very sick; they require intensive support to manage shock. Feeding must be stopped to allow the gut to heal. Analgesia is essential, because the condition is painful. Antibiotics, including those to treat anaerobic organisms, are given for 7–10 days.

> **Short bowel syndrome is significant malabsorption caused by extensive resection of the small intestine.**
> Patients require parenteral nutrition; factors influencing when they come off are the length of remaining bowel, which segments remain and intestinal adaptation to enteral feeds. In general, patients with an ileal remnant have better outcomes than those with a jejunal remnant.

Surgery

If bowel perforation has occurred, the baby needs to be assessed by paediatric surgeons. The perforation is managed either conservatively with peritoneal drainage or with surgery to remove the affected bowel and create a temporary stoma to allow the bowel to heal.

Figure 3.8 Necrotising enterocolitis. (a) Abdominal distension and discolouration: a clinical sign of necrotising enterocolitis. (b) Radiograph showing dilatated loops of the bowel and the bubbly appearance of air in the bowel wall ① of necrotising enterocolitis. (c) Free air in the abdomen ②, suggesting intestinal perforation.

Necrotising enterocolitis: staging		
Stage 1: suspected	**Stage 2: confirmed**	**Stage 3: advanced**
Non-specific signs: ■ Lethargy ■ Temperature instability ■ Poor glucose tolerance ■ Gastrointestinal signs ■ Poor feeding ■ Increased gastric aspirates ■ Bilious vomiting ■ Mild abdominal distension ■ Abdominal tenderness ■ Faecal occult blood	All stage 1 features plus: ■ Abdominal tenderness and/or guarding ■ Marked abdominal distension ■ Periumbilical flare ■ Blood or mucus in the stool	All stage 1 and 2 features plus: ■ Clinical deterioration ■ Evidence of septic shock ■ Marked gastrointestinal haemorrhage ■ Abdominal wall discoloration
Abdominal radiograph findings: ■ Within normal limits	Abdominal radiograph findings: ■ Intestinal distension ■ Bowel wall oedema ■ Featureless bowel loops ■ Persistent or unchanging bowel loops ■ Pneumatosis intestinalis ■ Portal venous gas	Abdominal radiograph findings: ■ Stage 2 features plus pneumoperitoneum

Table 3.6 Bell's staging for necrotising enterocolitis

Prognosis

In babies with very low birthweight, necrotising enterocolitis increases mortality by 20–40%. In the short term, bowel strictures may occasionally develop, necessitating surgery to resect the narrowed bowel. Any stoma is usually reversed within a couple of months; many babies initially return home with the stoma still present. In the long term, there is increased risk of growth delay and neurodevelopmental disabilities. Very occasionally a large length of affected bowel is removed surgically in the initial presentation, leading to short bowel syndrome.

Retinopathy of prematurity

Retinopathy of prematurity is the abnormal proliferation of blood vessels in the retinas of premature babies. It typically begins at 34 weeks' gestational age and advances until 45 weeks' gestational age.

The main concern regarding babies with retinopathy of prematurity is that it can lead to visual problems, including blindness. Retinopathy of prematurity is seen in 35% of very-low-birthweight infants.

Epidemiology and aetiology

Its incidence and severity increase with decreasing gestational age at birth.

Risk factors are multiple, and in addition to prematurity include high blood oxygen saturation and prolonged oxygen therapy.

Clinical features and diagnostic approach

Retinopathy of prematurity is an asymptomatic condition. It is only detected through regular screening by ophthalmologists of neonates at high risk, i.e. those born at < 32 weeks' gestation or weighing < 1500 g.

The ophthalmologist examines the retina after the baby's pupils have been dilated with mydriatic (antimuscarinic) eye drops.

Retinopathy of prematurity is graded according to its severity; severe stages include vitreous haemorrhage and retinal detachment. It can progress rapidly.

Management

In most babies, retinopathy of prematurity resolves spontaneously. Treatment is required for severe stages, usually with laser therapy under a general anaesthetic to prevent blood vessel proliferation. Further progression may be treated with an intravitreal injection of bevacizumab (anti-vascular endothelial growth factor).

Prognosis

Timely treatment prevents severe impairment of vision. If untreated, severe disease leads to retinal detachment and blindness which occurs in 1% of very-low-birthweight infants, mostly those born <28 weeks' gestation.

Conditions affecting term neonates

Some conditions occur in term neonates that are rarely encountered when caring for preterm babies. These conditions occur when term babies are exposed to intrauterine hypoxia, or hypoxia during delivery or immediately after birth. Preterm babies are more resilient to the effects of hypoxia before or around delivery.

Meconium aspiration syndrome

Meconium is a thick, sticky, dark-green substance that the baby passes as the first stool. It comprises of swallowed skin, hair and other debris from the gut. Meconium is normally passed within 48 h of birth. However, if the baby experiences hypoxia in utero it passes meconium in utero as a result of vagal stimulation and starts gasping. Meconium is then inhaled into the lungs during delivery causing the inflammation and airway obstruction known as meconium aspiration syndrome.

Epidemiology and aetiology

Meconium is rarely found in the amniotic fluid before 34 weeks' gestation and therefore mainly affects term infants. It is passed before birth in 20% of babies, with meconium aspiration syndrome affecting 5% of these.

Meconium causes hypoxia in the newborn baby via:

- airway obstruction, leading to areas of over-inflation, collapse and consolidation
- surfactant dysfunction
- chemical pneumonitis (inflammation)
- persistent pulmonary hypertension of the newborn (PPHN); the baby does not cry at delivery so adaptations at birth do not fully occur (see page 17)

Clinical features

Clinical features include a history of meconium-stained amniotic fluid and signs of respiratory distress at birth (e.g. tachypnoea or grunting). Meconium aspiration syndrome is associated with hypoxia, so the baby may have signs of hypoxic ischaemic encephalopathy (see page 142).

Diagnostic approach

Diagnosis is based on clinical features and confirmed by a chest radiograph showing hyperinflated lung fields with areas of collapse or consolidation, resulting in a patchy appearance (**Figure 3.9**). Pneumothoraces can also occur in babies with meconium aspiration syndrome, as a result of lung damage. Other causes of respiratory distress should also be considered (see **Table 3.4**).

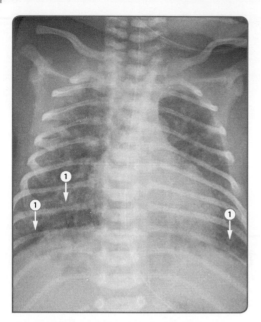

Figure 3.9 Chest radiograph showing patchy changes in the lung fields ① in a baby with meconium aspiration syndrome.

Management

Mechanical ventilation and surfactant may be required to ensure adequate ventilation and gas exchange. Oxygen therapy is given to maintain oxygen saturation at > 95% and to help reduce pulmonary artery constriction.

For babies with severe PPHN, treatment with inhaled nitric oxide is required to reduce pulmonary arterial pressures. Large pneumothoraces are treated by inserting a chest drain to remove air from the pleural space.

Prognosis

The outcome of meconium aspiration syndrome varies depending on its severity and whether the baby also has PPHN or hypoxic ischaemic encephalopathy. These associated conditions increase the mortality rate.

Hypoxic ischaemic encephalopathy

Hypoxic ischaemic encephalopathy is an acute or subacute brain injury caused by systemic hypoxaemia and/or reduced cerebral blood flow in the fetus.

Epidemiology and aetiology

Hypoxic ischaemic encephalopathy is diagnosed when a term neonate shows neurological abnormalities. The resultant brain injury affects the basal ganglia, thalami, brainstem and central cortex. It is caused by primary neuronal death at the time of the initial insult or reperfusion injury with secondary neuronal death.

In developed countries, hypoxic ischaemic encephalopathy is diagnosed in 0.5–1 per 1,000 live born term neonates, of which a third have a resulting significant neurological disability. In developing countries, it accounts for 23% of all neonatal deaths worldwide.

Clinical features

Neurological abnormalities are noticeable at birth and evolve over 72 h. Hypoxic ischaemic encephalopathy is graded clinically (**Table 3.7**).

Hypoxic ischaemic encephalopathy: grading			
Clinical characteristic	Mild	Moderate	Severe
Level of consciousness	Hyperalert	Lethargic or obtunded	Stuporous
Muscle tone	Normal	Mild hypotonia	Flaccid
Posture	Mild distal flexion	Strong distal flexion	Intermittently decerebrate
Suck reflex and Moro's reflex	Weak	Weak or absent	Absent
Seizures	None	Common: focal or multifocal	Uncommon
Outcome	No increased risk of death or disability	15–25% risk of death or severe disability	75–100% risk of death or severe disability

Table 3.7 Clinical grading of hypoxic ischaemic encephalopathy

Diagnostic approach

Diagnosis is based on a history of fetal distress in utero or during delivery, along with the clinical features. A cerebral function monitor is used to assess baseline brain activity and detect seizures, which occur in certain grades of hypoxic ischaemic encephalopathy (see **Table 3.7**). Abnormal results from serum liver or renal function tests suggest multiorgan damage. MRI carried out around day 7 is used to determine the location and extent of brain damage.

Management

The neuronal death from the primary insult cannot be reversed. However therapeutic hypothermia reduces the effect of the reperfusion injury. It is started within 6 h of birth and continued for 72 h; the neonate's body temperature is actively cooled to 33–34°C by a whole-body cooling mattress. Anticonvulsants are used to control seizures. Ventilation is necessary to achieve adequate gas exchange, which is impaired by the brain insult and the sedative effects of any anticonvulsants.

Prognosis

The presence and severity of neurological abnormalities and MRI findings are the best indicators of prognosis. A full recovery is expected in mild hypoxic ischaemic encephalopathy. Therapeutic hypothermia reduces the risk of death and severe disability in moderate encephalopathy, but severe encephalopathy has a mortality rate of 30–40% and >80% of survivors have neurodevelopmental disabilites such as cerebral palsy. A poor prognosis is associated with a requirement for nasogastric feeds or neurological abnormalities on discharge.

Neonatal jaundice

Jaundice is a yellow discoloration of the skin and sclera (white of the eye) caused by hyperbilirubinaemia, i.e. excess bilirubin in the blood. The priority in neonatal jaundice is to determine the underlying cause and to treat it as necessary.

Bilirubin is a yellow compound formed by the breakdown of haemoglobin from red blood cells (**Figure 3.10**).

Ultimately, it gives stool its dark, brown colour.

Aetiology

Hyperbilirubinaemia has many causes (**Table 3.8**). It is classified as:

- **Unconjugated hyperbilirubinaemia**, caused by increased production of unconjugated bilirubin or failure of bilirubin conjugation in the liver
- **Conjugated hyperbilirubinaemia**, caused by reduced excretion of bilirubin from the liver or biliary tract, or chronic illness affecting the liver (e.g. hepatitis)

Jaundice affects up to 50% of babies born at term and a higher percentage of premature babies. In the majority the cause is physiological (see separate section below).

Clinical features

Babies with jaundice are usually asymptomatic, so it is noted on examination. The presence of other clinical features depends on the cause of the jaundice. For example, a baby with sepsis may be irritable or abnormally quiet, or the baby may have a large cephalohaematoma secondary to birth trauma. If the jaundice has an obstructive cause, for example biliary atresia, the baby passes pale, clay like stools and dark urine.

> **Left untreated, neonatal jaundice can lead to kernicterus (bilirubin encephalopathy), which has the potential to cause deafness and cerebral palsy.** The lipid-soluble unconjugated bilirubin is able to cross the blood–brain barrier; kernicterus is caused by its accumulation in the basal ganglia.

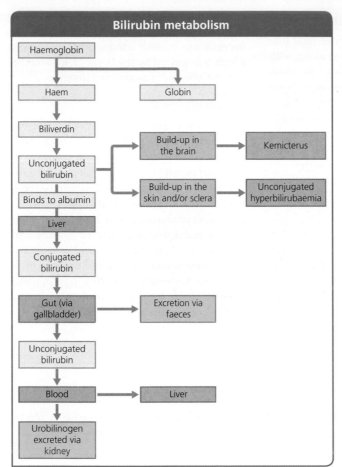

Figure 3.10 Bilirubin metabolism. If circulating levels of unconjugated bilirubin become sufficiently high it becomes detectable in the skin and sclera, producing the yellow, jaundiced appearance. If the unconjugated level is very high it crosses the blood–brain barrier and accumulates in the brain, producing kernicterus (see text box).

Diagnostic approach

The severity of jaundice cannot be judged by visual inspection alone; the total serum concentration of both unconjugated and conjugated bilirubin must be measured. A transcutaneous bilirubinometer can be used in term babies, but the serum test is the most accurate method of measurement. Once it has been established whether the jaundice is caused by conjugated or unconjugated bilirubin, determination of the underlying cause can begin. Jaundice within 24 hours of birth is always abnormal.

Management

Management depends on whether the hyperbilirubinaemia is unconjugated or conjugated.

Unconjugated hyperbilirubinaemia

If the serum concentration of unconjugated bilirubin reaches a certain threshold (determined by chronological age and gestational age at birth), the baby is placed under a phototherapy unit to speed up bilirubin metabolism.

Regular blood tests are required to check that levels of unconjugated bilirubin is decreasing. If the level is extremely high and increasing, for example in a case of haemolysis, and there is therefore a risk of kernicterus, an exchange transfusion may be required. In this procedure, the baby's blood is replaced with donor blood to reduce haemolysis.

Conjugated hyperbilirubinaemia

This has many causes, and the advice of a paediatric gastroenterologist is usually

Neonatal jaundice: classification by cause

Type	Category	Cause
Unconjugated hyperbilirubinaemia	Physiological jaundice	Excess red blood cell breakdown, decreased liver conjugation
	Acute intravascular haemolysis	Haemolytic disease: blood group incompatibility (e.g. Rhesus, ABO)
		Red blood cell enzyme defects: glucose 6-phosphate dehydrogenase deficiency, pyruvate kinase deficiency
		Red blood cell membrane defects: spherocytosis, ellipsoidosis
		Viral infection: cytomegalovirus, herpes, toxoplasmosis
		Bacterial infection: sepsis, urine infection
	Extravascular blood collections	Excessive bruising, cephalhaematoma, intraventricular haemorrhage
	Decreased conjugation	Sepsis
		Crigler–Najjar syndrome (deficiency of glucuronyltransferase enzyme)
	Increased enterohepatic circulation (resulting from decreased gut movement)	Delayed feeding, constipation or bowel obstruction
	Breast milk jaundice	Inhibition of conjugating liver enzymes, increased enterohepatic circulation of bilirubin
Conjugated hyperbilirubinaemia	Obstruction of bile flow	Biliary atresia, duodenal atresia, choledochal cyst
	Chronic illness	Cystic fibrosis, hypothyroidism, hypopituitarism
	Iatrogenic	Prolonged total parenteral nutrition, use of certain drugs
	Liver disease: cirrhosis	Hepatitis A, B or C
		Congenital viral infections: rubella, cytomegalovirus, herpes
	Metabolic problems	Alpha-1 antitrypsin deficiency
		Galactosaemia

Table 3.8 Classification of neonatal jaundice by cause

required to investigate the cause and plan the treatment. In conjugated hyperbilirubinaemia, an abdominal US scan is required to rule out biliary atresia, because this warrants prompt surgical intervention to avoid permanent liver damage.

> **In prolonged jaundice, serum 'split bilirubin' is measured to rule out conjugated hyperbilirubinaemia.** This is because biliary atresia, a cause of conjugated jaundice, requires prompt treatment.

Prognosis

This depends entirely on the underlying cause. However, prompt recognition and treatment will increase the likelihood of a good outcome.

Physiological neonatal jaundice

The commonest cause of neonatal jaundice in a term baby is physiological jaundice, which affects 50% of term and 80% of preterm infants. It is the result of unconjugated hyperbilirubinaemia secondary to the accelerated physiological breakdown of excess red blood cells in the neonate, and the low activity of the bilirubin conjugating enzyme uridine diphosphoglucuronyltransferase (UDPGT) in the liver. Levels of unconjugated bilirubin gradually increase after 24 h of age, reaching a peak at about day 5 before returning to normal levels by 2 weeks. In 80% of cases the hyperbilirubinaemia does not reach the threshold level for phototherapy and resolves on its own. Active management, if required, is as described above.

Jaundice in a term baby aged ≥ 2 weeks is known as prolonged jaundice and is abnormal. It should always be investigated, but there is usually no underlying cause other than physiological jaundice (which will be unconjugated) that is taking time to resolve.

> **Breastfed neonates are more prone to prolonged jaundice than those receiving formula milk.** If no cause is found, as is often the case, 'breast milk jaundice' is diagnosed, the cause of which is multifactorial and not clearly understood. This resolves without treatment.

Neonatal infection

Neonates acquire infection in one of three ways:

- in utero (congenital infection)
- during birth (perinatal infection)
- after birth (postnatal or late-onset neonatal infection)

Congenital infection occurs when the mother contracts an infection, for example rubella, to which she is not immune and the infection then passes to the fetus. Perinatal infections are contracted by the baby by vertical transmission from the mother's genital tract. Perinatal infection typically occurs during or within 72 h of birth. Postpartum (or late-onset) neonatal infection occurs after 72 h of life and is the result of direct contact with organisms from the mother, family or inanimate objects. Neonates have a higher risk of acquiring a serious invasive bacterial infection such as sepsis or meningitis than at any other point in childhood.

Congenital infection

Congenital infections are contracted by the fetus while in utero. Congenital infections can have serious effects on fetal growth and development; they can result in congenital abnormalities, spontaneous abortion or stillbirth. Causes and signs of congenital infection are shown in **Table 3.9**.

The finding of a congenital abnormality on an antenatal US scan prompts investigations to determine whether the cause is a congenital infection, thereby leading to a diagnosis. If there is a suspicion of congenital infection after birth, a blood sample is sent for serological tests.

Management depends on the cause of the infection. For example, cytomegalovirus infection is treated with antiviral agents, but there is no treatment for rubella. Children affected by congenital infection have neurodevelopmental difficulties and require follow-up by community paediatricians to ensure that their developmental needs are met.

Perinatal infection

The most common risk factors for perinatal neonatal sepsis are:

- maternal Group B *Streptococcus* (GBS) colonisation
- prolonged rupture of membranes (>12 hours predelivery)
- maternal urinary tract infection

Congenital infection: causes and signs

Infection	Signs
Rubella	Congenital heart disease
	Sensorineural hearing loss
	IUGR
	Hepatosplenomegaly
Cytomegalovirus	Intrauterine growth restriction
	Hepatosplenomegaly
	Jaundice
	Thrombocytopenia
	Microcephaly
	Intracranial calcification
	Sensorineural hearing loss
Toxoplasmosis	Jaundice
	Hepatosplenomegaly
	Intrauterine growth restriction
	Chorioretinitis
	Sensorineural deafness
Chickenpox	Skin lesions
	Eye defects
	Intrauterine growth restriction
	Limb abnormalities
Parvovirus	Severe anaemia leading to hydrops fetalis (severe fetal oedema)

Table 3.9 Causes and signs of congenital infection

■ maternal chorioamnionitis (fever due to infected amniotic fluid)

Group B *Streptococcus* (GBS) infection affects 0.7 out of 1000 live births. An estimated 25% of women in the developed world have GBS colonisation in their genital tract; the bacteria are present but cause no harm.

Most babies born to mothers colonised with GBS do not become infected. GBS infection occurs as the neonate travels down the birth canal or, less commonly, by haematogenous spread. About 90% of babies with GBS infection present at birth or within the first 12 h of birth, with clinical features of respiratory distress, apnoea, lethargy, poor feeding, irritability and sometimes seizures.

Diagnosis is based on clinical features and confirmation of GBS in blood or cerebrospinal fluid cultures.

Treatment is with high doses of intravenous antibiotics. If the baby is in shock, fluid, inotropes (to improve contraction of heart muscle) and ventilation may be needed. Mothers known to be colonised with GBS can be given intrapartum penicillin to reduce the risk of neonatal infection.

Group B streptococcal infection can result in serious complications and death. Overall mortality is 5–15% in developed countries.

Postnatal infection

Postnatal (late-onset) infection presents with non-specific signs of sepsis, including poor feeding, vomiting, jaundice, apnoea, respiratory distress and irritability. Although these infections are uncommon in term infants, neonatal meningitis has a mortality of up to 50%, with one-third of survivors having serious sequelae.

Maternal conditions and treatments affecting the neonate

Some pregnant women have, or take medication for, a pre-existing medical condition which affects the fetus and/or neonate. Mothers may also develop pregnancy-related complications that affect the growing fetus.

Maternal medical conditions

Maternal medical conditions can affect the fetus in many ways, depending on the condition (**Table 3.10**). Drugs that women take to treat certain conditions can also harm the fetus (**Table 3.11**). Some drugs act as teratogens; they affect embryogenesis, thereby resulting in congenital anomalies.

The best outcome for the baby is achieved when the pregnancy is planned for a time when the condition is well managed, for example when a mother with diabetes has good control of her blood glucose levels, or when a woman with drug addiction is receiving a morphine substitute rather than heroin. If a particular medication is known to be harmful to the fetus, it is changed to avoid causing congenital anomalies if it does not also cause the mother harm. For example, the antiepileptic drug sodium valproate is associated with many anomalies, but changing the medication during pregnancy predisposes the mother to seizures that can be more harmful to the mother and baby.

> **Alcohol readily crosses the placenta, and excessive consumption of alcohol in pregnancy can cause fetal alcohol syndrome and fetal alcohol spectrum disorders.** Associated features include dysmorphism, learning difficulties, attention deficit and behavioural problems.

Regular follow-up of the mother's health is needed throughout pregnancy. The baby needs to be monitored for the complications known to be associated with the mother's illness or the medication she takes.

Maternal conditions: effects on the fetus or neonate	
Maternal condition	Effect on fetus or neonate
Diabetes mellitus	Macrosomia (large baby)
	Hypoglycaemia caused by neonatal excess insulin production
	Respiratory distress as a result of immature surfactant production
	Congenital anomalies: congenital heart disease, sacral agenesis, microcolon
Maternal Graves' disease	Affects neonate during first 2 weeks of life
	Thyrotoxicosis in neonate: tachycardia, tremors, poor feeding, weight loss, goitre. Treated with antithyroid medication
Systemic lupus erythematosus	Complete heart block: autoantibodies (anti-Ro) cross placenta to damage the fetal cardiac conduction system, causing congenital heart block
Drug misuse	Withdrawal symptoms in neonatal period: tremors, high-pitched cry, temperure instability
	Long-term effects on cognitive development
Alcohol misuse	Fetal alcohol spectrum disorder including fetal alcohol syndrome

Table 3.10 Maternal conditions affecting the fetus or neonate

Congenital anomalies: associations with prescribed medications	
Drug	Anomalies
Antiepileptic drugs	Two- to threefold increase in major malformations, especially neural tube defects, with more established drugs (e.g. sodium valproate, phenytoin)
	Sodium valproate or polytherapy are most teratogenic
	Lamotrigine appears to have a lower risk
Isotretinoin	Craniofacial abnormalities, neural tube defects, cardiovascular defects, cleft palate, thymic aplasia
Tetracycline	Stained teeth, hypoplasia of teeth enamel
Thalidomide	Abnormal limb development, facial anomalies, cardiac and kidney defects
Warfarin	Nasal hypoplasia, hypoplastic phalanges, eye anomalies, intellectual disability

Table 3.11 Congenital anomalies associated with use of prescribed medications

Surgical emergencies in the neonate

Many congenital anomalies require prompt surgery for survival, for example congenital diaphragmatic hernia, bowel atresia, choanal atresia and malrotation of the gut. Neonatal surgery is carried out in special centres by paediatric surgeons.

Congenital diaphragmatic hernia

In congenital diaphragmatic hernia, the bowel, spleen and liver herniate through the diaphragm into the thorax. The hernia results from a defect in the diaphragm, which arises during antenatal development.

Congenital diaphragmatic affects 1 in 3000 live births. Boys are twice as likely to be affected than girls. Congenital diaphragmatic hernia occurs mostly as a result of defects in the posterolateral segment of the diaphragm and are on the left side. The lungs become underdeveloped (pulmonary hypoplasia), because some of the space where they should be is occupied by the herniated organs.

Clinical features

Congenital diaphragmatic hernia is diagnosed on antenatal US scans in 60–80% of cases; the remainder are detected clinically at birth. At birth, the baby has severe respiratory distress and a scaphoid (concave) abdomen. No breath sounds are audible on the affected side. If the hernia is on the left side, heart sounds may be displaced to the right because of pressure pushing against the heart.

Diagnostic approach

Antenatal fetal anomaly US scans (18–21 weeks) may show the presence of bowel in the thorax. Diagnosis at birth is based on chest radiograph findings: loops of bowel visible in the hemithorax, and mediastinal shift (**Figure 3.11**).

Management

Newborns with congenital diaphragmatic hernia require immediate intubation and ventilation. A large nasogastric tube is inserted into the stomach to enable air to escape rather than dilatate the bowel and thereby further compromise lung expansion by pressing against the lung. Ventilation is necessary because the hypoplastic lungs are unable to provide adequate gas exchange.

Surgery

Congenital diaphragmatic hernia is treated by surgery to repair the diaphragm defect. The procedure is delayed until the baby's respiratory status has been stabilised.

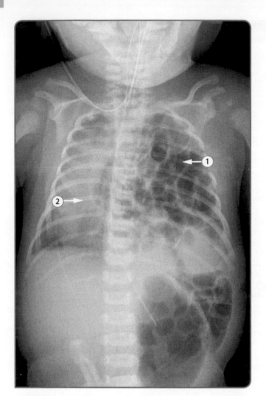

Figure 3.11 Chest radiograph showing a left-sided congenital diaphragmatic hernia with bowel loops in the thorax ① and a pressure effect pushing the heart over to the right ②.

Prognosis

Mortality is high, about 50%. The prognosis is better if the baby survives the first 24 h after birth.

Craniofacial anomalies

Craniofacial anomalies are defined as abnormalities of structures of the face or skull. The most commonly encountered problems are cleft lip and palate, and craniosynostosis.

Cleft lip and palate

A cleft defect can be isolated or involve both the lip and the palate.

- A cleft lip is a split in the upper lip
- A cleft palate is a split in the hard palate, the soft palate or both

The cleft can be unilateral or bilateral.

Epidemiology and aetiology

A cleft occurs when tissues of the upper lip and/or palate fail to fully fuse during embryological development. The cause is believed to be a combination of environmental and genetic factors. A minority of clefts (15%) are associated with genetic conditions, such as Pierre Robin syndrome, trisomy 13 (Edwards' syndrome) and trisomy 18 (Patau's syndrome).

Cleft lip and palate affects 1 out of 700 children.

Clinical features and diagnostic approach

The clinical features depend on the extent of the cleft (**Figures 3.12** and **3.13**). A cleft lip, with or without cleft palate, is either diagnosed on an antenatal US scan or at birth, when the defect is obvious. Isolated cleft palate is not detectable on antenatal US scans and is usually diagnosed during the examination of the newborn.

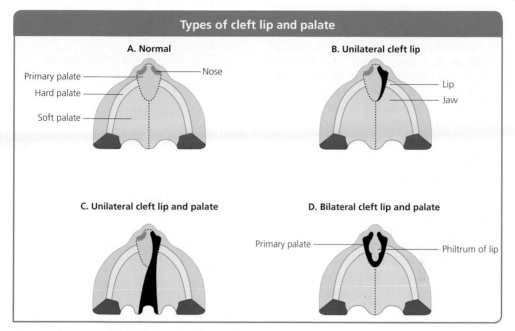

Types of cleft lip and palate

A. Normal

Primary palate — — Nose
Hard palate
Soft palate

B. Unilateral cleft lip

Lip
Jaw

C. Unilateral cleft lip and palate

D. Bilateral cleft lip and palate

Primary palate — — Philtrum of lip

Figure 3.12 The different types of cleft lip and palate, ventral view (in the mouth looking upwards).

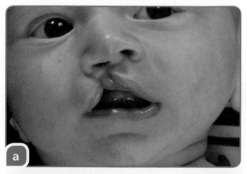

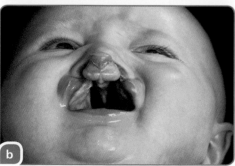

Figure 3.13 (a) Unilateral cleft lip. (b) Bilateral cleft lip and palate.

Management

Treatment is provided by a multidisciplinary specialist cleft team including surgeons, nurses, paediatricians, audiologists (cleft palate is associated with persistent middle ear effusion), dentists, and speech and language therapists. Feeding may be difficult in newborns because the baby may be unable to feed adequately at the breast; many babies require specialised squeezable bottles and soft teats to enable them to achieve the seal necessary for good suction.

Cleft lip is repaired at 4 months of age. Cleft palate is usually repaired at 1 year to ensure it is done before speech development but avoids the complications of early closure of the palate (midface hypoplasia with decreased dimensions of the dental arch).

Prognosis

Surgery has excellent functional and cosmetic results. Long-term complications include ear infections and glue ear, dental problems and speech difficulties, including nasal speech (mainly with cleft palate).

Craniosynostosis

In craniosynostosis, some of the sutures of the skull fuse prematurely; the aetiology is unknown. The sutures are fibrous tissue seams between the different skull bones. It is normal for the sutures to fuse (turn into bone) once the brain nears its full size (18–24 months), thereby forming the adult skull. In craniosynostosis only one or two sutures fuse early, so the head continues to grow in some planes (at right angles to the non-fused sutures) resulting in an abnormal head shape. It is unusual for this to cause restricted brain growth and increased intracranial pressure.

Craniosynostosis affects about 6 out of every 10,000 live births worldwide. Craniosynostosis tends to occur in isolation, but it can be associated with a syndrome, including Crouzon's syndrome and Apert's syndrome.

Clinical features

Clinical features vary because the condition affects different skull sutures (**Figure 3.14**). However, essentially the child has an abnormal head shape.

> The term **craniosynostosis** is made up from *cranio*, meaning 'skull'; *syn*, meaning 'joined'; and *ostosis* meaning 'bone'.

Management

Skull imaging, for example by radiography or CT, is used to identify the fused suture. Surgery is required to improve the shape of the head and very occasionally to relieve pressure on the brain. Surgical treatment for craniosynostosis is a highly specialised service; it is carried out in special centres only.

Plagiocephaly

Postural (positional) plagiocephaly is diagnosed when a baby has an asymmetrical head shape that has the appearance of plagiocephaly, i.e. flattening on one side with protrusion on the diagonally opposite side (**Figure 3.15**), but is not caused by premature fusion of the sutures. Instead, it is caused by external pressure, for example from lying on the affected side of the head preferentially.

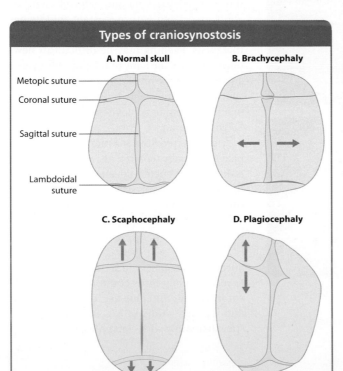

Types of craniosynostosis

A. Normal skull

Metopic suture
Coronal suture

Sagittal suture

Lambdoidal suture

B. Brachycephaly

C. Scaphocephaly

D. Plagiocephaly

Figure 3.14 The different types of craniosynostosis. The skull grows at right angles to the suture line. If the suture fuses prematurely, the skull will not grow in this direction. (a) Normal sutures. (b) Brachycephaly: a flat back of the head, secondary to fusion of both coronal sutures. (c) Scaphocephaly: a long, narrow head, secondary to premature closure of sagittal suture. (d) plagiocephaly: asymmetrical head, secondary to closure of one coronal suture.

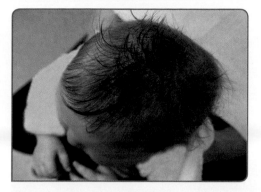

Figure 3.15 Postural plagiocephaly.

Investigations are not required. Parents are advised to vary their baby's position to minimise pressure on the flattened part of the head and thereby even out the appearance. This improves the appearance of the head over a few months, but some mild flattening occasionally remains.

Metabolic disorders

Metabolic disorders are problems with the child's metabolism at a biochemical or cellular level. A common but transient metabolic problem in neonates is hypoglycaemia. Inborn errors of metabolism are rare conditions that are lifelong.

Hypoglycaemia

Infants with a high risk of hypoglycaemia include (**Table 3.12**):

- infants of diabetic mothers
- infants whose mothers have taken beta-blockers
- infants with intrauterine growth restriction

In developed countries, the incidence of symptomatic hypoglycaemia is 1.3–3 per 1000 live births.

Symptoms of hypoglycaemia are lethargy, drowsiness, jitteriness, irritability, apnoea and seizures. If prolonged, symptomatic hypoglycaemia can cause permanent neurological disability.

Management aims to prevent hypoglycaemia. Babies at risk are identified at birth, fed soon after and at regular intervals to prevent the condition developing. For the first 24 hours, the blood glucose concentration is measured before feeds and prompt treatment given if it falls too low. In neonates at risk of developing hypoglycaemia blood glucose levels are kept above 2.6 mmol/L.

> **Buccal dextrose gel** is massaged into the baby's cheek, where it is directly absorbed into the blood. This treatment quickly increases the blood glucose concentration in patients with hypoglycaemia.

Hypoglycaemia is treated with a combination of oral and nasogastric feeds. If the hypoglycaemia is severe (> 1.4 mmol/L), or if it persists despite feeding, the baby is given intravenous dextrose.

Neonatal hypoglycaemia: causes	
Pathogenesis	Causes
Increased demand for glucose with decreased supply available	Prematurity
	Intrauterine growth restriction
	Hypothermia
	Infection
	Hypoxic ischaemic encephalopathy
Hyperinsulinism (excess insulin in the blood)	Diabetes in the mother
	Transient neonatal hyperinsulism
	Beckwith–Wiedemann syndrome
Endocrinopathies (endocrine abnormalities)	Pituitary: growth hormone deficiency
	Adrenal: congenital adrenal hyperplasia
Carbohydrate metabolism disorder	Glycogen storage disease
	Galactosaemia

Table 3.12 Causes of neonatal hypoglycaemia

Inborn errors of metabolism

Inborn errors of metabolism are the hundreds of rare genetic diseases that impair the individual's ability to metabolise substances at a biochemical level.

Children who have an inborn error of metabolism usually present shortly after birth (once they have been given milk) with lethargy, poor feeding and abnormal neurological signs. Because the signs are non-specific, it is important that this diagnosis is considered and appropriate blood and urine analysis requested promptly (see page 347).

Answers to starter questions

1. Preterm infants' arterial saturations should not go above 94% (unless they are in air) because this is associated with retinopathy of prematurity. If supplemental oxygen is required the lowest concentration needed is given because oxygen damages the lungs by triggering an inflammatory cascade causing long-term lung injury.

2. Jaundice in the first 24 hours of life indicates a haemolytic cause (such as an incompatibility in blood groups between the mother and fetus) that leads to a rapid and dangerous rise in bilirubin within days. The baby's blood–brain barrier is not yet mature, putting them at risk of encephalopathy or permanent neurosensory hearing

3. Pregnant women are advised to avoid gardening (or wear gloves and avoid then touching their mouths) and to avoid contact with kittens and cat litter trays. This is to avoid ingesting the protozoan *Toxoplasma gondii*, which cause miscarriage, stillbirth or congenital toxoplasmosis (blindness, neurodisability, seizures and deafness developing during childhood). Toxoplasmosis can also be contracted from eating raw or undercooked meat, handling raw meat, drinking raw milk or eating raw unwashed vegetables.

4. Term infants with hypoxic ischaemic encephalopathy are given therapeutic hypothermia for 72 hours to prevent secondary brain insult from brain oedema and cytokines. Term infants that require on-going resuscitation at 10 minutes of age are passively cooled (turn off the overheat heater, remove the hat) and, once admitted to the neonatal intensive care unit, actively cooled on a cooling mattress and their brain function monitored with a cerebral function monitor.

Chapter 4
Respiratory and ear, nose and throat disorders

Starter questions

Answers to the following questions are on page 174.

1. Why do children with cystic fibrosis need a high-calorie and high-fat diet?
2. Why are chest radiographs not helpful in infants with bronchiolitis?
3. Why are gastric aspirates used instead of sputum samples to diagnose tuberculosis in small children?
4. Why are children with Down's syndrome monitored for obstructive sleep apnoea?

Introduction

Respiratory conditions are common in children, being responsible for 50% of all acute paediatric admissions. Several chronic disorders, including cystic fibrosis and asthma, are associated with significant morbidity.

The vast majority of acute respiratory problems can be managed in the community by parents and the general practitioner (GP). Chronic respiratory disorders are managed by the paediatric respiratory team.

Case 3 Night-time cough in a 4-year-old

Presentation

Daniel is 4 years old. He has a 6-month history of coughing almost every night. The cough is dry and non-productive. It can be so forceful or prolonged that it makes him vomit. Daniel's cough is disturbing the whole family's sleep, and his concerned parents have taken him to see his GP.

Initial interpretation

Chronic cough in children aged 1–6 years is most commonly chronic non-specific cough of childhood or asthma. Many children of this age easily vomit with a cough due to the increased intra-abdominal pressure when coughing and the immaturity of the lower oesophageal sphincter in young children (see page 206).

Further history

Further questioning reveals that Daniel has had dry skin since he was a few months old, especially on his cheeks and more recently on the flexures of his elbows and knees. At 4 months of age, he had bronchiolitis that required admission to hospital and oxygen therapy.

His parents describe his breathing as 'chesty' when he has an upper respiratory tract infection. He sometimes coughs during the day when running around with friends, especially when he is excited, such as at birthday parties. There is no choking with eating or drinking, and Daniel has not vomited during coughing, so gastro-oesophageal reflux can be ruled out as a cause.

Daniel is an only child. There is no family history of asthma, but his father gets severe hay fever. No-one smokes at home, and the family have no pets.

Examination

On examination, Daniel is shown to be well grown, with his height and weight on the 75th centile. Examination is unremarkable; in particular, he has no finger clubbing, no chest deformity and no intercostal recession or tachypnoea. His chest is found to be clear on auscultation, and his heart sounds are normal.

Interpretation of findings

Cough is a common symptom in children. Daniel has a dry cough at night, as well as a cough associated with exercise. He has eczema and a strong family history of atopy. The nature of the cough and the atopy make asthma the most likely diagnosis. The 'chesty' episodes with upper respiratory tract infections are probably wheeze.

Investigations

Daniel is too young for lung function testing to produce reliable results, although such tests can be carried out for older children. Instead he is asked to run as fast as possible in the playground next to the clinic for 10 minutes. This causes him to cough, and auscultation finds wheeze throughout the lung fields.

Diagnosis

Asthma is diagnosed based on the history and examination findings: the presence of cough and wheeze on exercise, a history of eczema and the absence of faltering growth. Daniel is started on twice daily inhaled steroid and also a bronchodilator. He and his parents are taught correct inhaler technique by the respiratory nurse. With this treatment the night-time and exercise-induced coughing resolve over the next few weeks.

Case 4 Cough and weight loss in an 11-month-old

Presentation

Millie is an 11-month-old with a persistent cough. She has been referred to the paediatrician by her health visitor. At the ages of 2 and 5 months, Millie had several episodes of bronchiolitis that required prolonged admissions to hospital. The current referral is prompted by the health visitor noting that Millie's weight has decreased from the 50th centile at birth to the 9th centile. Millie is brought to the clinic by her mother and grandmother.

Initial interpretation

It is not unusual for children under 1 year to require more than one admission to hospital with bronchiolitis, but in this case the main concerns are the persistent cough and the faltering growth (her weight moving down the weight centile chart). It is acceptable to lose weight during an acute illness, but this should be regained promptly once the child has recovered.

Further history

Millie is the first child of non-consanguineous (unrelated) parents. The pregnancy was normal, and Millie was born at term. She has had all her immunisations. Millie has three meals a day as well as formula milk, and there is no vomiting. Her grandmother says that Millie has loose, offensive-smelling stools, which is 'normal' for her. The parents are non-smokers, and there is no family history of chest problems.

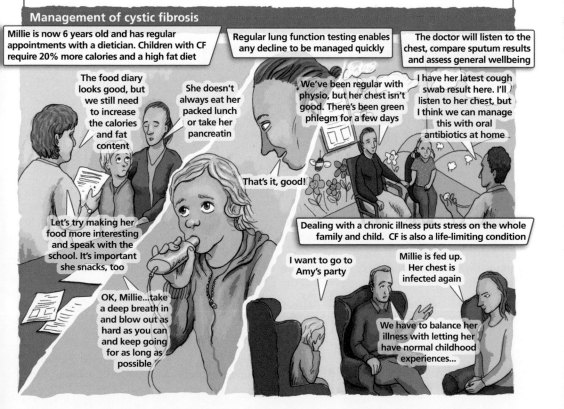

Case 4 *continued*

Examination

Millie is thin and looks undernourished. She is alert. She has no finger clubbing or eczema. She has Harrison's sulci; crackles and wheeze are heard throughout her chest. She is not tachypnoeic but has mild subcostal recession.

Interpretation of findings

The combination of chest signs and symptoms (evidence of chronic respiratory distress, crackles and wheeze, loose stools), along with faltering growth, must prompt consideration of cystic fibrosis as a possible diagnosis. Finger clubbing is not always seen, especially at younger ages. Other causes of failure to thrive should be considered, for example bowel conditions such as coeliac disease, but primary bowel conditions are not associated with chronic cough and chest infections. The fact that Millie's parents are not known to be even distantly related does not rule out cystic fibrosis: the recessive allele for cystic fibrosis is carried by 4% of people of northern European ethnicity, for example.

Investigations

A chest radiograph shows markedly increased streakiness in the lung fields, which suggests inflammation. A sweat test is arranged (see page 106).

Diagnosis

The result from the sweat test is positive for cystic fibrosis, and genetic testing confirms the presence of a mutation known to cause the condition. Millie is referred to the specialist multidisciplinary cystic fibrosis team. The cystic fibrosis nurse visits the family at home to discuss the condition at length.

Millie starts regular physiotherapy, a high-energy diet with pancreatic enzyme replacement and prophylactic antibiotic therapy. Her parents are offered genetic counselling regarding further pregnancies. Millie will attend clinic regularly throughout her life to monitor her lung function and growth.

Congenital respiratory tract anomalies

The development of the respiratory tract that starts in utero continues until 8 years of age. Oligohydramnios (deficiency of amniotic fluid) reduces lung growth in utero. External compression or internal masses also affect the growth and development of the lungs after birth. The varied congenital anomalies of the respiratory tract are shown in **Table 4.1**.

Choanal atresia

In choanal atresia, the nasal passages are blocked by bone or tissue. It occurs in 1 in 10,000 births and can be associated with other anomalies, for example CHARGE syndrome (see Table 11.2). Bilateral atresia presents with respiratory distress or cyanosis at birth, which improves on crying (when the mouth is open). Early surgery is required to open the blockage; nasal stents are inserted until the nasal passage heals.

Congenital cystic lung disease

Abnormal intrapulmonary development may lead to several congenital cystic lung diseases, including:

Congenital anomalies of the respiratory tract				
Ear, nose and throat	Trachea or bronchi	Extrinsic airway	Intrapulmonary	Extrapulmonary
Choanal atresia	Stenosis	Compression	Congenital lobar emphysema	Ribcage defects
Larynx	Tracheomalacia	Vascular ring	Cystic adenomatoid malformation	Neuromuscular disease
Laryngomalacia	Bronchomalacia	Bronchogenic duplication cyst		Chest wall deformities
Laryngeal cleft	Tracheo-oesophageal fistula		Lobar sequestration	
			Pulmonary hypoplasia	
			Diaphragmatic hernia	

Table 4.1 Congenital anomalies affecting the respiratory tract

- congenital pulmonary airway malformation
- pulmonary sequestration
- congenital lobar emphysema

Congenital cystic lung disease is sometimes identified on the maternal antenatal US scan. However, the exact type can be difficult to diagnose, so further imaging is needed after birth, for example with chest radiograph, CT or MRI. Congenital cystic lung diseases present most commonly in the neonatal period, with signs of respiratory distress.

Congenital pulmonary airway malformation

Congenital pulmonary airway malformation (CPAM), formerly known as congenital cystic adenomatoid malformation (CCAM), occurs in 1 per 10,000 live births. It is caused by unilateral non-functioning cystic pulmonary tissue.

- In symptomatic babies, i.e. when there is respiratory distress, the affected tissue is resected soon after birth
- In asymptomatic babies, an elective procedure later in life is required to remove the tissue, because of the risk of malignant change

Bronchopulmonary sequestration

Bronchopulmonary sequestration occurs in 0.8 per 10,000 live births. It is characterised by non-functioning pulmonary tissue that has become separated from the bronchial tree during fetal development but has preserved

an arterial blood supply from the aorta (**Figure 4.1**). It can become infected or compress the healthy lung. Symptomatic lesions require embolisation or surgical removal.

Congenital lobar emphysema

Congenital lobar emphysema is a congenital problem affecting a lobe of the lung. The lobe becomes hyperinflated, because air inflating the lung becomes trapped. The hyperinflated lung pushes against other lobes, thereby

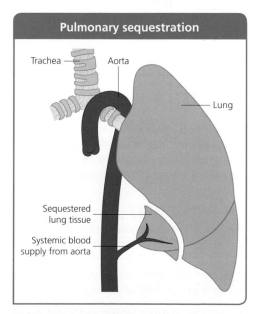

Figure 4.1 In pulmonary sequestration the sequestered tissue may become infected or compress the lung.

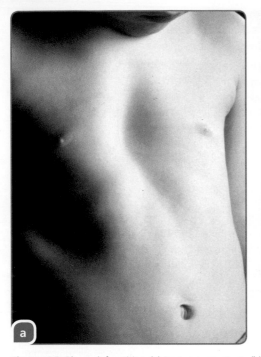 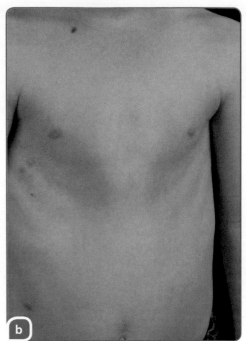

Figure 4.2 Chest deformities. (a) Pectus excavatum. (b) Pectus carinatum.

causing respiratory distress. Congenital lobar emphysema is rare, occurring in 1 per 90,000 live births. Symptomatic patients require a lobectomy.

Chest wall deformities

Pectus excavatum (concavity) and pectus carinatum (pigeon chest) (**Figure 4.2**) are congenital deformities in which the ribs and sternum grow abnormally.

Asthma

Asthma is a reversible, obstructive, chronic inflammatory disease of the airways, with increased bronchial sensitivity to various stimuli, and bronchoconstriction in consequence.

Epidemiology

Asthma is the commonest cause of wheeze in children. It affects 1 in 10 children aged > 5 years; boys are affected more commonly than girls. Children may grow out of asthma, or it may persist into adulthood.

Aetiology

The precise cause of asthma is unknown, but it is associated with atopy (allergic disease

such as eczema) in the child or their immediate family. Other risk factors for asthma include parental smoking (especially maternal smoking during pregnancy), prematurity and previous bronchiolitis infection.

Clinical features

The main clinical features of an asthma attack or exacerbation are:

- wheeze
- shortness of breath
- chest tightness
- cough

These features occur in response to a trigger. Triggers for asthma exacerbations are unique to the individual but the most common are:

- exposure to allergens or irritants, for example from house dust mites, moulds, pets and cigarette smoke
- upper respiratory tract infection
- exercise
- exposure to cold air
- certain emotions, such as anxiety or excitement

Children with symptoms that occur on most days, including at night, between the severe attacks/acute exacerbations of asthma are described as having interval symptoms.

During an acute exacerbation of asthma, the child is short of breath, has difficulty talking in full sentences and shows signs of respiratory distress, with wheeze heard throughout the lung fields (see page 405).

Examination of children between attacks rarely elicits any wheeze. Features associated with asthma may be present, including Harrison's sulci (**Figure 4.3**), nasal blockage (suggesting allergic rhinitis) and eczema.

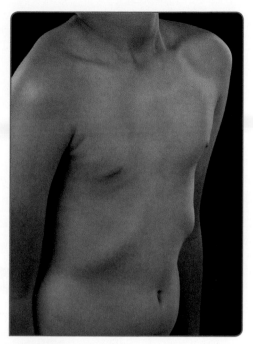

Figure 4.3 Harrison's sulci, a rib deformity at the insertion of the diaphragm muscle caused by chronic respiratory difficulty.

> **Acute asthma exacerbations occur during thunderstorms,** when large amounts of pollen, in very small particles, are released into the air. This phenomenon is reflected in an increase in hospital admissions for acute asthma exacerbations in stormy weather.

Diagnostic approach

In children, the diagnosis of asthma is based on clinical information obtained by thorough history taking. A symptom diary kept by the child or their parents can be helpful; it is used to record what the child was doing when they had their symptoms, and the allergens or irritants to which they may have been exposed.

Children who are unable to undergo lung function tests, because it is too complex for their developmental age, are given a trial of medication (e.g. a steroid inhaler for a few weeks). Asthma is diagnosed if the trial drug relieves their symptoms.

> **Transient early wheeze is diagnosed when a child aged between a few months to 3 years presents with multiple episodes of wheeze associated with an upper respiratory tract infection.** It is probably the result of pre-existing narrow small airways, which are easily obstructed by inflammation. Risk factors for transient early wheeze are maternal smoking (particularly in pregnancy), prematurity and male sex. It is not associated with a family history of atopy; the child is less likely to have interval symptoms and more likely to grow out of the symptoms than with true asthma.

Older children can undergo lung function tests (see page 104). Asthma is diagnosed if the results show airway obstruction. Lung function tests can also be used to help determine if the airway obstruction is reversible with the use of a bronchodilator.

Management

The aims of treatment for asthma are to control interval symptoms, decrease the frequency and severity of exacerbations, reduce sleep disturbances and minimise the number of school days missed because of exacerbations.

Asthma is treated with medications, which are increased in dose and variety in a stepwise manner until control of symptoms is achieved (**Figure 4.4**). Drugs used to treat asthma (**Table 4.2**) are inhaled or taken orally.

Inhalers are grouped according to their action on the lungs.

- Relievers reverse the bronchoconstriction by causing bronchodilation; they are short acting
- Protectors are longer acting bronchodilators
- Preventers are inhaled steroids that reduce inflammation and reduce the likelihood of bronchoconstriction

Oral medications can also be considered to be preventers. These include oral steroids and leukotriene receptor antagonists.

Monoclonal antibody therapy is very rarely used when symptoms are very difficult to control and are strongly associated with

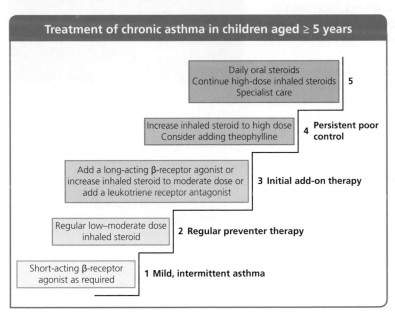

Figure 4.4 The five steps for the treatment of chronic asthma in children aged ≥ 5 years. Medications should be increased or reduced according to response.

Asthma treatments		
Action	Class of drug	Examples
Relievers (bronchodilators)	β_2 agonists	Salbutamol, terbutaline
	Muscarinic receptor antagonist	Ipratropium bromide
Protectors	Long-acting β_2 agonists	Salmeterol, formoterol
Preventers	Inhaled corticosteroids	Budesonide, beclometasone, fluticasone
	Leukotriene receptor antagonists	Montelukast, zafirlukast
	Methylxanthines	Theophylline, aminophylline
	Oral steroids	Prednisolone
Antiallergy	Injectable monoclonal antibodies	Omalizumab

Table 4.2 Different types of medication for asthma

allergic triggers. If treatment reaches step 5 (see **Figure 4.6**), support from a specialist respiratory paediatrician is required because this shows that the child's asthma is difficult to manage.

Education has an essential role in the management of asthma: children are taught the importance of taking medication regularly, inhaler technique and managing exacerbations.

At every clinic appointment, the respiratory nurse checks inhaler technique, i.e. how the child uses the inhaler, to ensure that this is adequate. Younger children need to have their inhaled medication given through a spacer and mask (see page 116), because they are unable to coordinate inhalation with activation of the device. Also at every clinic appointment, a peak flow meter is used to measure peak expiratory flow rate if the child is able (>5 years of age). This enables peak flow readings obtained during an exacerbation to be compared with the child's best measurement when well, thereby determining the severity of the attack.

Smoking cessation advice is given to parents who smoke. The child's growth is monitored, particularly if they are receiving steroids; both high-dose inhaled and regular oral steroids may impair growth. Compliance with treatment is also enquired about.

Prognosis

Current treatments for asthma enable most children to lead normal, active lives, and many grow out of the condition. Deaths in childhood from asthma are rare but unfortunately still occur (for example, up to 40 deaths per year in the UK).

Cystic fibrosis

Cystic fibrosis is an inherited genetic disorder that affects the lungs and digestive system for the whole of the affected individual's life and is associated with shortened life expectancy.

> **More than 2000 different gene mutations are known to cause cystic fibrosis.** In northern Europe, the delta F508 mutation is the most common of these.

Epidemiology and aetiology

Cystic fibrosis affects 1 in 2500–3000 live births in northern Europe (including the UK), being very rare in native Africans and Asians. It is an autosomal recessive disease that results from defects in the cystic fibrosis conductance transmembrane regulator (CFTR) gene. The CFTR gene encodes a protein that regulates chloride movement, and hence water, across epithelial surfaces.

Defects in the *CTFR* gene cause mucous, sweat and pancreatic cells to produce thick, sticky secretions that damage the lungs and affect the digestive system. One in 25 people of Northern European descent carry one abnormal copy of the gene responsible for cystic fibrosis, but two abnormal copies are needed for an individual to have the disease.

Clinical features

Cystic fibrosis has many clinical features, all of which are related to the abnormally thick mucus in the lungs and digestive tract (**Table 4.3**).

Respiratory problems associated with cystic fibrosis include recurrent chest infections and persistent wheeze, because the child is unable to cough up the thick secretions. The persistent mucus leads to bronchiectasis (widened airways).

Children with cystic fibrosis can present with bowel problems from birth; 20% of babies with cystic fibrosis have meconium ileus, i.e. bowel obstruction as a result of thickened meconium that cannot be passed. Thick secretions from the pancreas prevent absorption of

Cystic fibrosis: associated problems				
General	Respiratory	Gastrointestinal and nutritional	Metabolic	Other
Failure to thrive	Persistent wheeze	Meconium ileus	Hyponatraemic and hypochloraemic dehydration	Infertility in males
Salty taste to skin	Bronchiectasis: chronic cough and sputum production (Figure 4.5)	Loose, offensive-smelling stools		Subfertility in females
Clubbing		Bloating and abdominal pain		
	Nasal polyps	Rectal prolapse	Diabetes mellitus	
		Pancreatitis (acute and chronic)		
		Neonatal hyperbilirubinaemia		
		Cholelithiasis, cholestasis		
		Fat-soluble vitamin deficiency (vitamins A, D, E and K)		

Table 4.3 Problems associated with cystic fibrosis

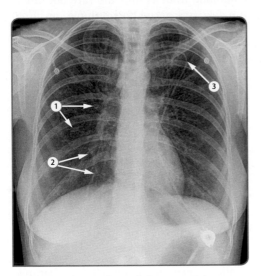

Figure 4.5 Chest radiograph from an adolescent with cystic fibrosis, showing the marked fibrotic changes ② and ring shadows ① typical of the condition. In the left upper thorax ③, a central line is visible; this is used to administer intravenous antibiotics.

fat-soluble vitamins (A, D, E and K) and other nutrients, leading to malnourishment and failure to thrive. Children with cystic fibrosis also have loose, offensive-smelling stools. If not detected on newborn screening, most children with cystic fibrosis present in the first year of life with these problems.

Diagnostic approach

If both expectant parents are known to carry the CFTR mutation, for example if they already have a child with cystic fibrosis, amniocentesis can be carried out to determine if the fetus has the disease. Cystic fibrosis can also be diagnosed in the neonatal period, if the parents opt to have newborn screening (see page 425).

Cystic fibrosis partially blocks pancreatic ducts, preventing the pancreatic enzyme trypsinogen from draining effectively, increasing its concentration in the blood. The serum concentration of immunoreactive trypsinogen (IRT) is therefore measured when screening for cystic fibrosis. Finding a high concentration along with cystic fibrosis DNA mutations prompts further investigation using a sweat test (the gold-standard test for cystic fibrosis). Cystic fibrosis is diagnosed when a high chloride concentration (> 60 mmol/L) is detected in sweat from the skin.

> **Any child with a history suggesting cystic fibrosis should be referred for a sweat test, regardless of the result from newborn screening for the disease.** This is because the newborn blood spot screening test can give a false negative result for babies with a falsely low measurement of immunoreactive trypsinogen.

Management

The management of cystic fibrosis requires a multidisciplinary approach, with support from paediatricians, specialist nurses, physiotherapists, dieticians, social workers, psychologists and pharmacists, and with structured annual reviews. The aims are:

- to prevent bacterial colonisation of the airways
- to prevent chest infections and promptly treat any that do occur
- to preserve pulmonary function
- to prevent non-pulmonary complications of cystic fibrosis

> **Genetic counselling is undertaken by specially-trained health professionals.** Once a genetic condition has been identified they help the family understand information about the condition, the inheritance pattern and risk of recurrence, and help them make informed decisions appropriate for them (i.e. non-directive). They also help adjust the family to living with the disorder or the risk.

Physiotherapy

Exercise is encouraged to help clear the thick respiratory secretions and thereby prevent chest infections. Chest physiotherapy is given daily, usually by the parents, to aid expectoration of phlegm. Adjuncts to sputum expectoration are mucolytics, which help break down the mucus, and inhaled hypertonic saline. Bronchodilators also help open the airways to facilitate the clearance of mucus.

Nutrition

Good weight gain and nutrition correlate with better lung function and improved survival. Children with cystic fibrosis have malabsorption and abnormal pancreatic secretions. Therefore they need a high-fat, high-calorie diet with pancreatic enzyme replacement and supplementation with fat-soluble vitamins (A, E and D) and salt. There is a risk that the child will develop cystic fibrosis-related diabetes because of their impaired pancreatic function; this complication is treated with insulin therapy.

Antibiotics

When cystic fibrosis is diagnosed, children are started on prophylactic flucloxacillin to prevent staphylococcal chest infection. The use of antibiotics in established chest infections is guided by the results of cultures from cough swabs. Patients with cystic fibrosis need antibiotics (often delivered intravenously), in high doses and for a long duration, to ensure that the sputum is infiltrated with the antimicrobial.

Chronic *Pseudomonas aeruginosa* infection is associated with deterioration of lung function and a poorer prognosis, so it is treated aggressively when the organism first presents. Chronic *Pseudomonas* infection is treated with nebulised antibiotics used daily.

Gene therapy

This is an exciting area of research. The goal of gene therapy is to replace the abnormal or defective gene in a patient's cells with a normal one, and thereby obviate the need for surgery or medication to treat the disease caused by the mutation. Much more research is needed to determine whether this is an effective option for cystic fibrosis.

Prognosis

Many patients with cystic fibrosis now live well into adulthood, but the median lifespan (about 40 years old) is shorter than that for an adult without cystic fibrosis. Lung transplantation can improve survival and quality of life for those with end stage lung disease (forced expiratory volume in 1s, FEV_1, < 30%). However, this is normally carried out in adulthood because lung function deteriorates with age.

> **The fungus *Aspergillus fumigatus* colonises up to 60% of patients with cystic fibrosis.** In 15% of these patients, it triggers allergic bronchopulmonary aspergillosis, a condition that causes inflammation in the lungs, secondary to hypersensitivity to the aspergillus. Management is with systemic corticosteroids and antifungal medication to prevent further lung damage.

Respiratory infections

Respiratory tract infections are very common in children, responsible for 50% of all illnesses in children younger than 5 years old. Most respiratory tract infections involve the upper respiratory tract only; about 5% affect the lower respiratory tract and are most frequently encountered in the winter months.

The vast majority of children can be treated at home or with advice from their GP. However, severe infections necessitate hospital admission.

Upper respiratory tract infections

Upper respiratory tract infections are infections of the ears, nose and throat. They are known to the layperson as the 'common cold'. Upper respiratory tract infections occur frequently in children; the average child has up to 12 such infections per year. The peak incidence is before 6 years of age. Viruses, typically rhinoviruses, are responsible for ≥ 90% of cases.

Diagnosis is based on clinical features.

- Symptoms of an upper respiratory tract infection are nasal discharge, sneezing cough, sore throat and earache
- Signs include fever, a red pharynx and bilateral redness of the tympanic membranes

Upper respiratory tract infections are treated symptomatically with paracetamol (acetaminophen), ibuprofen or both, as well as adequate fluid intake. Symptoms resolve in 7–10 days.

Bronchiolitis

Bronchiolitis is a viral infection of the lower respiratory tract that affects the bronchioles and alveoli. It is the commonest acute low respiratory tract infection in infancy, affecting about a third of children younger than 2 years at some time.

Epidemiology and aetiology

Respiratory syncytial virus causes 80% of cases of bronchiolitis. Other causes include adenovirus, influenza and parainfluenza virus.

Clinical features

Typical symptoms of bronchiolitis are a characteristic moist cough; difficulty breathing, with signs of respiratory distress; poor feeding, because of the respiratory distress; and audible wheeze. Apnoea sometimes occurs in very young babies (< 6 weeks of age) and preterm children. The clinical signs are shown in **Table 4.4**.

Risk factors for the development of severe bronchiolitis i.e. bronchiolitis requiring admission to hospital, are:

- age < 6 weeks
- preterm birth and neonatal chronic lung disease
- other pre-existing lung disease (e.g. cystic fibrosis)
- congenital heart disease
- immunocompromise
- neuromuscular problems

Bronchiolitis: clinical signs	
Region	Signs
Head and neck	Nasal flaring*
	Nasal discharge
	Tracheal tug*
Chest	Tachypnoea (rapid breathing)*
	Tachycardia (rapid heart rate)
	Oxygen requirement
	Widespread fine crepitation
	Prolonged expiratory phase with wheeze
	Intercostal recession*
	Subcostal recession*
Abdomen	Palpable liver edge due to lung hyperinflation
Whole body	Fever (< 38.5°C)
*Signs of respiratory distress.	

Table 4.4 Clinical signs of bronchiolitis

The natural history of bronchiolitis is a worsening of symptoms up until day 5–7, followed by gradual improvement and resolution at about day 10.

Diagnostic approach

The diagnosis is a clinical one. The virus causing the symptoms of bronchiolitis may be detected on testing of nasopharyngeal aspirate. A chest radiograph is not indicated, because it does not add useful information to the clinical diagnosis.

Management

Management of bronchiolitis is supportive. Children who are unable to take half of their normal feeds need to be admitted to hospital. Oxygen is given if hypoxia occurs. Babies are given small amounts of feeds at frequent intervals, and usually via a nasogastric tube to reduce the effort it takes for them to feed.

Feeding is stopped for children with significant respiratory distress, because a full stomach increases the work of breathing and leads to milk aspiration if the child vomits with the cough and exhaustion. To prevent dehydration, they are given intravenous fluids instead.

Continuous positive airway pressure or mechanical ventilation is required by children with worsening hypoxia, exhaustion or apnoeas.

Prognosis

Children with bronchiolitis, even those with severe symptoms, recover well. They may continue to cough and wheeze for many weeks, or when suffering from viral upper respiratory tract infections over the following year. The incidence of subsequent asthma is slightly increased.

Obliterative bronchiolitis (bronchiolitis obliterans) is an infrequent complication of bronchiolitis caused by adenovirus infection. There is chronic inflammation and scarring of the bronchioles, with cough and wheeze, and ongoing oxygen treatment is required, often for many years.

Pneumonia

Pneumonia is infection of the parenchyma of the lung. It is termed community-acquired pneumonia if it is contracted outside hospital.

Epidemiology

In Europe, the prevalence of pneumonia is 40 per 1000 children under the age of 5 years.

Aetiology

Community-acquired pneumonia is typically caused by bacteria, most commonly *Streptococcus pneumoniae*, but viruses are also responsible (**Table 4.5**).

Clinical features

The most frequently seen clinical features are tachypnoea, fever, cough and difficulty breathing. Crepitations over the site of the pneumonia are heard on auscultation. With more severe infections, the child may have signs of respiratory distress, reduced air entry and dullness to chest percussion. Oxygen saturation may be low.

> **Beware! Abdominal pain may be the only symptom of pneumonia.** Always consider the diagnosis of pneumonia before diagnosing appendicitis in a child. A chest radiograph is obtained in a child with high clinical suspicion for pneumonia, even in the absence of chest signs for the disease.

Community-acquired pneumonia in children: causative organisms	
Category	Subtype
Viruses	Respiratory syncytial virus
	Parainfluenza virus
Bacteria	*Streptococcus pneumoniae*
	Mycoplasma
	Haemophilus influenzae
	Staphylococcus aureus

Table 4.5 Organisms causing community-acquired pneumonia in children

Diagnostic approach

Diagnosis of pneumonia is based on clinical signs and symptoms. A chest radiograph is not necessarily required in children with clinical signs of pneumonia, unless there are concerns about parapneumonic effusion (pleural effusion), i.e. fluid in the pleural space as a consequence of inflammation in the adjacent lung, or if the child is very unwell. A chest radiograph, if obtained, shows an area of consolidation, which appears as a white patch (**Figure 4.6**).

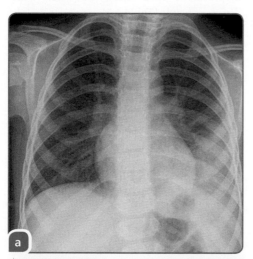

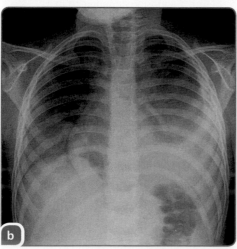

Figure 4.6 Chest radiographs from patients with pneumonia. (a) Left lower lobe consolidation. (b) Bilateral pneumonia.

Management

Children who do not require oxygen and have no respiratory distress can be treated at home with oral antibiotics and antipyretics and/or analgesics. Children with hypoxia, respiratory distress or parapneumonic effusion need to be admitted to hospital for treatment with oxygen and intravenous antibiotics.

If a child remains pyrexial 48 h after starting antibiotics, the presence of a parapneumonic effusion must be excluded by chest radiograph; chest US can also identify an effusion. There is a risk that the parapneumonic effusion will become infected and lead to an empyema. If this occurs, the infected fluid needs to be removed with a chest drain.

Prognosis

Most children recover fully from pneumonia, with no long-term sequelae. A follow-up chest radiograph is required only if symptoms or signs remain at 6 weeks; it is done to check for resolution or rule out a structural cause for the pneumonia.

Pertussis

Pertussis, also known as whooping cough, is a bacterial respiratory infection caused by *Bordetella pertussis*. Pertussis vaccines have significantly reduced the incidence and severity of pertussis in young children, where morbidity and mortality is highest. However, it still often occurs, yet is under-diagnosed, in older children because the effectiveness of the vaccine wanes and they have less severe symptoms. Transmission is by infected respiratory droplets.

Clinical features

The main clinical feature of pertussis is cough. Pertussis is known as 'the 100-day cough', because the cough often persists for > 3 months.

The cough is protracted, which makes the child turn red or even blue. The deep inspiration at the end of the coughing bout sounds like a 'whoop'. After incubation, the illness has three stages: catarrhal, spasmodic and convalescent (**Figure 4.7**).

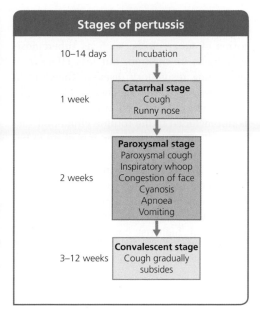

Stages of pertussis

10–14 days	Incubation
1 week	**Catarrhal stage** Cough Runny nose
2 weeks	**Paroxysmal stage** Paroxysmal cough Inspiratory whoop Congestion of face Cyanosis Apnoea Vomiting
3–12 weeks	**Convalescent stage** Cough gradually subsides

Figure 4.7 The three stages of pertussis.

Diagnostic approach

Diagnosis is made clinically on hearing the protracted cough and whoop. Lymphocyte count is usually markedly increased. *Bordetella pertussis* is usually detected on testing of a perinasal swab or nasopharyngeal aspirate, but only if the sample is taken in the first 3 weeks of the illness.

Management

Management is supportive, with oxygen therapy if hypoxia develops. No medication improves the clinical course. However, clarithromycin can be given to the child to prevent the spread of the disease, or given to vulnerable close contacts as prophylaxis

Prognosis

Major complications and deaths occur, mainly in those under 6 months of age. Complications include bronchopneumonia, severe weight loss caused by vomiting, cerebral hypoxia, cerebral haemorrhage and pneumothorax as a consequence of protracted coughing. Death is more likely in developing countries and is rare elsewhere, for example fewer than 1 death per 2 years in

New Zealand and around 10 per year in the UK (90% being under 4 months old).

Tuberculosis

Tuberculosis is an infection caused by *Mycobacterium tuberculosis*. Europe has about 16,000 new cases annually, most of which occur in Eastern Europe.

Tuberculosis is spread from person to person by respiratory droplets

- If a child has good immune function, their body fights the infection and they will have no symptoms
- If a child is unable to fight the infection, they will have active tuberculosis with characteristic clinical features

Some children have latent tuberculosis. They are infected but have no clinical symptoms; their immune system has prevented the development of clinical symptoms but is unable to completely eradicate the infection. Latent tuberculosis can be reactivated to cause symptoms of active tuberculosis, particularly if the child becomes immunocompromised.

Clinical features

Clinical features of active tuberculosis infection include:

- fever
- weight loss and loss of appetite
- chronic cough
- malaise
- night sweats

Examination may show cervical lymphadenopathy, chest signs (crepitations, bronchial breathing and signs of a pleural effusion) and hepatosplenomegaly.

Diagnostic approach

Active tuberculosis is diagnosed when *M. tuberculosis* is cultured from sputum, cerebrospinal fluid, urine or lung tissue samples obtained by bronchoscopic biopsy. Younger children swallow sputum, so early morning gastric aspirates are collected. A chest radiograph may show calcification or mediastinal lymphadenopathy. Latent tuberculosis is usually detected by the finding of a positive result from a Mantoux test (see page 106) during the screening of close contacts of an index case patient or the targeted screening of new immigrants from countries with a high incidence of tuberculosis (>40 per 100,000), such as India and eastern Europe.

Management

Tuberculosis is treated by a combination of oral antibiotics (isoniazid, rifampicin, pyrazinamide and ethambutol) taken daily for ≥ 6 months. Prompt treatment of the index case patient and contact tracing, carried out by public health professionals, helps to reduce outbreaks.

The BCG (bacillus Calmette–Guérin) vaccine 70–80% effective against the most severe forms of tuberculosis, such as tuberculosis meningitis in children, but less effective at preventing respiratory disease. Therefore in countries with a low incidence of tuberculosis, for example in Northern Europe and the UK, it is not included in the routine childhood vaccination schedule. However, it is given to babies born in low-risk countries if their parents migrated from countries with a high incidence of tuberculosis (>40 per 100,000), and to all babies born in cities in low-risk countries if a high percentage of the population has migrated from high-risk countries, for example London.

Ear, nose and throat conditions

Ear, nose and throat conditions are commonly encountered in paediatric medicine, because children have so many upper respiratory tract infections that affect these structures. The nose, throat and middle ear are closely related. Therefore a problem with one can lead to a problem in another nearby, for example in the case of acute otitis media and mastoiditis.

Tonsillitis

Tonsillitis is inflammation of the tonsils caused by infection with either a virus, for example adenovirus, or a bacterium, for example group A *Streptococcus*.

Clinical features and diagnostic approach

Clinical features include a sore throat, fever and bad breath.

Diagnosis is made clinically, when large red tonsils are seen. The tonsils may or may not be coated in a tonsillar exudate. A sample from a throat swab can be cultured to determine the type of bacterial infection.

Management

Management is supportive, with analgesia being most helpful. Antibiotics can be given if a bacterial infection is considered likely or confirmed by culture. Tonsillectomy is considered for children who have six or more episodes annually that are severe enough for them to miss school.

> **A rare complication of tonsillitis is the formation of a peritonsillar abscess known as quinsy.** The child presents with an extremely painful throat, finds it difficult to swallow and has difficulty opening their mouth. The treatment is surgical drainage of the abscess under general anaesthesia.

Acute otitis media

Acute otitis media is acute inflammation of the middle ear secondary to either viral or bacterial infection. It is common in the first 3 years of life, peaking in winter. Inflammation results in ear pain, fever and irritability.

Diagnosis is made when inspection of the tympanic membrane with an auroscope shows it to be red and bulging. Acute otitis media is very painful, and management includes analgesia. The infection usually settles without antibiotics, but amoxicillin is usually given if the child remains unwell beyond 48 h.

> **Mastoiditis, i.e. infection of the mastoid bone, is a severe complication of acute otitis media.** It presents with mastoid swelling, and the ear on the affected side is displaced, protruding forwards. The condition is treated with intravenous antibiotics and drainage of the abscess. Mastoidectomy, i.e. removal of mastoid bone, may be needed if the infection is severe.

Otitis media with effusion

Otitis media with effusion, also known as glue ear, is a middle ear problem in which there is a chronic effusion lasting > 3 months. The condition is associated with recurrent upper respiratory tract infections and acute otitis media, and inadequate drainage of the fluid that accumulates as a result of the inflammation.

Clinical features and diagnostic approach

Clinical features include difficulties with hearing and speech. Diagnosis is made when otoscopy shows loss of the normal tympanic membrane translucency, giving a dull appearance to the tympanic membrane. The effusion also impairs the motility of the tympanic membrane, thereby causing conductive hearing loss.

Management

Otitis media with effusion usually resolves over 4–6 months. For impaired hearing, tympanostomy tubes (grommets) can be inserted surgically to allow ventilation of the middle ear and promote drainage of the effusion. However, a conservative approach is favoured, with management more likely to be based on promoting hearing by giving children hearing aids to overcome the conductive hearing loss associated with the condition.

Laryngomalacia

Stridor is the term given to an upper airway noise made during inspiration. It can be acute, for example in croup (see page 401), or chronic, for example in laryngomalacia.

Laryngomalacia is diagnosed when the soft cartilage of the larynx collapses inwards during breathing, thereby narrowing the airway and causing a soft inspiratory stridor. It is the commonest cause of chronic stridor in infants; other causes shown are shown in **Table 4.6.**

Chronic stridor: causes	
Cause	Aetiology
Collapsing wall of the airway	Laryngomalacia or tracheomalacia
Subglottic stenosis (narrowing below the glottis)	Usually in children born before term, secondary to prolonged intubation
Vocal cord paralysis	Congenital As a consequence of cardiac surgery
Extrinsic airway compression	Vascular ring Mediastinal mass Enlarged thyroid
Pharyngeal or laryngeal mass	Papillomas Haemangiomas
Tracheoesophageal fistula	Tracheal stenosis after repair

Table 4.6 Causes of chronic stridor

Clinical features and diagnostic approach

An inspiratory stridor presents in the neonatal period up to several weeks of age. The stridor often becomes more marked when the baby is upset or has an upper respiratory tract infection. It can be intermittent.

Diagnosis is made clinically and can be confirmed by laryngoscopy.

Management

In most children, laryngomalacia resolves spontaneously by 12 months of age. If there is severe airway compromise, surgery may be required and occasionally includes a tracheostomy (**Figure 4.8**). The tracheostomy is usually temporary until the airway cartilage matures and becomes firmer.

Obstructive sleep apnoea

Obstructive sleep apnoea is diagnosed when partial airway obstruction occurs during sleep. The obstruction presents as snoring and can progress to full airway obstruction, which presents as an apnoea (a pause in breathing). The apnoea triggers the child to wake frequently during the night, resulting in poor sleep. It affects an estimated 1 in 20 children, and is associated with obesity, large adenoids and neuromuscular conditions.

Clinical features

Obstructive sleep apnoea can present with many symptoms related to poor sleep (**Table 4.7**), as well as higher levels of carbon dioxide in the blood, secondary to impaired ventilation.

Examination may find obesity, or mouth breathing if enlarged adenoids are a contributing factor (**Figure 4.9**). Ear, nose and throat examination may find large tonsils.

Diagnostic approach

If obstructive sleep apnoea is suspected overnight pulse oximetry is the first-line investigation. It can be done at home and shows desaturation clusters with associated increased heart rate. However, pulse oximetry produces many false negatives, so if the results are negative and symptoms persist, full polysomnography is carried out in a specialist centre.

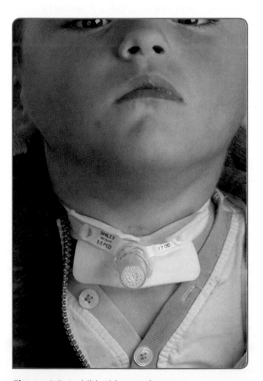

Figure 4.8 A child with a tracheostomy.

Obstructive sleep apnoea: symptoms	
Timing	Symptoms
During sleep	Snoring, with periods of apnoea and waking
	Restless sleep
	Unusual sleeping posture
On waking	Difficult to rouse in the morning
	Morning headache
	Irritability on waking
During the day	Mouth breathing
	Excessive daytime sleepiness
	Difficulties with learning or memory
	Hyperactivity or behavioural disturbance
	Poor growth

Table 4.7 Symptoms that suggest obstructive sleep apnoea

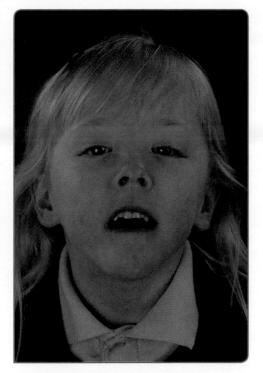

Figure 4.9 Adenoidal facies in adenoidal hypertrophy. Children are unable to breathe without their mouth open.

Management

Most children who snore have adenotonsillar hypertrophy. Adenotonsillar hypertrophy with obstructive sleep apnoea usually warrants adenotonsillectomy. Children without adenotonsillar hypertrophy, but with obstructive sleep apnoea are treated with non-invasive ventilation at night, in the same way that ventilatory support is provided for children with muscle weakness (**Figure 4.10**). Weight loss measures are implemented for obese children.

Prognosis

With adenotonsillar hypertrophy, removal of the adenoids and tonsils resolves the obstructive sleep apnoea, as will sufficient weight loss in obesity. In children who tolerate the non-invasive ventilation prognosis is also good. If obstructive sleep apnoea remains untreated, pulmonary hypertension, behavioural problems, failure to thrive and neurocognitive impairment are significant risks.

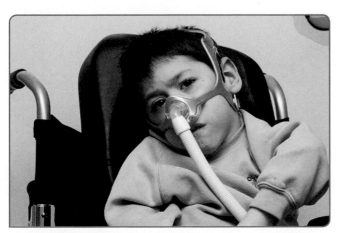

Figure 4.10 Non-invasive ventilation for a child with a neuromuscular condition. The same device may be used overnight to treat obstructive sleep apnoea.

Answers to starter questions

1. Cystic fibrosis results in malabsorption of fat and protein due to the insufficiency of pancreatic digestive enzymes secreted. There is also an increased calorie requirement due to the increased respiratory effort. Fat provides more calories than other foods and the body uses less oxygen to convert into energy than proteins or carbohydrates, so a high-fat diet is recommended for children with cystic fibrosis.

2. A chest radiogram in an infant with bronchiolitis will show hyperinflation and patchy consolidation. These features are misleading because they prompt doctors to start antibiotics thinking there is a bacterial infection (pneumonia); in fact they are due to the respiratory syncytial virus so antibiotics will be ineffective, with only support treatment required.

3. Young children cannot give a sputum samples because they usually swallow the sputum they cough up. Instead, to detect *Mycobacterium tuberculosis* three early morning gastric aspirates are collected: a nasogastric tube is inserted the night before and the samples collected the following morning.

4. Children with Down's syndrome have a large tongue which can obstruct their upper airway when asleep. This is exaggerated by the hypotonia and small airways seen in children with Down's syndrome. If obstructive sleep apnoea is left unnoticed the child can underperform at school and develop pulmonary hypertension and behavioural problems in the long term.

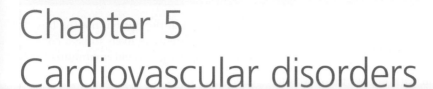

Chapter 5
Cardiovascular disorders

Starter questions

Answers to the following questions are on page 195.

1. Why does a large ventricular septal defect not usually produce a murmur in the first few days of life?
2. Why is prostaglandin given to babies born with congenital heart disease?
3. Why would an ice-pack be placed against the face of an infant?

Introduction

The primary cardiovascular disorder in children is congenital heart disease, which in most children presents in the first year of life. Cardiac failure in children with congenital heart disease is usually caused by either volume or pressure overload, which places an excessive and ultimately unsustainable demand on the heart. Occasionally, cardiac failure is the result of ventricular failure alone, for example in patients with cardiomyopathy and myocarditis.

Cardiac disease in children also includes less common conditions such as arrhythmias (supraventricular tachycardia and complete heart block), infections and inflammatory disease (infective endocarditis, Kawasaki's disease and acute rheumatic fever), and heart muscle disease (cardiomyopathies). Some of these conditions are responsible for the devastating outcome of sudden cardiac death (cardiac arrest in a person under 35 years of age).

Case 5 Blue lips in a seemingly well baby

Presentation

Ahmed is a 16-hour-old baby born at term in a district general hospital. The paediatric registrar carrying out the newborn examination thinks that Ahmed may have blue lips. However, it is difficult to tell with the poor lighting on the ward. The baby has been breastfeeding, and no concerns have been raised by the midwives.

Initial interpretation

Cyanosis (bluish discoloration) in a term baby is usually the result of either respiratory or cardiac problems, but sepsis and polycythaemia also need to be considered. Central cyanosis, involving the core, lips and tongue, is likely to be caused by an underlying condition, whereas peripheral cyanosis of the digits (acrocyanosis) and perioral cyanosis (duskiness of

the skin around the lips but not the lips themselves) are more likely to be a consequence of being in a cold environment.

Further history

Ahmed's mother has no medical problems. She had an uneventful pregnancy, with normal antenatal US scans. Ahmed was born by spontaneous vaginal delivery. He had good Apgar scores (9 at 1 minute and 10 at 5 minutes) and no resuscitation was required. There is no family history of cardiac problems.

Examination

Ahmed is well perfused with a capillary refill time of < 2 seconds, reflecting good cardiac output. He is neither tachypnoeic nor tachycardic, and he has no chest recession. His peripheral pulses are

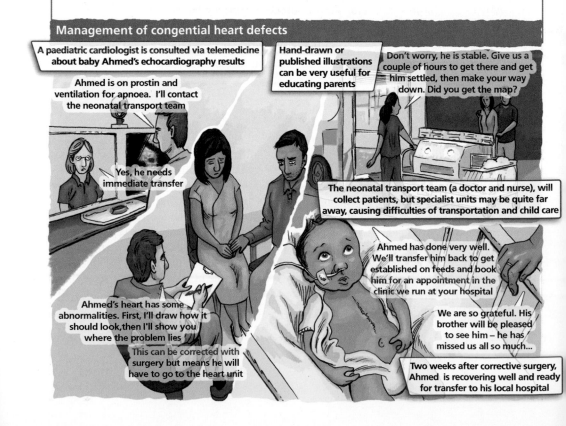

normal. There is no heave or murmur. As part of the examination, Ahmed's oxygen saturation is measured; it is 84% in air, with a consistent pulsatile trace indicating good skin contact. His blood pressure is also measured; the result, 60/40 mmHg, is normal.

Interpretation of findings

An oxygen saturation reading of 84% in air is low (normal > 96%). Therefore Ahmed is centrally cyanosed.

In the absence of respiratory signs, the most likely cause of cyanosis (low oxygen saturation) in Ahmed is cardiac. Sepsis as a cause is unlikely because it would result in poor perfusion and Ahmed would look unwell with pallor, floppiness etc. The normal blood pressure also rules out sepsis.

Investigations

Because of Ahmed's low oxygen saturation, he is immediately taken to the neonatal unit. The hyperoxia test (see page 111) is applied to distinguish a cardiac cause of cyanosis from a respiratory one. Ahmed is given 100% oxygen via a face mask and his oxygen saturation monitored, but his oxygen saturation only increases to 89%. His oxygen saturation would increase into the high 90s if he had a respiratory cause, but not in congenital heart disease (an especially useful distinction if the baby has tachypnoea). Here, the small rise in oxygen saturation

supports a diagnosis of congenital heart disease. A chest radiograph is obtained which shows a narrowing of the upper mediastinum and an 'egg on side' cardiac outline, increased pulmonary vascular markings and no consolidation. A cardiac cause, particularly transposition of the great arteries, is suspected. The narrow upper mediastinum appearance is due to the aorta being in front of the main pulmonary artery.

An echocardiogram obtained by the local cardiac technician confirms transposition of the great arteries. Electrocardiography (ECG) is normal. Causes of cyanotic congenital heart disease ('blue baby') are shown in **Table 5.1**.

Diagnosis

Transposition of the great arteries is a cyanotic congenital heart abnormality in which the aorta arises from the right ventricle and the pulmonary artery from the left ventricle. It is a duct-dependent lesion; the patent ductus arteriosus allows blood to pass between the two parallel circulations.

Ahmed is started on a prostaglandin infusion to keep the patent ductus arteriosus open, and is transferred urgently to a cardiac surgical centre for balloon atrial septostomy and corrective surgery (see page 187). Transfer is managed by the neonatal transport service.

Cyanotic congenital heart disease: causes	
Increased pulmonary blood flow	Decreased pulmonary blood flow
Transposition of the great arteries	Tetralogy of Fallot
Common arterial trunk (truncus arteriosus)	Severe pulmonary valve stenosis
Total anomalous pulmonary venous drainage	Tricuspid atresia
	Pulmonary atresia with ventricular septal defect

Table 5.1 Causes of cyanotic congenital heart disease

Case 6 Heart murmur on routine examination of a 3-year-old

Presentation

Theo is a 3-year-old well-grown child who has been referred by his general practitioner, because a soft systolic murmur was heard for the first time on routine examination as part of his preschool development screening.

Initial interpretation

An innocent heart murmur is the most likely cause of the asymptomatic murmur in a young child who is well grown; its features are shown in **Table 5.2**, see page 75. Such murmurs are the result of high blood flow in a normal heart. They are heard on routine examination or with tachycardia associated with upper respiratory tract infections in 50% of children at some point in time (see page 75).

Further history

Theo was born at term after an uncomplicated pregnancy. He is his parents' second child, and there is no family history of cardiac problems. He has not had a significant number of respiratory infections, averaging 3–4 per year.

Examination

Theo's height and weight are both on the 75th centile. He is difficult to examine because he is upset. He is pink and well perfused, with normal oxygen saturation on pulse oximetry. His blood pressure is slightly increased, at the 95th centile for his age and height.

There is no heave or thrill, and his heart sounds are normal. However, a soft grade 2/6 ejection systolic murmur in the second intercostal space is heard, lateral to the sternal border and audible through to the back. Theo's femoral pulses are difficult to feel, and there is slight radial-femoral delay.

Interpretation of findings

This is not an innocent murmur on clinical grounds. Distress would be expected to increase blood pressure, but the finding of radial-femoral delay means that Theo's high blood pressure is most likely a consequence of coarctation of the aorta.

Investigations

A chest radiograph shows a large aortic arch but no rib notching. ECG shows mild left ventricular hypertrophy, and echocardiography confirms mild coarctation of the aorta.

Diagnosis

Theo's murmur is the result of coarctation of the aorta. There is no rib notching,

Innocent heart murmurs: features	
Feature	Characteristics
Still's murmur	Vibratory quality
	Left lower sternal border and towards apex
Soft systolic ejection murmur	High left sternal border or high right sternal border (pulmonary area)
Venous hum	Continuous under clavicles and side of neck
	Usually loudest when sitting, and disappears in supine position or varies with turning of head
Carotid bruits	Murmur over carotids (not heard in aortic area, unlike aortic stenosis)

Table 5.2 Features of innocent heart murmurs

Case 6 continued

because the limited degree of narrowing in him means that collateral vessels have not developed. Coarctation presenting in this way does not need urgent treatment, unlike when it affects children presenting with shock in the neonatal period. However, assessment by a cardiologist is required (see page 184).

Rib notching, occasionally seen in coarctation of the aorta if severe and untreated for a few years, is caused by erosion of the underside of the ribs by enlarged collateral vessels (enlarged intercostal arteries), which develop to bypass the obstruction.

Congenital heart disease

Congenital heart disease is an umbrella term for abnormalities in the structure of the heart that develop between day 20 and day 50 of embryogenesis. Congenital heart disease is usually idiopathic, but specific types of the disease occur secondary to fetal exposure to teratogens (agents that interrupt normal embryogenesis), chromosomal abnormalities and other factors (**Table 5.3**).

Congenital heart disease occurs in 8 out of every 1000 live births, and the incidence of each type of underlying defect varies considerably (**Table 5.4**). Congenital heart disease is categorised as follows.

Congenital heart disease: risk factors		
Category	Risk factor	Associated congenital heart disease
Fetal exposure to teratogen	Maternal high-alcohol consumption	ASD, VSD
	Maternal lithium use	Apical displacement of tricuspid valve leaflets (Ebstein's anomaly)
Maternal condition	Maternal rubella	Patent ductus arteriosus, peripheral pulmonary stenosis
	Maternal systemic lupus erythematosus	Complete heart block
	Maternal diabetes	Hypertrophic cardiomyopathy
Syndrome or chromosomal abnormality	Chromosome 22q11 deletion (DiGeorge's syndrome)	Coarctation of the aorta or interrupted aortic arch
	Marfan's syndrome	Dilatation of ascending aorta, aortic valve insufficiency
	Noonan's syndrome	Pulmonary valve stenosis, ASD, cardiomyopathy
	Turner's syndrome (45XO karyotype)	Coarctation of aorta, bicuspid aortic valve (stenosis)
	Williams' syndrome	Supravalvar aortic stenosis, peripheral pulmonary artery stenosis
	Down's syndrome (trisomy 21)	AVSD, VSD
	Edward's syndrome (trisomy 18)	ASD, VSD
	Patau's syndrome (trisomy 13)	VSD

ASD, atrial septal defect; AVSD, atrioventricular septal defect; VSD, ventricular septal defect.

Table 5.3 Risk factors for congenital heart disease

Commonest congenital heart defects		
Category	Defect	Percentage
Acyanotic (left-to-right shunt)	Ventricular septal defect	25–30
	Patent ductus arteriosus	10–15
	Atrial septal defect	10–12
	Atrioventricular septal defect (complete or partial)	1–3
Acyanotic (obstructive)	Pulmonary stenosis	7
	Aortic stenosis	4
	Coarctation of the aorta	3–5
	Hypoplastic left heart syndrome	1–2
Cyanotic	Transposition of the great arteries	10–15
	Tetralogy of Fallot	5

Table 5.4 The 10 most common congenital heart defects by percentage of total newly diagnosed cases of congenital heart defect

- Acyanotic (no central hypoxia)
  - Left-to-right shunt
  - Obstruction of blood flow
- Cyanotic (central hypoxia)

Congenital heart disease with left-to-right shunt

In congenital heart disease with left-to-right shunt, a defect in the wall (septum) of the heart causes blood to shunt (flow) through the defect from the left side to the right side, or there is persistence of the fetal ductus arteriosus, which results in blood flowing from the aorta into the pulmonary artery.

> In congenital heart disease, **blood flow follows the path of least resistance from an area of high pressure to an area of low pressure.** As a general rule, the louder the murmur, the smaller the defect.

Types

Ventricular septal defect

This is a defect (hole) in the ventricular septum and is the most common congenital heart defect (see **Table 5.4**). Most ventricular septal defects (VSDs) are small, single defects in the membranous portion of the ventricular septum, but there can also be multiple defects in the muscular septum (**Figure 5.1a**).

Atrial septal defect

This type of defect (hole) is present in the atrial septum (**Figure 5.1b**). Atrial septal defects (ASDs) are typically located in the central septum.

Atrioventricular septal defect

There are two types of atrioventricular septal defect (AVSD): complete and partial. In a complete AVSD, a defect in the atrial and ventricular septa involves the atrioventricular valves, which creates one valve between the atria and ventricles instead of two (**Figure 5.1c**). A partial AVSD is a defect (hole) in the lower part of the atrial septum, but no ventricular defect.

> **Down's syndrome is associated with particular cardiac lesions,** including VSDs and AVSDs. Therefore all babies with Down's syndrome undergo echocardiography within the first few days after birth, even with a normal cardiovascular clinical examination.

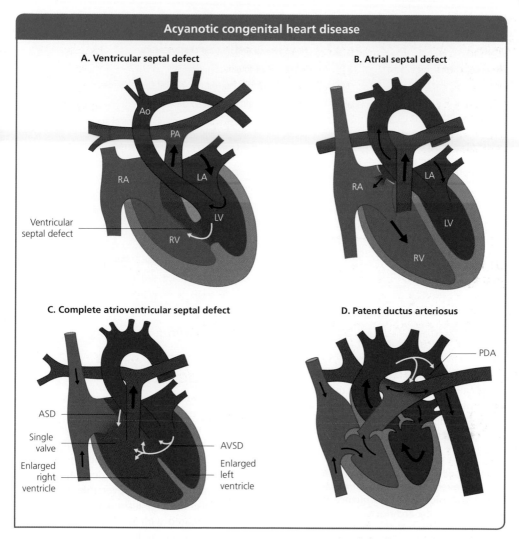

Acyanotic congenital heart disease

A. Ventricular septal defect

Ao
PA
RA
LA
Ventricular
septal defect
LV
RV

B. Atrial septal defect

RA
LA
LV
RV

C. Complete atrioventricular septal defect

ASD
Single
valve
Enlarged
right
ventricle
AVSD
Enlarged
left
ventricle

D. Patent ductus arteriosus

PDA

Figure 5.1 The four common types of acyanotic congenital heart disease with left to right shunt.

Patent ductus arteriosus

A ductus arteriosus is a vessel that is a remnant of the fetal circulation. Its function in utero is to shunt blood from the pulmonary artery to the aorta, thereby bypassing the non-functional lungs (see page 17).

The ductus arteriosus should close shortly after birth, because blood needs to flow to the lungs. If it fails to close, it is termed a patent ductus arteriosus (**Figure 5.1d**). In response to the decrease in pulmonary pressure at birth, the blood is shunted through the patent ductus arteriosus from left to right (aorta

to pulmonary artery), rather than continuing to shunt from right to left (pulmonary artery to aorta), as happens in utero.

Clinical features

Small congenital heart defects with left-to-right shunt are usually asymptomatic and only detected when a murmur is heard. The type of murmur heard can help distinguish the abnormality (**Table 5.5**).

Larger defects cause heart failure, i.e. failure to pump blood adequately (**Figure 5.2**). This occurs because the larger volume of blood

Acyanotic congenital heart disease with left-to-right shunt: examination findings		
Defect		Heart sounds and murmur characteristics
Ventricular septal defect	Small	Normal heart sounds
		Harsh pansystolic murmur at lower left sternal border
	Moderate to large	Loud pulmonary 2nd heart sound
		Thrill and loud, harsh pansystolic murmur maximal at lower left sternal border but all over precordium
		Apical mid-diastolic flow murmur (mitral)
Atrial septal defect		Right ventricle heave
		2nd heart sound widely and fixed split
		Ejection systolic murmur in 2nd intercostal space
		Mid-diastolic flow murmur (tricuspid) in large lesions
Atrioventricular septal defect		No murmur or as for atrial septal defect
		Frequently also apical pansystolic murmur of mitral regurgitation
Patent ductus arteriosus		Loud, continuous, harsh, low-pitched 'machinery quality' murmur below left clavicle
		Radiates to back

Table 5.5 Examination findings in acyanotic congenital heart disease with left-to-right shunt

flowing through the right side of the heart and lungs causes the right ventricle to become hypertrophied (enlarged) or dilatated. Increased blood flow through the lungs leads to pulmonary oedema.

> Increased blood flow through the lungs eventually causes pulmonary hypertension as a consequence of changes in the architecture of the pulmonary vessels. When pulmonary pressure is higher than systemic pressure, a left-to-right shunt becomes a right-to-left shunt and cyanosis develops as deoxygenated blood from the body bypasses the lungs; this is known as Eisenmenger's syndrome.

Investigations

Congenital heart disease with left-to-right shunt may be detected on an antenatal fetal anomaly US scan at 20 weeks' gestation. Diagnosis is confirmed by echocardiography. Congenital heart disease is not diagnosed by ECG, but the results may show complications of a left-to-right shunt, primarily right ventricular hypertrophy.

Management

Management of congenital heart disease with left-to-right shunt depends on the size of the defect. Small lesions are monitored every 6–12 months by echocardiography. Small ventricular and ASDs usually close spontaneously.

Large lesions require surgical repair before the development of irreversible pulmonary hypertension. Large lesions with cardiac failure are treated with medication to improve cardiac function and promote growth while the child is waiting for surgery.

Medication

Pulmonary oedema is treated with diuretics and fluid restriction. Oxygen is required if pulmonary oedema is causing hypoxia. High-calorie formula is given by nasogastric tube.

> The energy consumption and breathlessness associated with heart failure impairs the baby's ability to feed adequately, thereby limiting calorie intake. Nasogastric feeds with high-calorie milk are given to the baby with heart failure to promote their growth.

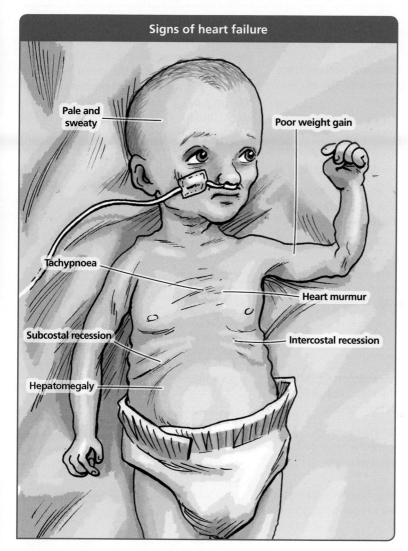

Signs of heart failure

Pale and sweaty

Poor weight gain

Tachypnoea

Heart murmur

Subcostal recession

Intercostal recession

Hepatomegaly

Figure 5.2 Common signs of heart failure in a baby.

Surgery

If the defect is large, or there is a risk of pulmonary hypertension, surgery is required to close the hole. This is carried out in specialist centres. Before definitive surgery, a pulmonary artery band procedure may be done to reduce lung blood flow and thereby prevent pulmonary hypertension. VSDs and ASDs are repaired by using a patch; in older children, the defect may be repaired with a cardiac catheter and umbrella device rather than open heart surgery. Complete AVSDs require surgery to the valves in addition to the defect. A patent ductus arteriosus is closed by a cardiac catheterisation occlusion device or ligation surgery.

Obstructive congenital heart disease

Obstructive congenital heart disease lesions occur when there is a narrowing of the heart valves or vessels leaving the heart. The narrowing causes resistance to blood flow, so the heart chamber proximal to the obstruction must pump harder to overcome the obstruction. As a consequence, the proximal chamber becomes hypertrophied.

Types

Aortic stenosis

This is narrowing of the aortic outflow tract, i.e. the exit of the left ventricle. The narrowing can occur at three levels:

- valvular (most common), i.e. when the aortic valve itself is narrowed
- supravalvular, i.e. above the aortic valve
- subvalvular, i.e. below the aortic valve

Typically, the aortic valve is narrowed because it is made up of two leaflets rather than the usual three (**Figure 5.3a**).

> **Exercise is generally encouraged in children with congenital heart disease.** However, strenuous exercise is avoided in severe aortic stenosis, because of the risk of sudden death.

Pulmonary stenosis

This is narrowing of the pulmonary outflow tract, i.e. the exit of the right ventricle. The narrowing can occur at three levels:

- valvular (most common), i.e. when the pulmonary valve itself is narrowed because of its abnormal structure (**Figure 5.3b**)
- supravalvular, i.e. above the pulmonary valve
- subvalvular, i.e. below the pulmonary valve

Coarctation of the aorta

In coarctation of the aorta, there is narrowing of the descending aorta. The narrowing is typically close to the site of the ductus arteriosus, distal to the left subclavian artery (**Figure 5.3c**). The coarctation is either present at birth or develops gradually in the weeks after birth.

> **Critical aortic stenosis or severe coarctation of the aorta** presents shortly after birth; the baby is very unwell as a consequence of poor systemic circulation. No femoral pulses are palpable.

> **Hypoplastic left heart syndrome is a rare obstructive congenital heart disease in which the left ventricle is severely underdeveloped.** The aortic and mitral valves can be very narrow or completely closed. Complicated surgery is possible, with a 60% survival rate.

Clinical features

Children with mild obstructive congenital heart disease lesions are usually asymptomatic and discovered only when a murmur is heard.

Larger lesions are associated with heart failure secondary to ventricular hypertrophy

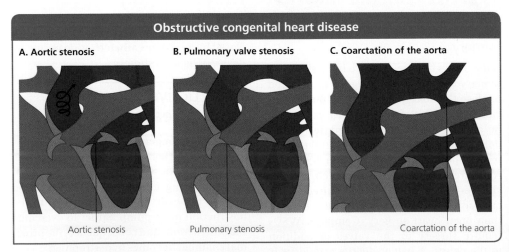

Obstructive congenital heart disease

A. Aortic stenosis   B. Pulmonary valve stenosis   C. Coarctation of the aorta

Aortic stenosis   Pulmonary stenosis   Coarctation of the aorta

Figure 5.3 The three types of obstructive congenital heart disease.

or dilatation, which make the heart unable to pump blood efficiently.

Older children with severe obstruction present with breathlessness (pulmonary stenosis) or syncope (aortic stenosis), as a result of poor cardiac output.

Examination findings in children with obstructive congenital heart disease are summarised in **Table 5.6**.

> **Coarctation of the aorta is associated with a radial femoral delay when the femoral pulse is palpated just after the radial pulse.** The delay is the result of the coarctation slowing the passage of blood to the femoral arteries.

Investigations

Obstructive congenital heart disease lesions are diagnosed by echocardiography (**Figure 5.4**).

Management

In children with mild obstructive lesions, annual echocardiograms are used to monitor the size of the stenosis and heart function. Monitoring continues into and throughout adulthood.

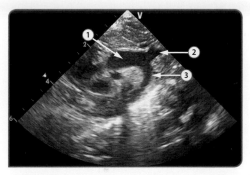

Figure 5.4 Echocardiogram showing coarctation of the aorta. The diameter of the arch of the aorta ① becomes narrower at the coarctation ③, distal to the left subclavian artery ②.

Obstructive congenital heart disease: examination and investigation findings				
Defect	Examination findings	Investigation findings		
		Chest radiography	Electrocardiography	BP measurement
Aortic stenosis	Slow rising carotid pulse Thrill over carotid arteries Left ventricular heave Ejection systolic murmur over aortic area, radiates to carotids	Prominent left ventricle Post-stenotic dilatation of ascending aorta	Left ventricular hypertrophy	Low systolic BP
Pulmonary stenosis	Right ventricular heave Thrill in pulmonary area Ejection systolic murmur in pulmonary area Wide split 2nd heart sound	Post-stenotic dilatation of pulmonary artery In severe cases, enlarged right atrium and right ventricle	Right axis deviation, right atrial hypertrophy, right ventricular hypertrophy	Normal BP
Coarctation of the aorta	Weak femoral pulses Radiofemoral delay Pansystolic murmur in left infraclavicular area, radiates to back	Prominent left ventricle Large aortic arch Rib notching (older children), caused by collateral vessels	Left ventricular hypertrophy	Increased systolic BP, upper body
BP, blood pressure.				

Table 5.6 Examination and investigation findings in obstructive congenital heart disease

Severe aortic or pulmonary stenosis requires balloon valvoplasty (widening of the valve by inflation of a balloon inserted via a cardiac catheter) or open valvotomy (cutting into the valve leaflets) to widen the valve.

Coarctation of the aorta is managed surgically in most neonates and infants by resection; the narrowed segment is cut out and the two healthy ends of the aorta are sewn back together. Recurrence of stenosis (fibrous tissue), which occurs in about 20% of patients as they grow, is treated with catheterisation and balloon dilatation of the narrowed segment (angioplasty). If required, an expandable metal mesh tube (a stent) is subsequently inserted to keep the narrowed area open after balloon dilatation. In older children, teenagers or adults diagnosed for the first time, balloon dilatation is the initial procedure.

Cyanotic congenital heart disease

Cyanotic congenital heart disease occurs when the abnormally-developed heart structure results in cyanosis (low oxygen saturation). This is a consequence of the abnormal structure causing one of two conditions:

- blood bypassing the lungs because of a right-to-left shunt (tetralogy of Fallot)
- blood flowing through the lungs but not into the systemic circulation (transposition of the great arteries)

Types

Tetralogy of Fallot

This type of cyanotic congenital heart disease has four typical features (**Figure 5.5a**):

- a large membranous VSD
- pulmonary stenosis
- overriding aorta
- right ventricular hypertrophy

Cyanosis results because the blood is preferentially shunted from the right ventricle to the left ventricle, rather than flowing through the narrowed pulmonary valve.

Transposition of the great arteries

In transposition of the great arteries, the aorta and pulmonary artery are 'transposed', meaning that the aorta comes from the right ventricle and the pulmonary artery from the left ventricle (**Figure 5.5b**). This results in two

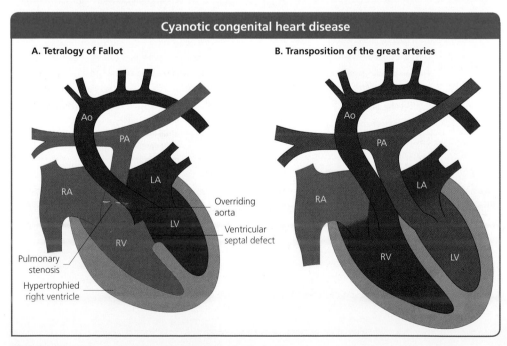

Figure 5.5 The two types of cynaotic congenital heart disease.

parallel circulations, which do not mix unless a VSD or patent ductus arteriosus is also present.

Clinical features

Babies with tetralogy of Fallot are usually pink at birth, with cyanosis developing during the first few weeks of life. Babies with transposition of the great arteries will appear cyanosed from birth.

A murmur is heard in tetralogy of Fallot (**Table 5.7**).

Investigations

Oxygen saturation is in the eighties or low nineties. There is also a difference between preductal and postductal saturation (see page 89).

The diagnosis may be suspected on the antenatal fetal anomaly US scan at 18–21 weeks, which picks up 25% of patients with either tetralogy of Fallot or transposition of the great arteries, but it is confirmed by echocardiography after birth. A chest radiograph and an ECG both have a typical appearance (see **Table 5.7**).

> **Digital clubbing** is associated with cyanotic congenital heart disease.

Management

Babies with tetralogy of Fallot tolerate low oxygen saturation well. They can be discharged from hospital, with regular cardiology follow-up until surgical correction is carried out at about 6–12 months of age. In this procedure, the section narrowed by pulmonary stenosis is widened and the VSD closed.

> **Administration of oxygen to babies with cyanotic congenital heart disease will not increase oxygen saturation.** It is the shunting of blood or presence of parallel circulations that is causing the cyanosis, not a problem with the lungs and oxygenation.

> **Oxygen can cause the ductus arteriosus to close.** Therefore its use is avoided in babies with cyanotic congenital heart disease as in some diagnoses it is vital to keep the duct open.

Babies with transposition of the great arteries need to be started immediately on a prostaglandin infusion; the prostaglandin ensures that the ductus arteriosus remains open and able to allow mixing of the pulmonary and systemic circulations. A balloon septostomy (formation of a hole in the septum) is carried out as soon as possible to enable the mixing to continue before an 'arterial switch' procedure is done.

Whether or not to close a patent ductus arteriosus depends on the type of congenital heart disease. A patent ductus arteriosus causing left-to-right shunt and secondary heart

Cyanotic congenital heart disease: examination and investigation findings			
Defect	Examination findings	Investigation findings	
		Chest radiography	Electrocardiography
Tetralogy of Fallot	Systolic thrill in pulmonary area Easily palpable right ventricular pulsation Ejection systolic murmur in pulmonary area Single 2nd heart sound	Boot-shaped heart Oligaemic lung fields	Right axis deviation, right atrial hypertrophy, right ventricular hypertrophy
Transposition of the great arteries	Cyanosis No murmur	'Egg-on-side' appearance of heart, narrow upper mediastinum	Normal

Table 5.7 Examination and investigation findings in cyanotic congenital heart disease

failure needs to be closed. Conversely, in some cyanotic congenital heart disease, such as due to transposition of the great arteries, the ductus arteriosus must stay open to allow mixing of blood, which helps keep the baby alive during the wait for more definitive surgical procedures.

Cardiac arrhythmias

A cardiac arrhythmia is an abnormal heart rhythm or rate caused by abnormalities in the electrical conducting system of the heart. Cardiac arrhythmias are uncommon in children. The arrhythmia most frequently encountered in paediatrics is supraventricular tachycardia (SVT).

Cardiac arrhythmias can lead to sudden cardiac death, so it is essential for all children presenting with collapse to undergo ECG to exclude arrhythmia. If the ECG is normal but clinical suspicion of an arrhythmia is high, then 24-h ECG is carried out.

Supraventricular tachycardia

An SVT is a paroxysmal rapid regular heart rate of > 220 bpm.

Epidemiology and aetiology

Supraventricular tachycardia presents at any age. However, it most frequently affects children under 3 months old, with another peak between 8 and 10 years and a further peak in adolescence.

It is caused by abnormal cardiac conduction at either the site of the atrioventricular node (atrioventricular node SVT) or via an accessory pathway connecting the atria and the ventricles. These areas of abnormal conduction mean that the electrical current passes immediately from the atria to the ventricles, rather than having the usual delay at the atriventricular node; the consequence is early excitation of the ventricles and a rapid heart rate. A retrograde current can pass through the abnormal connection back into the atria, thereby provoking early atrial contraction (re-entry SVT).

Clinical features

A baby with SVT presents with pallor, tachypnoea, irritability and poor feeding. If the SVT is prolonged, they can also have signs of heart failure. Older children describe palpitations or a 'funny feeling' in their chest for the duration of the SVT episode.

Investigations

Supraventricular tachycardia is characterised by a very fast regular heart rate, usually > 220 bpm. Diagnosis is made by the finding of a regular, narrow complex tachycardia on ECG. When the heart rhythm is not in SVT, the ECG shows normal sinus rhythm or occasionally abnormalities associated with Wolff–Parkinson–White syndrome (**Figure 5.6**).

> In Wolff–Parkinson–White syndrome, there is an accessory pathway between the atria and the ventricles. This pathway is a congenital abnormality of the conducting system. ECG may be normal or show typical features of the condition (see **Figure 5.6**).

Management

The priority is to terminate the SVT to prevent complications such as heart failure. Medical management includes vagal stimulation or administration of a rapid bolus of the drug adenosine (an antiarrhythmic drug with a very short duration of action). If unsuccessful, electrical cardioversion is used with synchronised direct current shock to convert the SVT back to a normal rhythm.

Once the SVT has been terminated, the aim is to prevent recurrence. Regular

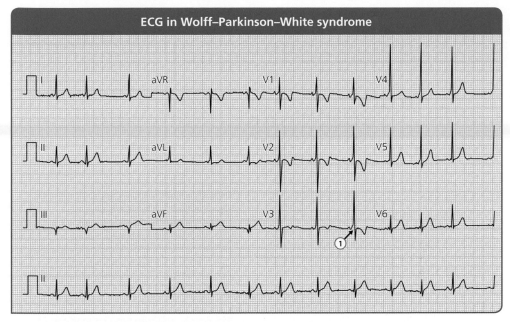

ECG in Wolff–Parkinson–White syndrome

Figure 5.6 Electrocardiogram from a patient with Wolff–Parkinson–White syndrome, showing the short PR interval and slurring upstroke at the start of the QRS complex (delta wave) ① and prolongation of the QRS complex.

antiarrhythmic medication, for example amiodarone or flecainide, is prescribed on a long-term basis. If an accessory pathway is identified that is resistant to medication, catheter-directed radiofrequency ablation is carried out. Radiofrequency ablation uses energy (heat) from a medium frequency alternating current directed to the precise area of the heart causing the arrhythmia, via cardiac catheterisation, destroying the abnormal electrical pathway. Radiofrequency ablation has a 90% success rate for SVT.

> There are many vagal stimulation manoeuvres, including submerging the child's face in ice cold water, applying an ice pack to their face, getting the child to strain as if opening their bowels and unilateral carotid sinus massage.

Atrioventricular heart block

Atrioventricular heart block occurs when conduction at the atrioventricular node is faulty and does not conduct electrical signals to the ventricles; this results in a very slow heart rate. Atrioventricular blocks occur in three degrees of severity:

- First degree: the impulse is conducted through the AV node, but delayed. The heart rate is not usually significantly slowed
- Second degree: not all impulses are conducted through the AV node
- Third degree: AV block is complete and no impulses are conducted across the AV node

In children, the cause is often congenital, either due to maternal autoantibodies with maternal systemic lupus erythematosus which affect the cardiac tissue, or associated with congenital heart disease, such as transposition of the great arteries. Acquired causes are an infection (such as viral myocarditis), post-surgery or are idiopathic.

The heart rate is usually about <60 bpm but may increase with exercise. Most children are asymptomatic, with complete heart block diagnosed on ECG; however, a minority have Stokes–Adams attacks (pallor associated with collapse). A pacemaker is indicated for second- or third-degree AV block with symptomatic bradycardia, ventricular dysfunction or low cardiac output. It is also indicated in children with congenital third-degree AV and a heart rate <50–55 bpm or with congenital heart disease and a heart rate <70 bpm.

Cardiac infections and inflammatory conditions

Cardiac infection is infection of heart tissue. The pericardium, endocardium and myocardium are all at risk of infection from bacteria and viruses. In children, pericarditis is encountered most commonly and is generally self-limiting. One of the most serious cardiac infections in children is endocarditis. The heart is also vulnerable to inflammatory processes, particularly as a result of autoimmune conditions.

Infective endocarditis

Infective endocarditis is bacterial infection of the endocardium (heart valve tissue).

Epidemiology and aetiology

The endocardium becomes infected when bacteria travelling in the bloodstream colonise the heart valve. Infective endocarditis is rare in children, particularly if they have a normal heart structure.

Infective endocarditis is typically encountered in children with pre-existing cardiac problems, including congenital heart disease, hypertrophic cardiomyopathy or prosthetic valves. In these conditions blood flow through the heart is more turbulent, with the blood moving in a way that makes it easier for bacteria to adhere to the cardiac tissue.

The bacteria that most commonly cause infective endocarditis are *Streptococcus viridans* (40% of cases) and *Staphylococcus aureus* (30% of cases).

Infective endocarditis can be prevented by avoiding bacteraemia (bacteria in the blood). Bacteria can enter the bloodstream during oral infections, dental treatment, body piercing and tattooing. Therefore children with congenital heart disease should maintain good oral hygiene and avoid body piercing (and tattooing later in life).

Previously, children with congenital heart disease were required to take antibiotics before dental treatment, to treat any resulting bacteraemia. However, this is no longer advised because it does not reduce the risk of infective endocarditis.

Clinical features

Table 5.8 shows the clinical features of infective endocarditis.

Investigations

The diagnosis of infective endocarditis is based on the echocardiographic finding of vegetations on the heart valves. The diagnosis is supported by the growth of bacteria in three separate sets of blood culture from samples taken within 24 h of presentation.

Management

High-dose intravenous antibiotics are given for ≥ 6 weeks. Cardiac surgery may be needed to remove the vegetations. Patients with

Infective endocarditis: clinical features	
Category (% of infective endocarditis patients with this feature)	Features
Infection (100% of cases)	Fever (> 90% of cases), malaise
	Increased inflammatory markers (erythrocyte sedimentation rate, C-reactive protein, anaemia, leucocytosis with neutrophilia)
	Splenomegaly
	Positive blood culture (> 85% of cases)
Destruction (> 90% of cases)	Change in character of cardiac murmur (valvular damage)
	Heart failure
	Conduction abnormality
Embolism and infarcts (20–50% of cases)	Systemic: brain, spleen, kidney (haematuria)
	Peripheries: petechiae, retinal haemorrhages, splinter haemorrhages, Janeway lesions (small painless nodules on soles), Osler's nodes (painful nodules on hands and feet)
	Pulmonary emboli
Immunological phenomena (25% of cases)	Arthritis and arthralgia
	Positive for antinuclear antibody and rheumatoid factor, low C3/C4
	Microscopic haematuria
	Roth's spots (retinal haemorrhages with white centres, caused by immune complex-mediated vasculitis)

Table 5.8 Clinical features of infective endocarditis

infective endocarditis can be extremely sick and occasionally need intensive care. Most recover well, but there is a risk of death and further episodes of infective endocarditis.

Kawasaki's disease

Kawasaki's disease, also called mucocutaneous lymph node syndrome, is an autoimmune disease of unknown aetiology that results in vasculitis (inflammation of blood vessels). The vasculitis affects medium-sized and small blood vessels; coronary arteries are particularly vulnerable.

The disease typically affects children younger than 5 years old, with a peak incidence at 10 months of age.

Clinical features

The diagnosis is based on particular clinical criteria (**Table 5.9**) and exclusion of diseases with a similar presentation, e.g. Staphylococcus infection (scalded skin syndrome or toxic shock syndrome, see page 359) or Streptococcus infection (e.g. scarlet fever).

Kawasaki's disease: clinical criteria	
Febrile illness + EITHER 4 or 5 of signs listed below* OR 3 of signs listed below IF coronary aneurysms present on echocardiography	
Region	Feature(s)
Mouth	Erythema of lips or oropharynx
	Fissured lips
	'Strawberry' tongue
Eyes	Bilateral non-purulent conjunctival infection
Hands	Oedema or erythema (in 1st week)
	Generalised or periungual peeling (days 14–21)
Whole body	Diffuse rash (in 1st week): macular, maculopapular, urticarial, scarlatiniform, morbilliform
Lymph nodes	Cervical lymphadenopathy: often painful solitary node
Heart	Coronary artery aneurysms

*with no other reasonable explanation.

Table 5.9 The clinical criteria for Kawasaki's disease

The diagnostic features may not all present at the same time. Infants without sufficient features for the diagnostic criteria, but who develop coronary aneurysms, are still considered to have Kawasaki's disease.

Kawasaki's disease has many complications, the most consequential being coronary artery aneurysms. They affect 25% of untreated children, usually within 8 weeks, and can lead to myocardial infarction and arrhythmias.

Other complications include aseptic meningitis, gall bladder hydrops, hepatitis, pancreatitis, arthritis, myositis, pericarditis and myocarditis. Peripheral aneurysms can cause gangrene or cerebral infarction.

Investigations

There is no particular test for Kawasaki's disease; diagnosis is usually based on clinical features. Inflammatory markers such as C-reactive protein and erythrocyte sedimentation rate may be increased, which would support the diagnosis. All children with Kawasaki's disease undergo echocardiography, at presentation and if negative again at 6-8 weeks, to identify any coronary artery aneurysms.

> **For any child presenting with more than 5 days of fever, consider Kawasaki's disease.**

Management

The aim of treatment is to prevent coronary artery aneurysms. Intravenous immunoglobulins are given until the high temperature resolves. Aspirin is prescribed to prevent formation of clots in the inflamed vessels. A repeat echocardiogram is obtained about 6 weeks later.

- If the echocardiogram is normal, the aspirin is discontinued
- If coronary artery aneurysms are present, regular cardiology follow-up is required to monitor them
- Mortality is low (0.1%).

Acute rheumatic fever

Acute rheumatic fever is an inflammatory condition, thought to be autoimmune-related, that affects the heart, joints and neurological system.

Epidemiology and aetiology

Acute rheumatic fever typically occurs 2 weeks after a throat infection caused by group A β-haemolytic *Streptococcus*. It is very rare in high-income countries, because such infections can be treated with penicillin; however, it remains common in the Middle East and Africa. Most children are diagnosed between the ages of 5 and 15 years.

Clinical features

Clinical features of acute rheumatic fever are shown in **Table 5.10**.

Investigations

The diagnosis of acute rheumatic fever is based on the Jones criteria. There must be evidence of a recent throat infection with group A β-haemolytic *Streptococcus* (increased anti-streptolysin O titre, anti-deoxyribonuclease B or positive throat swab result), along with either two major or one major and two minor criteria (see **Table 5.10**). Cardiac complications (pericarditis, myocarditis and endocarditis) are diagnosed by echocardiography.

Management

Penicillin is given to treat the group A β-haemolytic *Streptococcus* infection, and analgesia for pain. Steroids shorten the illness but do not prevent permanent heart damage. If there are cardiac complications, regular (every 6–12 months) cardiac follow-up into and during adulthood is needed for monitoring. There is risk of repeat infection and progressive valvular disease, so secondary penicillin prophylaxis for ≥ 5 years is advised.

Rheumatic fever: clinical features		
Feature	Jones criteria	Details
Fever and malaise (95%)	Minor	>38.5°C
Acute migratory polyarthritis (75%)	Major	Knees, ankles, wrists, elbows (for up to 2 months)
		Joints very tender, red and swollen
		< 1 week per joint, but switching to other joints
Pancarditis (50%)	Major	Pericarditis: friction rub or effusion, tamponade
		Myocarditis: tachycardia, cardiac enlargement, increased PR interval, arrhythmias, heart failure and death
		Endocarditis: systolic and diastolic murmurs resulting from valvular dysfunction
Skin rashes	Major	Erythema marginatum (5–10%): early, trunk and limbs, pink border with fading centre, macules spreading outwards
		Subcutaneous nodules (5–10%): painless, pea-sized, hard; mainly on extensor surfaces
Chorea (up to 15%) – Sydenham's	Major	Starts 2–6 months after infection
		Involuntary movements and emotional lability for up to 6 months
		Rarely associated with carditis
Polyarthralgia	Minor	Multiple joint pain
Increased inflammatory markers	Minor	Erythrocyte sedimentation rate, C-reactive protein, white cell count
Prolonged PR on electrocardiography	Minor	Indicates cardiac involvement

Table 5.10 The clinical features of rheumatic fever. Diagnosis is based on presence of two major or one major and two minor criteria, plus evidence of preceding group A streptococcal infection. Percentages indicate the proportion of children with rheumatic fever who meet these criteria

Cardiomyopathy

Cardiomyopathy is disease of the myocardium (heart muscle).

Epidemiology and aetiology

Cardiomyopathy has many different known causes (**Table 5.11**) but is usually idiopathic. It affects 1 in 100,000 children, and is less common in young children (< 2 years). Up to 30% of cases have a familial or genetic cause.

The three most common types of cardiomyopathy in children are as follows.

■ Dilated cardiomyopathy (58% of cases): the myocardium is thin and stretched and contracts inadequately, leading to heart failure
■ Hypertrophic cardiomyopathy (30% of cases): the myocardium is thickened and stiff, obstructing blood flow through the aortic

outlet, and the hypertrophy usually develops after puberty; 12 commonly associated genetic mutations have been identified, which are responsible for 60% of cases
■ Restrictive cardiomyopathy (5% of cases): the myocardium is stiffened and has abnormal relaxation

Clinical features

The clinical features depend on the type and severity of the cardiomyopathy. Most children with mild cardiomyopathy have no symptoms. Significant symptoms include dyspnoea on exercise, chest pain, palpitations and fainting.

Complications include arrhythmias (especially with hypertrophic cardiomyopathy), heart failure, thromboembolism, endocarditis and sudden death.

Causes of cardiomyopathy in children	
Category	Causes
Primary causes	Viral myocarditis, especially caused by Coxsackie B viruses
	Autosomal dominant genetic disease
	Kawasaki's disease
	Amyloidosis
	Haemochromatosis
	Noonan's syndrome
	Friedreich's ataxia
	Neurofibromatosis
	Lipodystrophy
	Glycogen storage disease
	Mucopolysaccharidoses
	Autoimmune disorders
Secondary causes	Use of certain therapeutic drugs (e.g. doxorubicin for cancer)
	Cystic fibrosis
	Muscular dystrophy
	Severe anaemia or nutritional deficiencies
	HIV
Causes in neonates	Temporary septal hypertrophy secondary to:
	■ maternal diabetes
	■ corticosteroid use in preterm babies
	■ severe neonatal illness

*Many cases of cardiomyopathy are idiopathic.

Table 5.11 Causes of cardiomyopathy in children. Many patients with cardiomyopathy have an idiopathic cause

Investigations

Echocardiography is used to confirm the diagnosis and evaluate cardiac function. Genetic investigations may detect particular genes associated with hypertrophic cardiomyopathy.

Management

Children with cardiomyopathy require 3–6 monthly echocardiograms and follow-up with a paediatric cardiologist. Treatment is with beta-blockers, calcium channel blockers and antiarrhythmic medication. A pacemaker to control heart rate or an implantable cardioverter defibrillator can be fitted to treat life threatening arrhythmias. Moderate, but not strenuous, exercise is beneficial.

> **Children with a parent who has cardiomyopathy undergo regular screening.** This is done by ECG and echocardiography, or genetic screening if there is a known genetic mutation. Such screening enables early identification of any developing cardiomyopathy.

Sudden cardiac death

Sudden cardiac (or arrhythmic) death is an umbrella term encompassing the many different causes of cardiac arrest in young people (those under 35 years old). It is associated with a number of cardiac conditions:

- cardiomyopathy
- myocarditis
- coronary artery disease and familial hypercholesterolaemia
- ion channelopathies, for example long QT syndrome
- Wolff–Parkinson–White syndrome
- coronary artery anomalies
- Kawasaki's disease
- Marfan's syndrome (which can cause aortic rupture)
- endocardial fibroelastosis

Sudden death is associated with other diagnoses, including asthma and epilepsy.

> **Sudden death in cardiomyopathy is caused by several factors,** including ventricular arrhythmia, myocardial ischaemia and outflow obstruction.

Answers to starter questions

1. Murmurs in ventricular septal defects are due to blood flow across the defect. Because of the high pulmonary resistance immediately after birth a murmur is often not heard because the pressure gradient between both ventricles is small, so there is not much flow of blood across the defect. By the end of the first week the pulmonary pressure has fallen enough for a murmur to be easily heard because the pressure in the right ventricle is much lower than in the left ventricle, so blood flows from left to right across the defect; this blood flow causes the murmur.

2. Prostaglandin is used to keep the patent ductus arteriosus open in cyanotic congenital heart disease until a more permanent procedure, such as an atrial septostomy, is carried out. Prostaglandin can be life-saving and allows babies to be transferred regional cardiac centres for surgery safely.

3. An ice-cold pack placed against an infant's face induces a vagal response that can stop an episode of supraventricular tachycardia (SVT). This can be applied at home by the parents to babies who have such episodes. Parents with infants known to have episodes of SVT are taught how to listen to the baby's heart rate with a stethoscope (which is given to them to take home) when the baby becomes unwell, to detect the very fast rate of SVT.

Chapter 6
Gastrointestinal and liver disorders

Starter questions

Answers to the following questions are on page 220.

1. Why are neurological examinations performed on patients presenting with vomiting?
2. Why is the spine examined in children with constipation?
3. Why is the chest examined in children with abdominal pain?

Introduction

Gastrointestinal conditions are common and affect children of all ages. Most congenital conditions are diagnosed antenatally or recognised shortly after birth. Some gastrointestinal diagnoses, for example pyloric stenosis, are specific to a particular age-range within childhood, whereas others, for example viral gastroenteritis, affect most children at some point in childhood.

Good nutrition, whether relating to the foods consumed or the efficiency of gastrointestinal uptake, is an essential requirement for normal growth and health. Excessive or deficient intake or absorption can lead to a wide range of clinical presentations.

Case 7 Vomiting and crying in a baby

Presentation

Alfie, a 6-week-old baby, is referred to the paediatric assessment unit with a history of crying and vomiting since birth. The frequency of the vomiting has been increasing over the past week, and his mother is concerned.

Initial interpretation

It is first necessary to explore what the mother means by 'vomiting', and thereby determine whether the baby is truly vomiting or simply posseting (the normal regurgitation of small amounts of milk by babies). In true vomiting, there may be a serious pathology or congenital abnormality. Infection, including meningitis,

or a surgical cause should be considered. Overfeeding is a common cause of vomiting in bottle-fed babies.

If the baby has been vomiting since birth, assessment of weight gain and hydration status is vital.

Further history

Alfie's mother explains that he has always been a 'whinging' baby. He has been formula-fed since birth and takes about 120 mL of formula every 4 h. He seems uncomfortable during and after his feeds. He arches his back and cries uncontrollably at times. Often the volume of vomit is high and it looks like milk. Alfie prefers to be held in an upright position; only then does he settle. After an hour he

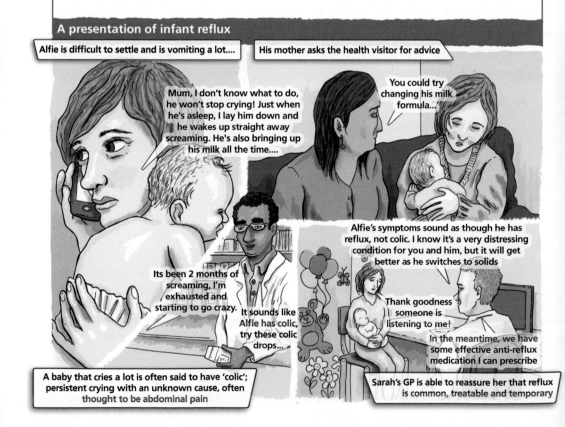

A presentation of infant reflux

Alfie is difficult to settle and is vomiting a lot....

Mum, I don't know what to do, he won't stop crying! Just when he's asleep, I lay him down and he wakes up straight away screaming. He's also bringing up his milk all the time....

Its been 2 months of screaming, I'm exhausted and starting to go crazy.

It sounds like Alfie has colic, try these colic drops...

A baby that cries a lot is often said to have 'colic'; persistent crying with an unknown cause, often thought to be abdominal pain

His mother asks the health visitor for advice

You could try changing his milk formula...

Alfie's symptoms sound as though he has reflux, not colic. I know it's a very distressing condition for you and him, but it will get better as he switches to solids

Thank goodness someone is listening to me!

In the meantime, we have some effective anti-reflux medication I can prescribe

Sarah's GP is able to reassure her that reflux is common, treatable and temporary

sleeps, and he is happy when he wakes. His mother dreads feeding times. Alfie's stools are normal.

Examination

Alfie's weight is on the 50th centile, the same centile as his birthweight. He is woken easily and smiles at his mother as she undresses him. His fontanelle feels soft and is not sunken. His capillary refill time is 2 s, and his tongue and lips look moist. His abdomen feels soft, and no masses are palpable. He vomits a small amount of milk-like fluid during the examination.

Interpretation of findings

The history of vomiting since birth suggests a chronic problem rather than an acute condition such as meningitis. Alfie's total feed volume is appropriate for his weight, which rules out overfeeding. Alfie's vomit is milky rather than green (bilious), which would have suggested a surgical problem (e.g. malrotation).

Vomiting in child of Alfie's age might suggest pyloric stenosis (which usually presents at 3–8 weeks); however, his symptoms are chronic and he does not have the projectile vomiting that is typical in babies with this condition. Importantly, Alfie is well, gaining weight appropriately and not dehydrated, making a serious underlying pathology unlikely.

Investigations

No investigations are indicated, because the history and examination are reassuring and a clinical diagnosis can be made.

Diagnosis

Gastro-oesophageal reflux is diagnosed based on the history of frequent vomiting associated with discomfort (whinging and feeling uncomfortable during feeds) due to the sensation of milk in the oesophagus and possibly acid from the stomach. This is supported by some improvement with the upright posture, which is likely to reduce the amount of milk refluxing up the oesophagus. Alfie is well, is gaining weight normally and shows no signs of dehydration, making more serious diagnoses such as pyloric stenosis (see page 207), much less likely.

His mother is advised to give Alfie smaller, more frequent feeds, and to try adding a thickener to the milk. Alfie is reviewed 4 weeks later in the outpatient clinic, and his symptoms are much improved.

Case 8 Abdominal pain in a 4-year-old

Presentation

Four-year-old Amy is referred to the paediatric assessment unit because she has had central abdominal pain for the past week. She is otherwise well.

Initial interpretation

The cause could be surgical or medical, such as appendicitis or mesenteric adenitis. Consideration of the location of the pain and any symptoms associated with the pain, for example vomiting or diarrhoea, will aid the diagnosis.

Case 8 *continued*

Further history

Amy has been well, with no other symptoms apart from a reduced appetite. Her usual diet consists of pizza and chips, with barely any fruit or vegetables. She has not lost or gained any weight. She opens her bowels every day, usually passing a small volume of watery stool but occasionally small pellets of hard stool after a period of straining.

Examination

Amy is happy and cooperative. Her abdomen is bloated. A bulky mass is palpable in the left iliac fossa, but there is no tenderness.

Interpretation of findings

A 1-week history of abdominal pain makes the diagnosis of acute appendicitis unlikely. Appendicitis has a shorter duration than Amy's symptoms, the child presents unwell and the abdomen is tender on palpation. There are no symptoms of fever or upper respiratory tract infection, so mesenteric adenitis is unlikely. Coeliac disease presents with a distended abdomen, but Amy has no other features of coeliac disease. The history of her current bowel habit suggests overflow diarrhoea, which is typical of constipation.

Investigations

No investigations are indicated at present. However, if Amy's symptoms become chronic, she should be tested for hypothyroidism, hypercalcaemia and coeliac disease.

Diagnosis

The diagnosis is idiopathic constipation. Amy is started on a faecal disimpaction regimen with a macrogol laxative, followed by maintenance laxative therapy. Her mother is given dietary advice by the dietician. At follow-up 2 months later, Amy's mother says that Amy is now passing normal stool on a daily basis.

> In children, faecal disimpaction is usually carried out by using an escalating dose of macrogol laxative (see Table 6.6). For example, the child might start on two sachets on the first day, and four sachets on the second and third day, increasing to six sachets from the 4th day, until the bowel is cleared.

Congenital anomalies

Many congenital anomalies affect the gastrointestinal system. These are listed according to embryological origin in **Table 6.1**. Most are the result of abnormal development during the first trimester, specifically with the separation of the foregut into the gastrointestinal tract and respiratory system, and the physiological herniation of the gut during 6–10 weeks' gestation. Diagnoses are usually made on antenatal US scans or in the neonatal period.

Oesophageal atresia and tracheo-oesophageal fistula

These defects usually (88% cases) occur together.

- Oesophageal atresia is a blind-ending oesophagus
- A tracheo-oesophageal fistula is an abnormal connection between the oesophagus and the trachea

Gastrointestinal tract anomalies	
Location	Anomaly
Foregut	Oesophageal atresia
	Duodenal atresia
	Extrahepatic biliary atresia
	Annular pancreas
Midgut	Stenosis, atresia and duplications
	Exomphalos
	Umbilical hernia
	Gastroschisis
	Malrotation
	Reversed rotation
	Ileal diverticulum (Meckel's diverticulum)
Hindgut	Imperforate anus
	Fistulae: rectum to urethra, bladder or vagina
	Hirschsprung's disease

Table 6.1 Anomalies of the gastrointestinal tract

There are several different types of oesophageal atresia and tracheo-oesophageal fistula (**Figure 6.1**).

Oesophageal atresia and tracheo-oesophageal fistula affect 1 in 3500 live births. It is caused by disruption of the normal division of the foregut into trachea and oesophagus at 6 weeks' gestation; the reason for the abnormal division is unknown. Oesophageal atresia and tracheo-oesophageal fistula may be associated with chromosomal anomalies, including trisomy 18 (Edward's syndrome) and Down's syndrome, or VACTERL association.

> **VACTERL association is a group of congenital anomalies that often present together:**
>
> ■ Vertebral anomalies
>
> ■ Anorectal anomalies
>
> ■ Cardiac anomalies
>
> ■ Tracheo-oesophageal anomalies
>
> ■ Renal anomalies
>
> ■ Limb anomalies, especially radial

Clinical features

Oesophageal atresia, or tracheo-oesophageal fistula associated with oesophageal atresia, may be suspected antenatally because of the finding of polyhydramnios (excess amniotic fluid in the uterus) on the antenatal ultrasound. A neonate with an oesophageal atresia or a tracheo-oesophageal fistula has saliva pooling in the mouth. They also have choking or dusky episodes (becomes cyanosed) when feeding as the milk spills into the lung due to the oesophageal atresia. An isolated narrow 'H-type' tracheo-oesophageal fistula (with no oesophageal atresia) may be diagnosed in an older child with recurrent chest infections.

Diagnostic approach

The diagnosis of oesophageal atresia is made postnatally if a nasogastric tube cannot be passed into the stomach.

■ In isolated oesophageal atresia, no stomach bubble is present on a chest radiograph

■ The presence of a stomach bubble on a radiograph from a baby with oesophageal atresia suggests that there is also a distal tracheo-oesophageal fistula (**Figure 6.2**)

■ Diagnosis of an isolated tracheo-oesophageal fistula (H type) requires a contrast swallow radiograph

Management

The baby must be designated nil by mouth until reanastomosis surgery is carried out, usually within 24 h. Continuous suction of the oropharynx is essential to prevent aspiration of saliva. Prognosis is good, although children frequently have a problem with gastro-oesophageal reflux. Strictures are a complication of surgery and present with dysphagia.

Gastroschisis and exomphalos

Gastroschisis and exomphalos are defects of the anterior abdominal wall that allow

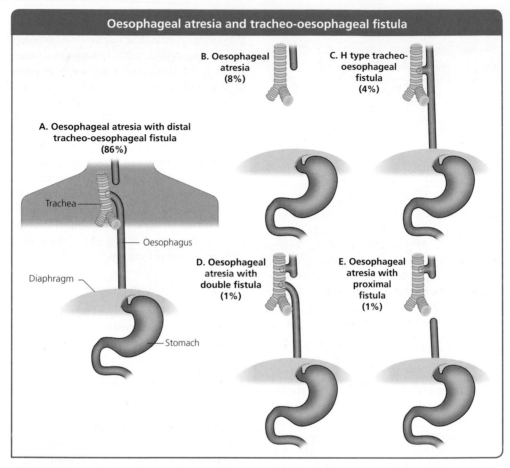

Figure 6.1 Types of oesophageal atresia and tracheo-oesophageal fistula.

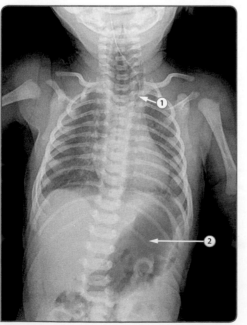

Figure 6.2 Chest radiograph showing a tracheo-oesophageal fistula. The coiling of the nasogastric tube in the oesophagus ① suggests an atresia. The presence of air in the stomach ② indicates a distal connection with the trachea.

herniation of the bowel from the abdominal cavity (**Figure 6.3**). The differences between the two conditions are described in **Table 6.2**. Over 90% of cases are diagnosed on antenatal US scan at 18–21 weeks gestation. After birth, careful attention must be taken to prevent heat and fluid loss, as well as infection at the defect, before surgery.

Malrotation

In malrotation, the bowel is fixed in an abnormal position in the abdomen (**Figure 6.4**). This occurs as a result of abnormal rotation of the midgut during embryological development (see page 9). The small bowel is fixed to the posterior abdominal wall via the mesentery, and the blood vessels (mainly originating from the superior mesenteric artery) supplying the small intestine run through it.

Malrotation affects about 1 in 2500 babies. Children with malrotation occasionally remain asymptomatic; however, symptoms and complications occur if they develop a volvulus (twisting of the intestine around the

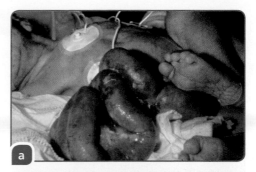
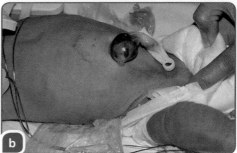

Figure 6.3 Gastroschisis and exomphalos. (a) Gastroschisis: there is no peritoneal covering. (b) Exomphalos: herniation through the umbilicus, with a peritoneal covering over the abdominal contents.

Comparison of gastroschisis and exomphalos		
Characteristic	Gastroschisis	Exomphalos
Incidence	5 in 10,000 live births	3 in 10,000 live births
Associated risk factors	Young maternal age Smoking Drug abuse	Smoking Drug abuse
Site of herniation	To right of umbilicus	Umbilical cord
Contents of herniation	Intestine	Intestine Liver
Covering of organs	No covering, loops of bowel exposed	Peritoneal membrane covering
Associated conditions	Rare ■ Cleft lip and palate ■ Heart defects ■ Intestinal atresia	Common (50%) ■ Beckwith–Weidermann syndrome ■ Trisomy 13 (Patau's syndrome), 18 (Edwards' syndrome), 21 (Down's syndrome)
Management	Surgery Bowel is surrounded by doughnut-shaped support to prevent vascular occlusion Abdomen is wrapped in cling film to prevent fluid loss	Surgery
Outlook	Good prognosis, but some babies have prolonged feeding difficulties	Good outlook if isolated defect Variable if associated with syndrome

Table 6.2 Differences between gastroschisis and exomphalos

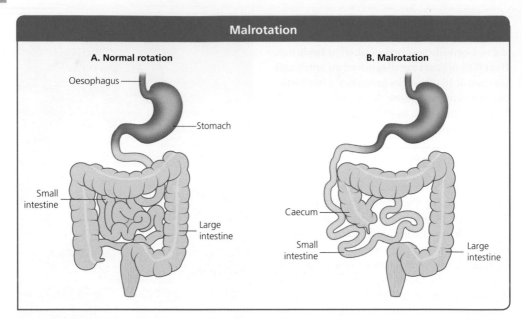

Figure 6.4 Malrotation compared with normal gut rotation. The normal fixation points of the mesentery are at the duodeojejunal flexure just to the left of the midline at the level of the L1 vertebra, and near the ileocaecal valve in the right lower quadrant. This gives it a wide, stable base that does not twist easily. In malrotation, the duodeojejunal flexure and caecum are close to each other in the right upper quadrant. Therefore, if the mesentery is also fixed at these points it has a narrow base that is prone to twisting on itself.

mesentery). Volvulus presents with bilious vomiting, especially in the neonatal period. Rarely, maltrotation presents with intermittent abdominal pain in older children.

Diagnosis is made by upper gastrointestinal contrast studies, which show an abnormal position of the duodeojejunal flexure. Volvulus is a surgical emergency, because the bowel can become necrotic as a consequence of occlusion of blood supply from the mesentery. Malrotation is treated by surgical fixation of the bowel which removes the risk of volvulus or other complications.

Hirschsprung's disease

In Hirschsprung's disease, there is a lack of parasympathetic innervation of the distal colon, which results in constant contraction of the affected segment of bowel. Obstruction and gross dilatation of bowel proximal to the affected segment occurs in consequence. The length of the affected bowel varies:

- the internal anal sphincter is always involved

- the sigmoid colon is frequently involved
- the descending colon is involved in 20% of cases

Hirschsprung's disease is caused by failure of the migration of neural cells to the bowel muscle. It occurs in 1 in 5,000 live births.

Clinical features

The typical presentation is a newborn who has failed to pass meconium within 48 h of birth. The baby also usually has a distended abdomen and vomiting. Typically, withdrawal of the finger at the end of a rectal examination triggers the explosive passage of stool, as a consequence of the temporary widening of the narrow opening.

Diagnostic approach

An abdominal radiograph shows dilatated loops of bowel (**Figure 6.5**). The diagnosis of Hirschsprung's disease is confirmed by a lack of ganglionic nerve cells in tissue obtained by rectal biopsy.

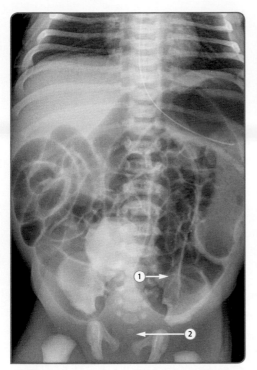

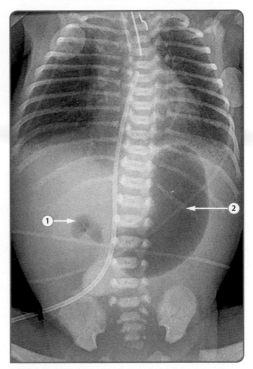

Figure 6.5 Abdominal radiograph showing the typical appearance of Hirschprung's disease. There is a lack of air in the rectum ②. Grossly dilatated loops of bowel are visible ①, proximal to the abnormal bowel.

Figure 6.6 Abdominal radiograph showing the double-bubble appearance of duodenal atresia. Dilatation of the stomach ② and the first part of the duodenum ① proximal to the obstruction is caused by the atresia.

Management

Surgery is required. The aganglionic section is resected and the colon is anastomosed to the anal canal. This may be possible to achieve in one operation, or a colostomy may be fashioned and the anastomosis carried out at a later date.

Prognosis is variable. Many children have long-term problems with continence and constipation.

Intestinal atresia

An atresia (blind-ending passage) can occur anywhere along the gastrointestinal tract as a result of abnormal embryological development. Duodenal atresia is the most common bowel atresia. Up to 30% of cases of duodenal atresia are associated with Down's syndrome.

Features of any type of bowel atresia include vomiting, which is bilious if the atresia is distal to the hepatopancreatic duct, and failure to pass flatus and faeces. Diagnosis is confirmed by an abdominal radiograph showing dilatated bowel loops proximal to the atresia. Treatment is surgical, with anastomosis of the proximal and distal ends.

> **Duodenal atresia typically has a 'double bubble' appearance on abdominal radiograph (Figure 6.6).** Air distends the stomach and the first part of the duodenum proximal to the atresia, which gives rise to two bubbles; there is a lack of air in the distal bowel.

Biliary atresia

Biliary atresia is a rare condition in which there is atresia of the common bile ducts or the hepatic ducts. Bile is produced, but it is unable to be secreted into the small intestine, which leads to inflammation of the bile ducts and liver. The condition affects about 1 in 15,000 live births. The cause of biliary atresia is unknown.

Clinical features

Biliary atresia presents in the first few weeks of life with prolonged jaundice (persisting beyond 14 days in a term infant), pale stools, dark urine and poor weight gain.

Diagnostic approach

Blood tests show conjugated hyperbilirubinaemia (conjugated bilirubin fraction > 20% of the total) and deranged liver function. Ultrasound may show the absence of the biliary tree. However, this finding is unreliable, so it is used mainly to exclude other causes of cholestasis in an infant. Diagnosis is confirmed by radioisotope scans showing no excretion of radioisotope-labelled bile from the liver.

Management

A hepatoportoenterostomy (Kasai's procedure) is carried out by specialist surgeons, with the aim of enabling bile to flow from the liver to the small intestine. The procedure is more successful the earlier it is done, so early diagnosis and referral of biliary atresia is essential. However, surgery is not curative, and many children require liver transplantation at a later date.

Vomiting

Vomiting can be a symptom of various acute and chronic conditions, and it may have surgical, medical and non-gastrointestinal causes. Causes of persistent vomiting are shown in **Table 6.3**. The age of the child, the type of vomiting and associated symptoms give clues to the cause; the presence or absence of bile in the vomit is particularly useful in this respect. An approach to an infant with vomiting is shown in **Figure 6.7**.

Persistent vomiting in children: causes	
Category	Underlying pathology
Intestinal	Gastro-oesophageal reflux
	Pyloric stenosis
	Malrotation and partial obstruction
	Cow's milk protein allergy
Infection	Urinary tract infection
Cerebral disorders	Increased intracranial pressure
Renal disorders	Renal failure
	Renal tubular acidosis
Metabolic-endocrine disorders	Adrenal failure

Table 6.3 The main categories of persistent vomiting in children and the most common underlying pathologies

Gastro-oesophageal reflux

In gastro-oesophageal reflux, there is non-forceful regurgitation of stomach contents (food and acid) back up into the oesophagus and sometimes out of the mouth. It is physiological in infants, but for some it can be more severe and cause troublesome symptoms, for example faltering growth. Infants are affected because they:

- have an immature lower oesophageal sphincter, which allows the easy passage of stomach contents into the oesophagus
- have a liquid diet until they are weaned
- are most often in the supine position

Overt regurgitation occurs at least daily in 50% of infants. Premature babies and children with severe neurodevelopmental problems are at increased risk of gastro-oesophageal reflux. Older children and adolescents can also be affected, but it is less common in this group, with only 2% of 3- to 9-year-olds experiencing symptoms more often than weekly.

Clinical features

Physiological reflux in infants can be asymptomatic. Those with symptomatic reflux are

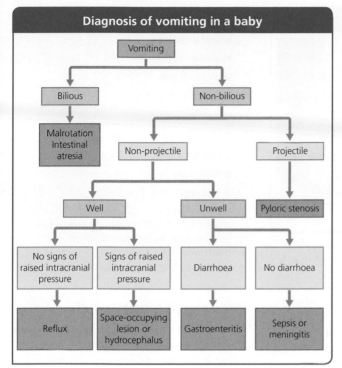

Diagnosis of vomiting in a baby

Vomiting
- Bilious
  - Malrotation Intestinal atresia
- Non-bilious
  - Non-projectile
    - Well
      - No signs of raised intracranial pressure
        - Reflux
      - Signs of raised intracranial pressure
        - Space-occupying lesion or hydrocephalus
    - Unwell
      - Diarrhoea
        - Gastroenteritis
      - No diarrhoea
        - Sepsis or meningitis
  - Projectile
    - Pyloric stenosis

Figure 6.7 An approach to diagnosis of the cause of vomiting in a baby. Some of these diagnoses also apply to older children; however, they can usually communicate their symptoms, unlike younger children.

typically uncomfortable during or after feeds; they may draw up their legs, arch their back or cry. Some infants have small possets or large vomits of milk shortly after a feed, and a minority appear to choke. With severe reflux, there is poor weight gain.

> **Reflux is a common problem, but it can cause significant parental anxiety.** Reassurance that the condition is benign and self-limiting is all that is required usually.

Diagnosis is clinical. Investigations are not indicated unless the symptoms are associated with growth failure.

> **In infants, there is considerable overlap between the symptoms of gastro-oesophageal reflux and those of cow's milk protein allergy** (see page 293). A trial of treatment of the alternative condition may be required if initial management is unsuccessful.

Management

Overfeeding is a common exacerbating factor in babies with reflux, especially in those who are formula-fed. Therefore reducing feed volumes to appropriate levels, or offering smaller, more frequent feeds, may be all that is required. Treatment options for symptomatic reflux include a sequential trial of feed thickeners, alginate therapy (thickens the stomach contents and may form a viscous gel layer which floats on the surface of the stomach contents) or antacids (in the form of an H_2 receptor antagonist or proton pump inhibitor). In children with severe neurodisability, reflux can lead to aspiration, so surgical management (fundoplication) may be required.

Symptoms usually improve once the infant is weaned and able to sit upright, and 90% of cases resolve by 1 year of age.

Pyloric stenosis

Pyloric stenosis is caused by hypertrophy of the pyloric muscle (**Figure 6.8**). It occurs in

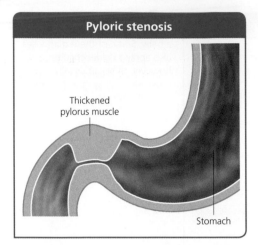

Pyloric stenosis

Thickened pylorus muscle

Stomach

Figure 6.8 In pyloric stenosis, thickening of the pyloric muscle narrows the gastric outlet.

> **Clinical signs of dehydration in an infant include:**
>
> - sunken fontanelle
> - mottled skin
> - cold hands and feet
> - sunken eyes
> - dry mucous membranes
> - capillary refill time > 2 s
> - tachycardia
> - lethargy
>
> Learn the clinical signs of dehydration in children; they are commonly requested as an answer to an examination question.

2–4 out of 1000 live births, in whites of northern European descent, less frequent in blacks and rare in those of Asian or Indian descent. It affects boys more than girls (ratio, 4:1). The cause is unknown, but there appears to be a genetic link.

Clinical features

A baby with pyloric stenosis typically presents between 3 and 8 weeks of age. Pyloric hypertrophy prevents emptying of gastric contents by peristalsis; forceful projectile vomiting results. The vomitus is non-bilious, because the obstruction is proximal to the hepatopancreatic duct. The baby appears hungry and dehydrated, and there may be a recent history of poor weight gain.

> **Be clear what a parent means when they say 'bile'.** Parents often mistakenly describe yellow vomit as bile, when bilious vomit is green.

Diagnostic approach

A test feed is carried out. In cases of pyloric stenosis, peristaltic waves can be seen travelling across the abdomen, and a small firm lump ('olive') may be palpable in the epigastric area. Blood tests show a hypokalaemic hypochloraemic metabolic alkalosis resulting from the loss of hydrochloric acid from the stomach. The diagnosis is confirmed by abdominal US scan.

Management

After correction of any electrolyte disturbance, a surgical procedure called Ramstedt's pyloromyotomy is carried out. The pylorus muscle is cut to the mucosal layer, thereby widening the abnormally narrow pylorus. Oral milk feeds can be reintroduced almost immediately, and prognosis is good.

Abdominal pain

Abdominal pain (stomach ache) is described by location, character, duration and associated symptoms, and as acute, persistent or recurrent. In most cases, a good history and examination will point to the most likely cause (see pages 58 and 76). Most episodes of abdominal pain are non-specific and self-limiting, but the following symptoms require further evaluation:

- severe abdominal pain
- pain that lasts a long time
- pain that is recurrent

Causes of abdominal pain are categorised as medical (infective or non-infective) or surgical (**Table 6.4**).

Appendicitis

Appendicitis is acute inflammation of the appendix, which occurs when the lumen of the appendix is obstructed by faecoliths. It can occur at any age and affects up to 10% of the population during their lifetime. It is most common in adolescence.

Clinical features

The classic presentation is with decreased appetite and central abdominal pain, which later migrates to the right iliac fossa. There may be vomiting and fever. Symptoms may be less specific in young children.

Examination finds localised tenderness and guarding over the right iliac fossa, and rebound tenderness. Generalised rigidity is present in peritonitis secondary to perforation of appendix.

> **Do not miss the diagnosis of appendicitis.** Delay can result in peritonitis and a seriously unwell child.

Diagnostic approach and management

Appendicitis is a clinical diagnosis. Increased infection and inflammatory markers can support the diagnosis. US may show an inflamed appendix. Appendicitis is treated surgically by appendicectomy.

Intussusception

Intussusception occurs when a section of bowel invaginates, like a telescope being closed (**Figure 6.9**). The usual site of

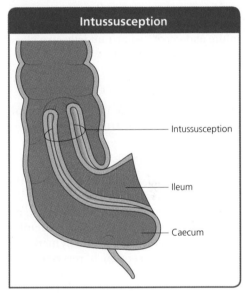

Intussusception

- Intussusception
- Ileum
- Caecum

Figure 6.9 Intussusception, with telescoping of the proximal bowel (ileum) into the distal bowel (caecum and colon).

Abdominal pain in children: causes		
Surgical	Infective	Non-infective
Appendicitis	Gastroenteritis	Constipation
Intussusception	Pneumonia (lower lobe)	Coeliac disease
Obstructed hernia	Urinary tract infection	Inflammatory bowel disease
Testicular torsion	Mesenteric adenitis	Diabetic ketoacidosis
		Non-organic abdominal pain
		Peptic ulcer (rare)

Table 6.4 Causes of abdominal pain in children

intussusception is the terminal ileum, which invaginates into the caecum, taking the mesentery with it; this causes oedema, ischaemia and eventually necrosis and perforation if the obstruction is not relieved. Less commonly, intussusception occurs at the site of a lymph node or a polyp.

Babies aged 6–12 months are most commonly affected, but intussusception can occur between 3 months and 6 years of age.

Clinical features

Intussusception typically presents with intermittent episodes of pain characterised by drawing up of the legs and inconsolable crying. Vomiting and pallor are common, and a sausage-shaped mass may be palpable in the abdomen. Redcurrant jelly–like blood in the stools is a late sign.

Diagnostic approach

The diagnosis can be confirmed by abdominal US scan or contrast studies.

Management

If the child is haemodynamically stable, the intussusception is reduced by air enema. An air enema is performed by a radiologist; air under pressure is delivered via a rectal tube, and then the air pressure gradually increased until the intussusception is reversed. This is successful in 70% of cases, while the others will require surgery. In about 1% the air enema may cause or reveal a perforation, which will require surgery and in 5% the intussusception may recur in the next few days, requiring repeat treatment or surgery. Surgery is required if there is suspicion of perforation or if the duration of symptoms is > 24 h, because of a higher risk of bowel necrosis by this time.

Meckel's diverticulum

Meckel's diverticulum is a remnant of the vitellointestinal duct (a connection between the yolk sac and the gut during embryonic development) in the small intestine, near the iliocaecal valve; it contains heterotopic mucosa, most commonly gastric (70%). It occurs in 2% of the population. Most children with a Meckel's diverticulum are asymptomatic; however, a minority (5%) experience complications, most commonly bleeding of the gastric tissue within the diverticulum. They present with fresh bleeding from the rectum or melaena. Haemoglobin levels may be low after an acute bleed, or there may be microcytic anaemia with chronic bleeding. Other complications include abdominal pain secondary to acute inflammation (similar to appendicitis), intussusception or intestinal obstruction.

The diagnosis is confirmed by identification of the ectopic mucosa on radioisotope scanning. The diverticulum is removed surgically.

> **Meckels diverticulitis can be remembered by the rule of 2s:** Affects 2% of the population; 2:1 boys:girls; 2 years is the most common age of presentation; usually 2 feet from the ileocaecal valve; 2 inches long; 2 cm wide.

Mesenteric adenitis

Mesenteric adenitis, i.e. inflammation of the mesenteric lymph nodes, is a common cause of abdominal pain in children. The nodes become enlarged secondary to infection. The infection is usually viral and can be at a distant site, such as the upper respiratory tract.

The condition is self-limiting and requires simple analgesia only. However, the pain can be very severe and mimic appendicitis.

> **Right lower lobe pneumonia typically causes referred abdominal pain.** This settles when the pneumonia is treated.

Non-organic abdominal pain

Non-organic abdominal pain is a common diagnosis in a child with recurrent abdominal pain, when the results of investigations are normal and no cause is identified. Typically, the pain is poorly localised or central. Growth is normal. Management consists of providing the child and parents with coping strategies to manage the pain.

A subset of children with recurrent episodes of abdominal pain receive a diagnosis of abdominal migraine. The pain is acute but poorly localised and may be associated with vomiting. There is frequently a family history of migraine. Investigation results are normal, and the child is well between attacks. The abdominal pain usually resolve as the child grows; however, many later develop the more classic migraine headaches.

Constipation

Constipation is the infrequent passage of hard stool. It affects up to 30% of children, possibly reflecting the lack of fibre in many families' diets. It can be very distressing for the child and their parents. Constipation is a symptom and has many causes. In children, it is most commonly idiopathic; however, other rarer underlying causes should be excluded.

Clinical features

Children typically present with generalised abdominal pain and poor appetite, with a history of infrequent bowel opening, straining and passage of small, hard stools. The passage of stool may be associated with pain, or blood if there is an anal fissure. The pain may make the child hold in stool, thereby exacerbating the problem. It is common for these children to later soil themselves, as a result of liquid overflow stool bypassing the faecal mass.

Diagnostic approach

The diagnosis is clinical. A thorough history and examination are required, including plotting growth to rule out any underlying disease that requires specific management. Features associated with non-dietary causes of constipation are shown in **Table 6.5**.

Abdominal examination usually finds a large faecal mass in the left iliac fossa. The anal area is inspected for fissures, but a digital rectal examination is unnecessary and distressing for the child. Neurological examination of the legs, including sensation, is required to exclude spinal neurological pathology.

Constipation: findings that suggest an underlying cause	
Finding	Underlying diagnoses
Presence since birth	Structural congenital anomaly
Delayed passage of meconium	Hirschsprung's disease
	Cystic fibrosis (meconium plug)
Failure to thrive	Coeliac disease
	Hypothyroidism
	Cystic fibrosis
Abnormal spine or weakness of the legs	Neurological problem (e.g. spina bifida occulta)

Table 6.5 History and examination findings that suggest an underlying cause for constipation

Investigations are guided by the history and examination. For example, thyroid function tests in a child who is lacking in energy, feels the cold and has gained excess weight. However, investigations are not routinely carried out.

> **Faecal loading** may be seen on abdominal radiograph, but abdominal radiographs are not obtained solely to diagnose constipation.

Management

If the constipation is idiopathic, information on appropriate diet and fluid intake is given. Parents are encouraged to develop a reward system to encourage good toileting behaviour. Laxatives can also be used, usually macrogols (**Table 6.6**). A small minority of

Types of laxative		
Type	Mode of action	Examples
Stimulant	Stimulates peristalsis	Senna
		Sodium picosulfate
Osmotic	Retains water in the gut to soften stool	Lactulose
Macrogols	Bulks the stool and has an osmotic action	Polyethylene glycol and electrolytes

Table 6.6 Different types of laxative

children may need to follow a laxative disimpaction regimen (see page 200) before starting maintenance therapy. With perseverance and adherence to advice and medications, the prognosis is good.

Diarrhoea

Diarrhoea is the frequent passage of stools that are looser than is normal for the child. By far the commonest cause in children is infection of the bowel, known collectively as gastroenteritis. However, diarrhoea can also be a symptom of other conditions, as a result of malabsorption, intestinal inflammation or accelerated transit times.

> **A thorough history of the child's long-term bowel habit is essential. This is** because many patients apparently presenting with diarrhoea actually have constipation, the 'diarrhoea' being liquid-overflow stool around impacted faeces.

Malabsorption

Malabsorption is failure of normal digestion and absorption of nutrients. In children, it is usually caused by:

- disorders affecting digestion in the lumen, for example pancreatic insufficiency in cystic fibrosis or reduced bile in cholestatic liver disease
- damage to the mucosal epithelium, for example in coeliac disease or after gastroenteritis

An accelerated transit time means that food passes more rapidly through the digestive tract, so that there is insufficient time for the normal digestive and absorptive processes to take place. This is the case in, for example, diarrhoea secondary to hyperthyroidism.

Gastroenteritis

Gastroenteritis is an infection of the gastrointestinal tract. It is extremely common, affecting almost all children at some point in their lives. Gastroenteritis is mostly caused by viruses, most commonly rotavirus (before the introduction of immunisation); bacteria are less commonly responsible (**Table 6.7**). The route of transmission is faeco-oral, and it is highly contagious. Peak incidence is at 9 months to 2 years of age. The incidence is reduced in breastfed babies due to the immuno-protective effect of breast milk (bottles can also become contaminated with infection).

> **The rotavirus vaccine was added to the routine immunisation schedule for infants in the UK in 2013.** This has prevented >70% cases of rotavirus gastroenteritis.

Gastroenteritis: viral and bacterial causes	
Viral (70%)	Bacterial (10–20%)
Rotavirus*	Campylobacter
Norovirus	Salmonella
Enterovirus	Escherichia coli

Table 6.7 Viral and bacterial causes of gastroenteritis in order of frequency.* Rotavirus has reduced in countries where it is included in the primary vaccination schedule

Clinical features

Clinical features include vomiting, loose stools, abdominal cramps and general malaise. The severity of the illness varies, and young children can become seriously dehydrated. The diagnosis is mainly clinical but can be confirmed by isolating the viral or bacterial pathogen from the stool.

Management

Management is supportive. If necessary, children can be treated with small, frequent amounts of oral rehydration solution. This contains glucose and electrolytes. The glucose provides energy and facilitates absorption of fluid and electrolytes across the intestinal mucosa. Babies and younger children may require nasogastric administration of oral rehydration solution. IV fluids are indicated only in children who are in shock, severely dehydrated or persistently losing their oral rehydration solution through vomiting.

Symptoms usually resolve after 48 h. Loose stools may continue for a week or two in children with rotavirus, and in a minority for a few months as a result of lactase deficiency secondary to damage to the intestinal villi.

Toddler diarrhoea

Toddler diarrhoea is diagnosed when a child of preschool age is frequently passing loose stools but is otherwise well and thriving, with no abnormal clinical findings. Parents describe the presence of undigested food, typically vegetables, in the stool, hence its name of the 'peas and carrots condition'. The cause is unknown.

The problem resolves gradually without intervention. Symptoms may be relieved by dietary changes, such as reducing the intake of fructose, especially in the form of fruit juices, or increasing the consumption of fat.

Coeliac disease

Coeliac disease is an autoimmune disease in genetically susceptible individuals, in which ingestion of gluten triggers inflammation and the production of autoantibodies, which damage the villi of the small intestine. Malabsorption develops as a consequence.

The estimated prevalence is 1 in 100, but many with minor symptoms remain undiagnosed. It was originally though to exclusively affect white Europeans, but with increased awareness in areas such as north Africa, the Middle East and Asia the prevalence in these areas is now thought to be similar to Europe. Coeliac disease does not occur in babies before weaning, but it can present at any age after the introduction of gluten into the diet.

Clinical features

Failure to absorb nutrients leads to many of the typical features of coeliac disease:

- poor weight gain or growth
- abdominal pain
- diarrhoea, constipation or both
- bloated abdomen
- gluteal muscle wasting
- iron deficiency anaemia

Diagnostic approach

Levels of the causative autoantibodies, anti-tissue transglutaminase antibodies, are high in coeliac disease, so their measurement is used as a screening test. The test is very sensitive and specific, but false negative results occur if the patient is immunoglobulin A-deficient or if their diet contains insufficient gluten at the time of testing.

A biopsy finding of villous atrophy in tissue from the small bowel confirms the diagnosis. However, the diagnosis can be confirmed without biopsy in a selected group of symptomatic children with a concentration of anti-tissue transglutaminase antibodies that is > 10 times the upper limit of the reference range. Further blood testing shows high levels of anti-endomysial antibodies and the human leucocyte antigen (HLA) DQ2 or DQ8 genotype.

Management

Treatment is a lifelong gluten-free diet. Support from a dietician is essential. Non-adherence to a gluten-free diet increases the risk of bowel malignancy in later life.

Inflammatory bowel disease

Inflammatory bowel disease mainly refers to two related but distinct conditions that affect the bowel: Crohn's disease and ulcerative colitis.

- Crohn's disease is a chronic, patchy, transmural inflammation of any part of the gastrointestinal tract
- Ulcerative colitis is diffuse mucosal inflammation limited to the colon

Inflammatory bowel disease has an incidence of 3–5 per 100,000, with Crohn's disease accounting for a higher percentage of cases than ulcerative colitis. The aetiology for both is unknown, but there appears to be a genetic link.

Clinical features

Patients can present with the following symptoms, of varying severity:

- abdominal pain
- diarrhoea
- blood-stained stools (more common in ulcerative colitis)
- weight loss or poor growth

Non-specific symptoms, such as lethargy and reduced appetite, are also common. There may also be associated extraintestinal manifestations (**Table 6.8**).

Diagnostic approach

Blood tests show increased levels of inflammatory markers (C-reactive protein and erythrocyte sedimentation rate), usually associated with anaemia and low albumin. Endoscopy of the upper and lower gastrointestinal tract can be used to identify the sites of any lesions and enables collection of tissue samples for confirmation of the diagnosis by biopsy. A barium follow-through can be used to identify lesions in the small bowel if Crohn's disease is suspected.

Comparison of Crohn's disease and ulcerative colitis		
Characteristic	Crohn's disease	Ulcerative colitis
Incidence (UK data)	3 per 100,000	1.5 per 100,000
Site affected	Anywhere from mouth to anus, particularly the terminal ilium	Large colon and rectum
Layer of intestine affected	Transmural	Mucosa
Associated features	Aphthous ulcers	Uveitis
	Perianal skin tags	Arthritis (seronegative)
	Anal fissures	Pyoderma gangrenosum
	Pyoderma gangrenosum	Erythema nodosum
	Erythema nodosum	
	Uveitis	
	Arthritis (seronegative)	
Biopsy findings	Granulomas	Crypt abscesses

Table 6.8 Differences between Crohn's disease and ulcerative colitis

Management

The aim of management of inflammatory bowel disease is to reduce the inflammation. The first-line treatment for Crohn's disease is exclusive enteral nutrition, for example with an elemental diet, in which the patient's complete nutrition is provided as a liquid in which the nutrients are predigested, making them easier to absorb. For patients who are unable to tolerate enteral nutrition, corticosteroids may be required. Corticosteroids are also the first-line treatment in ulcerative colitis. Ongoing maintenance is usually provided by:

- aminosalicylates, for example mesalazine, in ulcerative colitis
- immunosuppressants, such as azathioprine or methotrexate, in Crohn's disease
- Immunosuppressive therapy, monoclonal antibody treatment (antitumour necrosis factor), such as infliximab, in both conditions

Surgery may be required when the patient is refractory to medical treatment. Ulcerative colitis can be cured by total colectomy, but this is not a popular option for children as it requires a two or three-stage surgery over the course of 1 year, and complications can occur in up to 50% (pouchitis 40%, strictures with obstruction and fistulae). Total colectomy is therefore reserved for severe colitis which is not responsive to medication. Prognosis is variable, with many patients experiencing recurrent flare-ups of the condition.

Obesity

Obesity is defined as a body mass index (BMI) above the 98th centile. A child is classified as overweight when their BMI is between the 91st and 98th centile. Childhood obesity is a growing problem in many high-income countries, with nearly a third of children in these countries classed as overweight or obese. This has great implications for public health in the short and long term, because obese children are at high risk of becoming obese adults.

> A child's BMI is interpreted by plotting their height and weight centile on a dedicated section of the growth chart.

Obesity is caused by excessive intake of calories in relation to energy expended. Very rarely, an endocrine or a genetic condition may contribute. Complications of obesity in childhood include:

- hypertension (increased blood pressure)
- insulin resistance and type 2 diabetes
- sleep apnoea
- orthopaedic problems
- low self-esteem

In the long term, there is a risk of early onset cardiovascular disease and type 2 diabetes.

Severe obesity is managed by a multidisciplinary team. The child and their family are educated about diet and lifestyle changes, and support is provided to help them achieve any goals set. National prevention strategies to promote healthy eating and physical activity in schools are also beneficial.

> Unlike adults with obesity, obese children are generally not placed on a weight loss diet. The aim is to put in place a long-term healthy eating plan and allow children to 'grow into' their weight.

Undernutrition

In undernutrition, nutritional intake is insufficient to meet the body's requirements for normal physiological function and, in children, growth. Undernutrition is a major problem in many low-income countries, mainly because of lack of food. However, it is also present in higher income countries, where the insufficient nutritional intake is more usually secondary to chronic illness.

The two major classes of undernutrition are:

- macronutrient deficiency, for example protein-energy undernutrition
- micronutrient deficiency, i.e. insufficient intake of vitamins and minerals

Undernutrition secondary to chronic illness is caused by inadequate intake, malabsorption or excessive losses of nutrients, or increased metabolic demands (**Table 6.9**).

Symptoms of undernutrition in children include poor growth, lean body mass, lethargy, reduced activity and delayed development.

Severe protein-energy undernutrition is mainly the consequence of inadequate food supply in low-income countries. It is divided into two conditions: kwashiorkor and marasmus.

- **Kwashiorkor** is characterised by muscle wasting (with some preservation of subcutaneous fat) and peripheral oedema, and is secondary to a lack of protein
- **Marasmus** is characterised by severe wasting and an emaciated appearance; it is secondary to a total lack of calories and protein

Undernutrition results in a lack of energy for learning and playing, increased susceptibility to illness and infection, poor growth and generally poorer health outcomes.

Micronutrient deficiencies

Micronutrients, i.e. vitamins and minerals, play a vital role in children's general health and development. Deficiencies of particular micronutrients can cause a specific disease, for example rickets secondary to vitamin D deficiency, but there is growing evidence that micronutrients play an essential role in areas such as growth, immunity and chronic disease.

In many northern European countries (including the UK), the commonest micronutrient deficiencies are vitamin D deficiency and iron deficiency (see page 371). Many foods, such as breakfast cereals, are fortified with certain vitamins and minerals, but extra supplementation is required in groups at risk of deficiency.

Vitamin D deficiency

This vitamin promotes intestinal absorption of calcium, which is essential for normal bone mineralisation. Some of the body's vitamin D is obtained from the diet, such as oily fish, eggs and mushrooms, but most is synthesised in skin exposed to sunlight. Lack of exposure to ultraviolet rays from sunlight is the main cause of vitamin D deficiency, especially in people with darker skin.

Vitamin D deficiency is common (estimated 40% of children under 5 years in the UK). Supplementation of vitamin D is recommended for all pregnant and breastfeeding women, and all children aged 6 months to 5 years who are not drinking > 500 mL of milk daily.

Causes of undernutrition	
Immediate cause	**Underlying causes**
Inadequate intake of nutrients	Inadequate food supply
	Anorexia secondary to chronic illness or eating disorder
	Physical feeding difficulties, such as those associated with severe cerebral palsy
Malabsorption of nutrients	Gastrointestinal disease
	Pancreatic insufficiency secondary to cystic fibrosis
Excessive loss of nutrients	Chronic diarrhoea
increased metabolic demands	Congenital heart disease
	Cystic fibrosis
	Thyrotoxicosis

Table 6.9 A classification of the causes of undernutrition

One clinical manifestation of severe vitamin D deficiency in children is rickets, which is the consequence of inadequate mineralisation of the growth plates in addition to the matrix of bone. This leads to bony deformity with clinical manifestations (**Figure 6.10**), mainly:

- bowed legs
- rachitic rosary
- tender swollen joints, especially the wrists and ankles

Other presenting symptoms include a delay in walking or a waddling gait, poor growth, softening of the skull leading to frontal bossing, and symptoms of hypocalcaemia.

There are other causes of rickets that are unrelated to vitamin D status (**Table 6.10**) which present with similar signs and symptoms.

Vitamin D deficiency can also contribute to seizures and cardiomyopathy in infants and poor growth and muscle weakness in children of all ages.

Rickets: causes	
Category	Examples
Calcipenic rickets (caused by low calcium levels)	Nutritional deficiency, usually secondary to vitamin D deficiency
	Hereditary vitamin D-resistant rickets
	Conditions affecting vitamin D absorption or metabolism (e.g. coeliac disease, severe liver disease)
Phosphopenic rickets (caused by low phosphorus levels)	Renal phosphate wasting as a result of renal tubular disorders
	X-linked hypophosphataemic rickets

Table 6.10 Causes of rickets

Rachitic rosary is the name for a series of bead-like thickenings seen on the chest wall on examination as well as radiographically. It is the result of expansion of the costochondrial junctions, making the anterior rib ends more prominent.

Vitamin K deficiency

Because this vitamin is essential for the normal function of many coagulation factors, vitamin K deficiency usually presents with bleeding.

Newborn babies have low levels of vitamin K, and breast milk is also low in vitamin K. This means that the neonate is at risk of vitamin K deficiency bleeding, previously known as haemorrhagic disease of the newborn. Vitamin K deficiency bleeding presents with bleeding from puncture sites, mucous membranes, the umbilical stump and the gastrointestinal tract. It occurs most commonly in the first week of life but is now rare in developed countries because of the recommendation for all newborn babies to receive an intramuscular dose of vitamin K immediately after birth (see page 39).

Older children at risk of vitamin K deficiency are mainly those with liver disease and malabsorption states, such as unrecognised coeliac disease or inflammatory bowel disease.

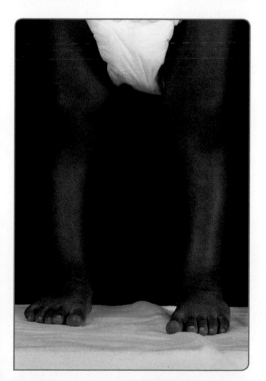

Figure 6.10 Nutritional rickets presents clinically with bowed legs and swelling at the epiphyses (knees and ankles).

Zinc deficiency

This deficiency is rare in healthy children. However, it can occur in children with conditions that reduce absorption of zinc from the small intestine, such as Crohn's disease and short bowel syndrome. The most common symptoms of zinc deficiency are poor growth, diarrhoea and impaired immunity.

Acrodermatitis enteropathica is an autosomal recessive condition leading to impaired absorption of zinc. It presents in infancy after weaning, with a rash (characteristically perioral and perineal), alopecia, chronic diarrhoea and faltering growth. It responds well to zinc supplementation.

Vitamin A deficiency

This is rare in higher income countries but common in low-income countries. It causes various problems, including immune deficiency. One of its most serious consequences is night blindness.

Liver disease

The liver carries out a wide range of functions for most systems of the body. It is responsible for glycogen storage, breakdown of red blood cells, synthesis of plasma proteins, hormone production, detoxification, and production of coagulation factors and bile. Acquired liver failure in children is primarily the result of hepatitis.

signs only after these irreversible changes have occurred (**Figure 6.11**). Depending on the cause, cirrhosis can develop over months or years.

Patients with acute fulminant hepatic failure or chronic liver disease are treated in specialist centres. Prognosis is variable. Liver transplantation is often required.

Hepatitis

Hepatitis is inflammation of the liver. It can be acute or chronic. There are many causes (**Table 6.11**), the most common being viral infection.

Acute hepatitis

This is defined as hepatitis that resolves within 6 months. Children may present with non-specific symptoms, including fever, diarrhoea and vomiting, and a flu-like illness. Most children become jaundiced. Hepatomegaly is present and splenomegaly in 20–30% of cases.

Blood tests show increased levels of liver enzymes. Viral serology is used to identify any specific causative virus.

Acute hepatitis is generally self-limiting. Rarely, however, it progresses to acute liver failure. Treatment is supportive.

Chronic hepatitis and chronic liver disease

In chronic hepatitis, inflamed liver cells are replaced by fibrous scar tissue and nodules (cirrhosis). Patients frequently present with

Causes of hepatitis in children		
Type of hepatitis	Acute hepatitis	Chronic hepatitis
Viral	Hepatitis A, B, C, D or E Epstein–Barr virus Cytomegalovirus	Hepatitis B, C or D
Bacterial	Leptospirosis	–
Fungal	*Aspergillus*	–
Parasitic	*Toxoplasma*	–
Drug-induced	Paracetamol (acetaminophen)	Isoniazid Methotrexate
Genetic	Wilson's disease	Wilson's disease alpha-1 antitrypsin deficiency Haemochromatosis
Autoimmune	Autoimmune hepatitis Systemic lupus erythematous	Autoimmune hepatitis

Table 6.11 Causes of acute and chronic hepatitis in children

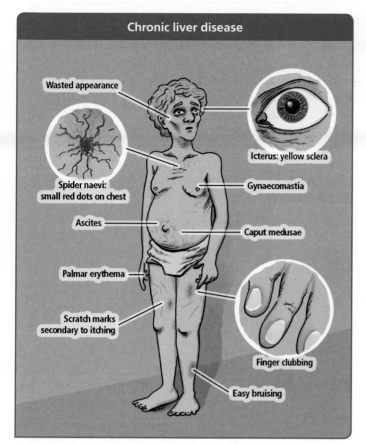

Figure 6.11 Features of chronic liver disease.

Chronic liver disease

- Wasted appearance
- Icterus: yellow sclera
- Spider naevi: small red dots on chest
- Gynaecomastia
- Ascites
- Caput medusae
- Palmar erythema
- Scratch marks secondary to itching
- Finger clubbing
- Easy bruising

> **Reye's syndrome is a rare disease that causes liver damage.** It has been associated with the use of aspirin in children, so aspirin is no longer prescribed to children, apart from for specific conditions such as Kawasaki's disease (see page 191)

Non-alcoholic fatty liver disease

Fatty liver disease is a spectrum of disease ranging from steatosis (accumulation of fat in liver cells) to cirrhosis . Non-alcoholic fatty liver disease is thought to be caused by environmental and genetic factors.

Non-alcoholic fatty liver disease is associated with obesity and insulin resistance. Therefore it is likely to become more common because of the increasing prevalence of childhood obesity. Management focuses on weight loss and lifestyle modification.

Answers to starter questions

1. In children with persistent vomiting associated with headaches, particularly in the morning, the possibility of a brain tumour is considered. It is rare, but must not be missed. The neurological examination, including fundi, looks for subtle signs of raised intracranial pressure.

2. Constipation is often idiopathic, but there are secondary causes of constipation, such as spina bifida occulta. The spine is examined to rule out neurological causes of constipation.

3. Abdominal pain can often be caused by right lower lobe pneumonia. This is picked up by observing the respiratory rate during a chest examination.

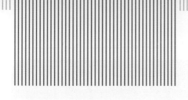

Chapter 7
Urogenital disorders

Starter questions

Answers to the following questions are on page 242.

1. Why should you investigate a newborn baby boy who has a poor urinary stream?
2. Why would you be concerned if a child known to have nephrotic syndrome presented with pleuritic chest pain?
3. Why is testicular torsion a surgical emergency?

Introduction

Urogenital disorders are a disparate group. Some are detected antenatally, for example hydronephrosis, whereas others can occur at any time during childhood, for example urinary tract infections. Awareness of the different presenting symptoms and different complications, depending on the age of the child, is crucial in the management of many of these conditions.

Some conditions such as vesico-ureteric reflux with scarring, even though they occur in children, cause long-term damage, others are more common in children than adults such as haemolytic uraemic syndrome, Henoch–Schönlein purpura and enuresis (bed wetting). Conditions that occur at all ages such as nephrotic syndrome and glomerulonephritis are generally caused by a less severe pathological process in children compared with adults. Chronic renal failure, although it can occur in childhood, is uncommon compared with adults.

Case 9 Fever and pain on passing urine

Presentation

Molly is 3 years old. Her mother visits their general practitioner (GP), because she is concerned that Molly has been generally unwell, with a fever for the previous 24 h. Molly also complains of pain when passing urine. Her mother describes the urine as smelly.

Initial interpretation

As always in the case of fever in a child, the source of infection must be considered. Dysuria and a high temperature put urinary tract infection high on the list of possible diagnoses. However, other foci of infection, including chest and meninges, must always be considered, particularly in younger children who cannot communicate their symptoms.

Further history

Molly has no cough, sore throat, headache, rash or other specific symptoms that would suggest a distant source of infection. The GP notes that this is the third attendance in 12 months with similar symptoms. On the previous occasions, Molly was treated for a urinary tract infection. She has never needed to be admitted to hospital, and she previously recovered quickly on oral antibiotics.

Examination

Molly looks flushed. Her temperature is 38.2°C, but all other observations are satisfactory. Her abdomen is soft on palpation, although there is some left loin tenderness. Her perineum is clean and not inflamed. Cardiovascular, respiratory and ear, nose and throat examination are normal.

Interpretation of findings

Pyrexia and loin tenderness in a child with a history of recurrent urinary tract infections suggests an upper urinary tract infection. There are no other concerning symptoms to suggest a focus of infection elsewhere.

Investigations

Dipstick urinalysis carried out by the GP gives a positive result for leucocyte esterase and nitrites. This finding is diagnostic of urinary tract infection in children > 3 years old. The urine is also sent for culture to establish the causative organism.

Diagnosis

Culture of urine samples during previous episodes had grown *Escherichia* coli sensitive to co-amoxiclav (amoxicillin/clavulanic acid), so Molly is prescribed a 10-day course of this antibiotic. She is also referred to the paediatric outpatient clinic for specialist advice in view of the recurrence of the infections. After 48 h, the most recent urine culture shows growth of *E. coli*, thereby confirming the diagnosis of a urinary tract infection.

Case 10 Swollen eyes

Presentation

Adam, aged 6 years, presents to the GP with a 7-day history of swelling around both eyes. In the previous week, he had seen another GP, who had diagnosed an allergic reaction and prescribed antihistamines. His mother became concerned this morning, when she noted that Adam's scrotum appeared swollen.

Initial interpretation

Periorbital swelling secondary to an allergic reaction is common, but an allergy would not cause scrotal swelling. Periorbital cellulitis should be considered, although bilateral infection is uncommon. Nephrotic syndrome is the most likely diagnosis (see Interpretation, below).

Further history

Adam had a cold recently but is otherwise healthy. The periorbital oedema is worse on waking. Adam's mother thinks he has gained some weight, because he is unable to button his trousers.

Examination

Adam's observations are stable. Examination confirms periorbital oedema and scrotal oedema. His abdomen appears distended, and there is a dull percussion note over both flanks. Pitting oedema is present at the ankles.

Interpretation of findings

The history of weight gain associated with periorbital, scrotal and ankle oedema, and testicular swelling, suggests a diagnosis of nephrotic syndrome. To confirm the diagnosis Adam is admitted to the paediatric unit for investigations.

Investigations

Blood testing shows low albumin levels (20 g/L). Dipstick urinalysis gives a ++++ result for protein. He has a high urine protein:creatinine ratio on a spot urine sample and analysis of urine collected throughout a 24-h period shows that Adam is passing > 3.5 g of protein daily.

Diagnosis

The examination and investigation findings confirm the triad of oedema, hypoalbuminaemia and proteinuria needed to make a diagnosis of nephrotic syndrome. Adam is started on oral steroids, in addition to penicillin (to protect against infection with encapsulated organisms) and ranitidine (to prevent gastritis caused by steroids).

Nephrotic syndrome is explained to Adam's parents, including how the urinary leakage of protein causes oedema. They are also told of the possible side-effects of steroid therapy, and that the steriod should not be stopped suddenly. The response to steroids is usually good (80% respond to the first course) but it often can come back (75% of cases) in the first few years after diagnosis, but Adam will relapse less frequently as he grows.

Adam's parents are shown how to test the first urine sample of the day with a urine dipstick; the colour on the dipstick will change if protein is present.

Adam is discharged after 4 days, once the protein content in his urine has begun to decrease and his parents are confident about checking his urine for protein at home.

Congenital anomalies

Congenital disorders of the renal tract are either detected antenatally on US scan or diagnosed postnatally. Most are minor structural anomalies in the complex embryological development of the urogenital system. Other, less common, anomalies result in renal failure, the most severe being incompatible with life. Congenital anomalies of the kidneys, bladder and genitalia are shown in **Table 7.1**.

Renal agenesis

Renal agenesis is failure to develop one or both kidneys. Unilateral renal agenesis occurs in 1 in 750 live births worldwide; bilateral renal agenesis occurs in 1.5 per 10,000 fetuses, many not surviving to birth. The aetiology is unknown.

Clinical features

In bilateral renal agenesis, no urine is produced in utero. The resulting oligohydramnios, i.e. abnormally low volume of amniotic fluid, leads to pulmonary hypoplasia (poor development of the lungs). At birth, the baby has classic features related to oligohydramnios and caused by compression in utero; these are known as the oligohydramnios sequence (Potter's sequence) (**Table 7.2**).

> **The oligohydramnios sequence (Potter's sequence) is not exclusively associated with bilateral renal agenesis.** It is a consequence of any pathology causing severe oligohydramnios.

Unilateral renal agenesis is asymptomatic, usually an incidental finding on antenatal US scan. There is usually compensatory hypertrophy of the other kidney.

Management

Bilateral renal agenesis has a very poor prognosis. There is an increased risk of intrauterine death, and babies who survive to delivery usually die soon after birth from respiratory insufficiency secondary to pulmonary hypoplasia.

Children with one kidney generally lead a normal life and require only monitoring of kidney growth and blood pressure.

Multicystic dysplastic kidney

A multicystic dysplastic kidney is a non-functioning kidney full of multiple cysts, the result

Urinary system anomalies	
Location	Anomaly
Kidneys	Duplications of the urinary tract (e.g. duplex kidney)
	Ectopic ureter
	Double ureter and supernumerary kidney
	Renal agenesis
	Ectopic pelvic kidney
	Horseshoe kidney
	Cystic kidney diseases
Bladder	Urachal fistula
	Exstrophy of bladder
Genitalia	Hypospadias
	Epispadias

Table 7.1 Anomalies of the urinary system

Oligohydramnios sequence (Potter's sequence): clinical features	
Location	Feature
Face	Flat-beaked nose
	Prominent epicanthal folds
	Micrognathia
	Low-set ears
Lungs	Pulmonary hypoplasia
Limb deformities	Talipes
	Dislocated hips
	Contractures

Table 7.2 Clinical features of oligohydramnios sequence (Potter's sequence)

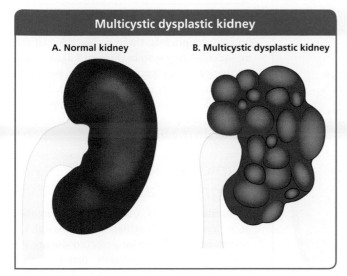

Multicystic dysplastic kidney

A. Normal kidney   B. Multicystic dysplastic kidney

Figure 7.1 Comparison of a normal kidney (a) and a multicystic dysplastic kidney (b).

of failure of normal development of the parenchyma in utero (**Figure 7.1**). It occurs in about 1 in 2500 children and is usually unilateral. The cause is unclear, but it is not hereditary.

Clinical features

The condition is usually detected on US in the antenatal period. An abdominal mass may be palpable in the neonate, but there are usually no other symptoms or signs.

Management

Multicystic dysplastic kidney is managed mainly by US monitoring of growth of the healthy kidney. The abnormal kidney usually involutes (shrinks in size until it is not visible), in 60% of cases by the time the child is 10 years old. However, if it does not, there is a risk of malignant change, so the abnormal kidney is monitored by ultrasound or some patients opt for preventative nephrectomy as the kidney is non-functioning.

Prognosis is good for unilateral multicystic dysplastic kidney. However, the normal kidney is at increased risk of vesicoureteric reflux (see page 227). This would require investigation, because the one remaining kidney is essential for the maintenance of normal renal function in children with multicystic dysplastic kidney.

Bilateral multicystic dysplastic kidney is incompatible with life.

Duplex kidney

A duplex kidney is a normal anatomical variant in which there is duplication of the pelvicalyceal and ureteric systems (**Figure 7.2**). It occurs in 1 in 750 children.

Clinical features

Many duplex kidneys are asymptomatic and present as an incidental finding. However, some children with duplex kidney present with recurrent urinary tract infections, because the duplicated ureter is prone to hydronephrosis and vesicoureteric reflux (see page 227). The condition is then identifiable on renal US when investigations into any underlying cause for the urinary tract infections are carried out.

Management

No intervention is required in children who are asymptomatic. However, children with recurrent urinary tract infection require monitoring and occasionally prophylactic antibiotics (see page 230).

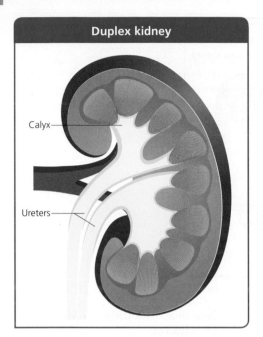

Duplex kidney

Calyx

Ureters

Figure 7.2 A duplex kidney: two ureters from one kidney.

A **horseshoe kidney** is diagnosed when the kidneys are found to be fused at the isthmus to form a horseshoe shape. A horseshoe kidney is usually located in the pelvis as the iliac vessels obstruct the kidney migrating up the abdomen during fetal development.

Hydronephrosis

In hydronephrosis, there is dilatation of the renal collecting system (**Figure 7.3**) as a consequence of blockage or reflux at positions along the urinary system (**Table 7.3**). The site of the blockage or reflux determines whether the hydronephrosis occurs unilaterally or bilaterally (**Figure 7.4**).

Clinical features and diagnostic approach

Hydronephrosis is usually asymptomatic. It is frequently identified on antenatal US scans, and may also be detected during US investigation for recurrent urinary tract infections. The underlying cause for the dilatation (reflux or blockage) is determined by other investigations, for example micturating cystourethrography for urinary reflux

Causes of hydronephrosis	
Cause	Site
Obstruction	Pelviureteric junction
	Vesicoureteric junction
	Bladder neck (posterior urethral valves)
Reflux	Vesicoureteric junction

Table 7.3 Causes of hydronephrosis

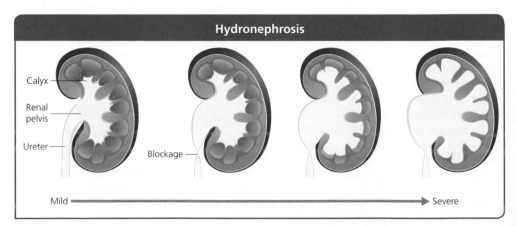

Hydronephrosis

Calyx

Renal pelvis

Ureter

Blockage

Mild ←——————————————————→ Severe

Figure 7.3 As hydronephrosis becomes more severe, the ureter, renal pelvis and calyces become increasingly dilatated.

(see below) or a radio-isotope scan for ureteric blockage.

Management

Management and prognosis depend on the underlying cause of the hydronephrosis and the damage sustained by the kidney. Posterior urethral valves and vesico-ureteric reflux are discussed below. Obstruction to the ureters rarely requires surgery, the narrowing improving with the child's growth.

> **Hydronephrosis is not always congenital.** It can occur later in adulthood as a result of various different causes, for example renal stones.

Posterior urethral valves

Posterior urethral valves are a congenital anomaly in which a membrane (valve) develops in the posterior neck of the urethra in the region of the prostate, thereby obstructing the flow of urine from the bladder. Posterior urethral valves are the commonest cause of bladder obstruction in male babies, occurring in about 1 in 8000 live births. Females are not affected due to their different anatomy. The cause for this embryonic anomaly has not been identified.

Clinical features

Obstruction of the flow of urine from the bladder results in:

- dribbling of urine and a poor urinary stream, and consequently an enlarged bladder
- hydronephrosis secondary to urinary obstruction and reflux (see **Figure 7.4**)
- recurrent urinary tract infections secondary to stagnation of urine

Antenatal detection of bilateral hydronephrosis in male fetuses raises suspicion of posterior urethral valves.

Diagnostic approach

Diagnosis of posterior urethral valves is confirmed by US scan, micturating cystourethrography and cystoscopy.

Management

A catheter is inserted to allow the urine to drain, after which the valve is surgically ablated. Prognosis depends on the severity of the damage sustained by the kidneys secondary to back pressure from the obstructed and refluxing urine.

Vesicoureteric reflux

Vesicoureteric reflux is the backward flow of urine from the bladder into the ureters and towards the kidneys, resulting in dilatation of the renal tract. It affects 1 in 100 children, girls more commonly than boys, and is frequently familial. It occurs as a result of anatomical anomalies at the vesicoureteric junction or secondary to conditions leading to bladder obstruction, such as posterior urethral valves. It can be unilateral or bilateral.

Clinical features

Vesicoureteric reflux is either detected following investigations for an antenatal diagnosis of hydronephrosis, or following a urinary tract infection in an infant or toddler. Reflux of the urine results in recurrent urinary infections or pyelonephritis, because the urine becomes stagnant and infected. Recurrent infections occasionally lead to scarring of the kidneys (reflux nephropathy) in children under 2 years of age.

Diagnostic approach

Vesicoureteric reflux is suspected in the presence of hydronephrosis detected antenatally (**Figure 7.4**), or recurrent or unusual organism urinary tract infections. Micturating cystourethrography is used to confirm the diagnosis and grade the severity of any reflux (**Figures 7.5** and **7.6**).

Management

Management depends on the severity of the reflux. Prophylactic antibiotics prevent infection or reduce the frequency of infections, thereby preventing or reducing damage to the kidney. Most children grow out of the problem. However, if a child continues to have recurrent urinary infections or severe reflux, or if

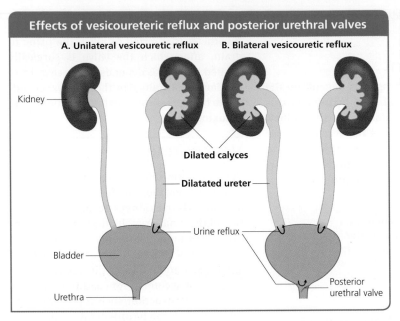

Effects of vesicoureteric reflux and posterior urethral valves

A. Unilateral vesicouretic reflux   B. Bilateral vesicouretic reflux

Kidney

Dilated calyces

Dilatated ureter

Urine reflux

Bladder

Posterior urethral valve

Urethra

Figure 7.4 Effects of (a) unilateral and (b) bilateral vesicoureteric reflux and posterior urethral valves on the urinary system.

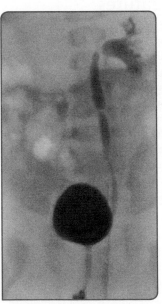

Figure 7.5 A micturating cystogram showing vesicouteretic reflux into the left kidney. Contrast inserted into the bladder via a urethral catheter shows retrograde flow (reflux) into the left kidney.

it is located anywhere along the ventral aspect of the penis. The condition occurs as a result of abnormal fusion of the urethral folds in the fetus. This leads to a proximally displaced urethral meatus (opening).

The cause of hypospadias is unknown but is likely to be a combination of different genetic and environmental factors, such as phytoestrogens in the mother's diet. It is common, occurring in 1 in 300 males in Europe (including the UK).

- Most cases (80%) are mild, with the urethral meatus still located in the glans of the penis
- In moderate hypospadias (15%), the urethral orifice is on the shaft
- In severe hypospadias (5%), the orifice is in the scrotum or perineum

There may also be an associated ventral chordee (downward curvature) of the penis. Surgical correction is required, unless the defect is mild and with no chordee.

the kidney shows signs of damage (scarring on US or radio-isotope scan), surgery may be required.

Hypospadias

Hypospadias is a congenital condition in which the opening of the urethra is not in its usual position at the tip of the penis; instead,

> **Babies with a hypospadias should not be circumcised.** This is because the foreskin may be required for the corrective surgery.

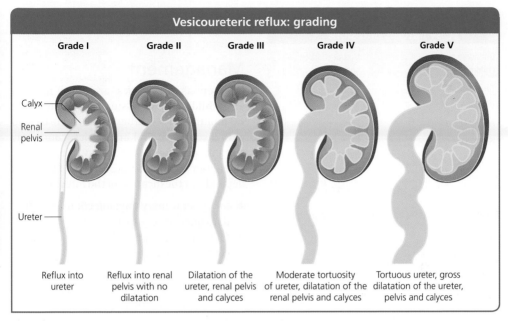

Figure 7.6 Grading of the severity of vesicoureteric reflux.

Urinary tract infections

A urinary tract infection is an infection in any part of the urinary system, i.e. the kidneys, ureters, bladder or urethra.

- Infection of the upper urinary tract causes acute pyelonephritis (inflammation of the kidney)
- Infection of the lower urinary tract causes cystitis (inflammation of the bladder)

Upper urinary tract infections are more serious than lower urinary tract infections, and are more likely to cause systemic symptoms.

The infection is usually bacterial, with the commonest pathogen being *E. coli* from the gut flora. Urinary tract infection is usually diagnosed when there is bacteriuria (bacteria in the urine) and pyuria (pus in the urine) in the presence of symptoms.

In the neonatal period bacteria reach the urinary tract via the blood stream, whereas later they ascend the urinary tract from the perineum. The risk of infection is increased with anatomic abnormalities such as vesicoureteric reflux and obstruction.

The prevalence of urinary tract infection varies markedly with sex and age. Symptomatic urinary tract infections occur in approximately 1.4 per 1000 neonates up to 3 months of age, and boys are more likely to be affected at this age. Thereafter it is much more common in girls due to their shorter urethra. By 6 years of age up to 8% of girls and 2% of boys have had a symptomatic urinary tract infection, with up to 30% having a recurrence within a year. By adolescence 1 in 10 girls and 1 in 30 boys will have been affected.

Clinical features

The clinical features of a urinary tract infection depend on the age of the child (**Table 7.4**) and which part of the urinary tract is affected.

> In babies, symptoms of urinary tract infection are very non-specific. Therefore a urinary tract infection needs to be actively excluded in any baby who presents 'unwell' or with an unexplained fever.

Urinary tract infection: symptoms and signs	
Babies and young (<4 years) children	Verbal children (>4 years)
Temperature	Dysuria
Vomiting	Frequency
Poor feeding	Loin and/or abdominal pain
Lethargy	Incontinence
Crying	Fever
	Vomiting

Table 7.4 Symptoms and signs of a urinary tract infection

Diagnostic approach

The diagnostic approach depends on the age of the child, but in all children the optimal method of urine collection is a 'clean catch' sample (see page 100).

■ In children older than 3 years, the diagnostic test is bedside dipstick urinalysis; a positive result shows the presence of both nitrites and leucocyte esterase
■ In children older than 3 years and with a history of recurrent urinary tract infection, after a positive result from dipstick urinalysis a urine sample is sent for culture before starting antibiotic treatment, to ensure that the bacterium is sensitive to the antibiotic used
■ In babies and other children younger than 3 years, the results of dipstick urinalysis

are unreliable, so diagnosis is based on microscopy and culture

Management

Intravenous antibiotics are used to treat any child who is systemically unwell or < 3 months old. All other children are treated with a course of oral antibiotics, commonly trimethoprim or co-amoxiclav (amoxicillin/clavulanic acid). The duration of treatment depends on the location of the infection:

■ for upper urinary tract infections, a 7–10 day course is required
■ for lower urinary tract infections, a 3-day course is adequate

In children older than 6 months, the prognosis for a first simple urinary tract infection is good, and no further action is required. In babies younger than 6 months, and children with recurrent or an atypical urinary tract infection, i.e. with an unusual organism, further investigations are required to rule out any renal tract abnormalities (e.g. vesicoureteric reflux) and to determine the need for prophylactic antibiotics.

> **In children with recurrent urinary tract infections, look at the previous results from urine culture.** Knowledge of the responsible pathogens and antibiotic sensitivity pattern in previous infections is used to direct antibiotic treatment for the current episode.

Nocturnal enuresis

Nocturnal enuresis (bed-wetting) is the involuntary voiding of urine while asleep.

■ In primary nocturnal enuresis, the child has never been consistently dry at night for a period of at least 6 months
■ In secondary nocturnal enuresis, the child has previously been dry at night, for at least 6 months

Epidemiology

Nocturnal enuresis is common. Its prevalence decreases with age; however, 2.6% of 7-year-olds still wet the bed on two or more nights per week. Boys are affected more than girls.

Aetiology

The cause of primary nocturnal enuresis is multifactorial. It is usually a combination of genetics (it is frequently associated with a family history), delayed maturation of bladder neurological control and small bladder capacity. A low level of vasopressin (anti-diuretic hormone) is a factor in some, causing overproduction of urine during the night. Secondary nocturnal enuresis is usually due to emotional issues or a urinary tract infection.

Clinical features

Although children with developmental delay are more likely to be affected, most children with nocturnal enuresis are neurodevelopmentally normal. Most children will have no other symptoms, but about 20% have associated symptoms of bladder dysfunction, such as daytime incontinence, frequency and urgency. Constipation can also contribute to the problem due to pressure on the bladder and incomplete bladder emptying during the daytime.

Diagnostic approach

Diagnosis is usually clinical and depends on a thorough history and examination. The most relevant points in the history are:

- the frequency and pattern of bed-wetting
- any daytime symptoms
- any associated symptoms, such as constipation
- the child's usual drinking and toileting habits

Questions to uncover a pathological cause, such as a urinary tract infection or diabetes, are also asked.

> **Noctural enuresis is rarely considered a problem in children younger than 5 years.** It is common in this age group but usually resolves over time. Families tend to seek help from their GP if the child is particularly distressed by the bed-wetting, or if it is causing social difficulties, for example when the child stays with friends overnight.

Urinalysis is carried out to screen for urinary tract infection or diabetes, unless the child has simple primary nocturnal enuresis only. Other investigations may be required if symptoms suggest an underlying pathology. For example, any abnormal neurology of the lower limbs suggesting a spinal cord lesion.

Management

Most children with nocturnal enuresis are managed with simple behavioural advice:

- encouraging the child to drink enough fluid during the day and use the toilet regularly, to prevent constipation; reward systems are helpful for this
- limiting the amount of fluid the child drinks immediately before bed, and reminding the child to use the toilet before going to sleep

If these measures are unsuccessful and the child is over 5 years and the bed-wetting is causing distress, a bed-wetting alarm system is considered. This consists of a moisture-sensitive pad, placed on either the child's night clothes or their mattress, which sounds an alarm if they start to wet the bed. Regular use of the alarm system helps to condition the child to wake, or inhibit bladder contraction in response to a full bladder.

Desmopressin, a synthetic hormone that mimics the action of antidiuretic hormone (vasopressin), is considered for children older than 7 years for whom an alarm system has been unsuccessful or is inappropriate (such as if the child shares a bedroom). It causes the kidneys to reabsorb more water, thereby reducing the amount of urine passed at night. It works well with up to 70% responding to some degree, but relapse is common (65%) on stopping and sustained effects are better when used in conjunction with rewards and the alarm.

> it is important that a child does not drink for 1 hour before and 8 hours after taking desmopressin as it can lead to fluid overload.

Prognosis

The prognosis is good. By 10 years of age 95% of children are dry at night, although estimated adult bed wetting rates are 0.5–2%.

Nephrotic syndrome

Nephrotic syndrome is the triad of proteinuria, hypoalbuminaemia and oedema caused by leakage of protein (mainly albumin) from the glomeruli into the urine. There may also be hyperlipidaemia as a consequence of increased production of lipoproteins which transport cholesterol and triglyceride, in conjunction with a general increased protein production by the liver in response to the hypoproteinaemia. There is also reduced lipid catabolism as a result of lower levels of the main lipoprotein breakdown enzyme, lipoprotein lipase (also a protein), and an increase in the hepatic synthesis of cholesterol.

The condition affects 1 in 50,000 children of European ethnicity, typically aged between 2 and 6 years. It is more common in children of Asian descent. Most childhood causes of nephrotic syndrome are idiopathic, but rarely it occurs secondary to systemic illness, such as systemic lupus erythematosus or Henoch–Schönlein purpura.

Nephrotic syndrome is classified histologically as follows.

- **Minimal change disease** (80% of cases): there is no glomerular inflammation and no changes are visible on normal light microscopy; however, electron microscopy shows effacement of the podocytes forming the filter in the Bowman's capsule in some glomeruli. The pathogenesis is unknown
- **Focal segmental glomerulosclerosis** (10% of cases): there is sclerosis of the podocytes in some glomeruli. There is a defined genetic cause in up to 25% of cases
- **Membranoproliferative glomerulonephritis** (6% of cases): there is inflammation and proliferation of the glomerular basement membrane and mesangium (the supporting structure of the glomerular capillaries) . It is is due to immune complex deposition or abnormalities of the alternative pathway of complement

Clinical features

The most common presenting feature in children is periorbital oedema. As the disease progresses, the oedema becomes more generalised, with scrotal swelling in boys.

The oedema is caused by leakage of fluid into interstitial spaces as the result of loss of intravascular oncotic pressure. Ascites and pleural effusions can occur in severe nephrotic syndrome. Some children with nephrotic syndrome can present in shock, because of low intravascular fluid volume.

> **Nephrotic syndrome presenting as bilateral periorbital oedema may be mistaken for allergy.** Dipstick urinalysis is used to test for proteinuria, unless there are other features of allergy.

Diagnostic approach

Diagnosis is based on clinical findings and investigations. Dipstick urinalysis shows a positive result for protein, and proteinuria is confirmed by a high early morning protein:creatinine ratio. It is taken after waking because proteinuria increases with upright posture and physical activity. Blood tests show low levels of protein, especially albumin, and hyperlipidaemia. Because the most likely cause in children is minimal change disease, which has a good response to steroids, a renal biopsy is only indicated if any of the following conditions apply:

- age < 1 year or > 8 years
- hypertension
- gross haematuria
- proteinuria > 4 weeks after starting steroids

Management

Terms used in the management of nephrotic syndrome are listed in **Table 7.5**. The condition is treated with steroids, which induce remission in most children (80–90%). However, many of these children (up to 75% of those who have remitted) experience a relapse within 2 years of the start of initial treatment, particularly when they are unwell such as with a viral infection (common cold).

Terms used in management of nephrotic syndrome	
Term	Definition
Remission	Trace or negative result for protein on dipstick urinalysis for ≥ 3 consecutive days
Relapse	3+ result for protein on dipstick urinalysis for ≥ 3 consecutive days
Steroid dependent	Proteinuria during tapering of steroids
Steroid resistant	Persistent proteinuria after 4 weeks of steroid treatment
Frequent relapses	More than two relapses within 6 months of diagnosis

Table 7.5 Definition of terms commonly used in the management of nephrotic syndrome

Of the 75% of children who experience a relapse, a minority are steroid dependent and therefore experience a relapse as soon as steroids are tapered or discontinued. These children, and those who do not respond to the initial steroid treatment, usually require treatment with other immunosuppressants, such as ciclosporin.

Other elements of management include a low salt diet and fluid restriction initially, to reduce the fluid retention (oedema). Children with nephrotic syndrome also lose other proteins, such as antithrombin III and immunoglobulins, through the kidney. This puts them at risk of venous thrombosis and infection with encapsulated organisms, so clinicians are advised to ensure that the child's pneumococcal vaccinations are up to date.

Prognosis

For children with minimal change disease, the prognosis is good; most will stop having relapses by adulthood. Patients with the other types of nephrotic syndrome have variable prognosis, ranging from most cases of minimal change nephropathy remitting spontaneously within 5 years, to 30% of membranous nephropathy progressing to end-stage renal failure. End-stage renal failure is managed with renal dialysis or renal transplant. Recurrence of membranous nephropathy post-transplant is common.

Glomerulonephritis

Glomerulonephritis is inflammation of the glomeruli. The inflamed glomeruli allow red blood cells and protein to leak into the urine, so kidney function is impaired. The exact cause of glomerulonephritis is not fully understood, but it is usually the result of an abnormal immune response to an infection or other disease, with antigen-antibody complexes trapped in the renal parenchyma leading to an inflammatory process and cell proliferation within the glomeruli.

The condition can be primary or secondary.

- In **primary glomerulonephritis**, the disease is isolated to the kidney, for example in immunoglobulin A nephropathy, in which there is abnormal deposition of immunoglobulin A in the glomeruli
- **Secondary glomerulonephritis** is caused by a systemic condition, such as Henoch-Schönlein purpura vasculitis (see page 234) or systemic lupus erythematosus

In children, glomerulonephritis is most commonly secondary to a group A streptococcal infection.

Clinical features

The main clinical findings are microscopic or macroscopic haematuria which manifests as red or brown, cola-coloured urine, and proteinuria. Associated features are decreased urine production, hypertension and oedema.

The history may suggest a recent streptococcal infection, such as sore throat or skin infection.

Diagnostic approach

Diagnosis is based mainly on urinalysis showing the presence of blood and variable levels of proteinuria. Renal function (serum urea and creatinine) is checked, because there can be renal failure. In post-streptococcal glomerulonephritis, the results of throat swab culture or blood test (anti-streptolysin titre, ASOT) may indicate a recent streptococcal infection, and concentrations of the C3 component of complement are low.

If the diagnosis is clearly post-streptococcal glomerulonephritis, based on the results of throat swab and blood ASOT, kidney biopsy is not indicated. However, biopsy is required for the diagnosis of all other causes of glomerulonephritis.

Management

Post-streptococcal glomerulonephritis usually starts to resolve spontaneously within a couple of weeks. Therefore its management is based on fluid and salt restriction, and monitoring of renal function and blood pressure. Diuretics and antihypertensives are also required to treat hypertension if present.

For other causes of glomerulonephritis, steroids or immunosuppressants are indicated to control the inflammatory process underlying the glomerulonephritis.

The prognosis for post-streptococcal glomerulonephritis is good; in the vast majority there is a complete recovery. However, many children with other causes of glomerulonephritis develop chronic kidney failure or hypertension.

Henoch–Schönlein purpura

Henoch–Schönlein purpura is a vasculitis that causes inflammation of small blood vessels in several systems in the body. It is the most common vasculitic disease of childhood, with an annual incidence in the order of 10–20 per 100,000 children between the ages of 2 and 11 years. Boys are more affected than girls.

The condition is thought to occur via an immune-mediated process triggered by an infection, usually of the upper respiratory tract.

Clinical features

Inflammation of the blood vessels causes blood to leak into the surrounding tissue, causing the characteristic palpable purpuric rash, mainly on the legs and buttocks (**Figure 7.7**). Associated symptoms include joint pain and swelling, particularly of the knees and ankles, and abdominal pain.

There may also be features of complications, such as glomerulonephritis, gastrointestinal bleeding or intussusception.

Diagnostic approach

Diagnosis is clinical, based on the rash and other symptoms. However, a full blood count and coagulation tests are usually carried out to rule out other causes of purpura, such

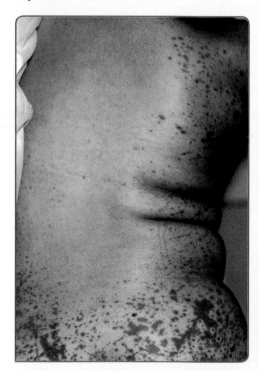

Figure 7.7 The typical purpuric rash in Henoch–Schönlein purpura, on the buttocks and back.

as thrombocytopenia. Urinalysis and kidney function tests are done to exclude renal impairment.

Management

Treatment for Henoch-Schönlein purpura is supportive, and includes analgesia for arthralgia, and monitoring of blood pressure and dipstick urinalysis to identify any renal involvement. Most children recover without problems, but the condition can recur and 1% of patients develop end-stage renal disease.

Renal failure

Renal failure is classed as acute kidney injury or chronic kidney disease.

- **Acute kidney injury** is the sudden or rapid decline of renal function, leading to retention of waste products; the impairment of renal function may be reversible, depending on the cause
- **Chronic kidney disease** is irreversible injury leading to renal function that is persistently reduced and may progress to below the critical level needed to maintain homeostasis

The differentiation of acute kidney injury from chronic kidney disease is usually straightforward. However, the diagnosis of acute-on-chronic kidney disease is more challenging.

Acute kidney injury

Acute kidney injury has prerenal, renal and post-renal causes (**Table 7.6**).

Clinical features

The clinical features of acute kidney injury depend on the cause, but the child will feel non-specifically unwell and be passing little or no urine. A detailed history and examination will usually identify the underlying cause, for example diarrhoea and vomiting with signs of hypovolaemia or hypovolaemic shock, or starting a new medication.

Diagnostic approach

The diagnosis of acute kidney injury is made on the basis of a detailed history, examination and investigations. Blood tests show increased levels of urea and creatinine, and sometimes electrolyte disturbances, including hyperkalaemia and hyponatremia. Metabolic acidosis is occasionally also present.

Management

Management depends on the underlying cause but always includes monitoring of electrolyte levels and fluid balance and correction of any abnormalities. Children with severe acute kidney injury need to be cared for in a specialist renal unit or intensive care unit and occasionally dialysis may be required. Prognosis depends on the severity of the renal failure and its underlying cause.

Acute kidney injury: categorisation of causes		
Prerenal	Renal	Post-renal
Hypovolaemia, for example as a result of: ■ diarrhoea ■ vomiting ■ haemorrhage ■ burns	Haemolytic uraemic syndrome	Posterior urethral valves
	Glomerulonephritis	Renal stones
	Use of or overdose of certain drugs, for example: ■ aminoglycosides ■ amphotericin B	Blocked catheter
Heart failure		
Renal artery stenosis		
Use of or overdose/accidental ingestion of certain drugs, for example: ■ non-steroidal anti-inflammatory drugs ■ angiotensin-converting enzyme inhibitors	Autoimmune disease (i.e. systemic lupus erythematosus)	

Table 7.6 Prerenal, renal and post-renal causes of acute kidney injury

Chronic kidney disease

Chronic kidney disease is generally defined as a glomerular filtration rate of:

- < 60 mL/min/1.73m^2 in the absence of any other kidney abnormalities
- < 90 mL/min/1.73m^2 if there is a known structural defect or abnormality on urinalysis

However, these definitions do not apply to children under 2 years old, because their glomerular filtration rate is physiologically lower. Chronic kidney disease can be further staged at decreasing levels of glomerular filtration rate.

Chronic kidney disease is uncommon in childhood. It is normally caused by congenital or structural problems with the kidneys, occasionally acquired or inherited conditions. The most common causes are:

- Hypoplastic or dysplastic kidneys
- Reflux nephropathy
- Obstructive uropathy
- Focal segmental glomerulosclerosis
- Polycystic kidney disease

Clinical features

The presenting symptoms of chronic kidney disease depend on the underlying cause, for example haematuria, proteinuria or oedema in glomerular disease; however, it is asymptomatic in its early stages. As the disease advances, symptoms include lethargy, anorexia, nausea and vomiting. Clinical findings include hypertension, poor growth, anaemia, and metabolic or biochemical disturbance leading to metabolic acidosis.

Management

Management is based on regular monitoring and the attempted preservation of existing renal function via control of blood pressure and the avoidance of any triggers for further deterioration, for example dehydration or the use of nephrotoxic drugs.

Management of complications (**Table 7.7**) is also important for growth and wellbeing, overseen by a paediatric nephrologist and a dietician.

Dialysis or kidney transplantation is usually needed if glomerular filtration rate

Chronic kidney disease: complications and their management		
Complication	Cause	Management
Poor nutrition	Anorexia and vomiting associated with chronic kidney disease	Calorie supplements Ensure adequate nutrition (sufficient intake of protein for growth to avoid accumulation of toxic metabolites)
Renal osteodystrophy	Reduced activation (1-hydroxylation) of vitamin D leading to secondary hyperparathyroidism (leads to phosphate retention and hypocalcaemia)	Phosphate restriction (reduce milk intake) Calcium carbonate (phosphate binder) Activated vitamin D supplements
Acidosis	Urinary bicarbonate wasting	Bicarbonate supplements
Salt and water balance	Structural malformations and dysplasia associated with salt and water loss	Adequate access to water and sodium chloride supplement
Anaemia	Decreased production of erythropoietin Low-grade haemolysis	Recombinant human erythropoietin injections, oral iron and folic acid
Hormone abnormalities	Growth hormone resistance (high circulating levels) Delayed puberty	Recombinant human growth hormone injections
Hypertension	Sodium and water overload Excessive renin production	Angiotensin-converting enzyme inhibitors

Table 7.7 Complications and management of chronic kidney disease

decreases to < 15 mL/min/1.73 m² (end-stage renal failure).

Haemolytic uraemic syndrome

Haemolytic uraemic syndrome is the triad of:

- haemolysis of red blood cells, causing anaemia and jaundice
- acute kidney injury, which increases urea levels
- low levels of platelets

It affects about 1 in 100,000 children, mainly Caucasian and under 5 years of age (UK data). Boys and girls are affected equally. It is typically secondary to exposure to Shiga-like toxin produced by *E. coli* O157. The *E. coli* O157 infection is most commonly acquired via consumption of contaminated meat. The Shiga-like toxin binds to specific receptors on the glomerular endothelial cells. The resulting damage to the endothelial cells leads to microthrombi in the arterioles and capillaries (thrombotic microangiopathy), platelet activation, widespread inflammation and red blood cell fragmentation. About 5% of childhood cases are not secondary to exposure to Shiga-like toxin; their causes include nonenteric infections, drugs and a familial type.

Clinical features

There is a recent history of vomiting and diarrhoea, which is often bloody, 3–7 days before the onset of haemolytic uraemic syndrome. The child is generally unwell, pale or jaundiced, with reduced urine output. There may be haematuria. A minority, mainly non-Shiga type, have neurological features; encephalopathy, stroke and seizures.

Diagnostic approach

Full blood count shows anaemia and thrombocytopenia, and there is evidence of haemolysis on blood film. The haemolysis is not autoimmune (as it is Coombs test negative); it is microangiopathic haemolysis, the thrombi in the vessels physically destroying the red blood cells. Renal function is impaired, with features of acute renal failure (see above) in 70% of children. Microbiological analysis of a stool sample will confirm the presence of *E. coli* O157 if this is the cause.

Management

Management is supportive and includes correction of fluid and electrolyte imbalances. Dialysis or transfusion may be required to manage the acute renal failure and the haemolytic anaemia. Most children (70–85%) with typical haemolytic uraemic syndrome make a full recovery, but regular follow-up is needed to monitor renal function. If the renal failure continues (end-stage or chronic renal failure) the child will need renal dialysis or a renal transplant. Overall mortality is 5–15%, but of those with non-Shiga disease 25% die during the acute phase, and 50% will have end-stage renal failure.

Genital disorders in boys

Although hernia, hydrocele and undescended testes are morphological abnormalities, they are classed as normal variants or reflections of underlying weakness rather than congenital anomalies. Development of all three conditions is linked, and can be traced to problems with the in utero descent of the testes from their initial position near the kidneys to their final position within the scrotum (see page 14).

- Herniae or hydroceles result from failure of closure of the processus vaginalis and resulting weakness in the abdominal wall
  - If the passage is wide, a hernia develops
  - If it is narrow, a hydrocele is more likely
- Undescended testes are the consequence of their incomplete descent

Other common problems of the male genitalia are testicular torsion and inflammation, usually associated with infection, of the epididymis (epididymitis) and testicle (orchitis). Tightness of the foreskin (phimosis) can lead to infection of the penis (balanitis), managed by circumcision, although some boys are circumcised for religious or cultural beliefs.

Hernia

A hernia is the protrusion of an internal organ or tissue through a weakness in its containing cavity. In children the commonest type is an inguinal hernia (**Figure 7.8**), which results from protrusion of the intestine through the abdominal wall via the inguinal canal. It is present in 3% of term newborns in a male:female ration of 9:1. Its incidence rises with increasing prematurity.

Clinical features

Features include a painless swelling, which may be intermittent, in the inguinal region or the scrotum. The swelling is impalpable from above. At this stage, the hernia can be reduced by gentle sustained pressure on the swelling up towards the abdomen.

An incarcerated (unable to be reduced, therefore 'stuck' outside the abdominal cavity) hernia presents as a painful firm and irreducible mass. Symptoms of obstruction, such as abdominal distension and vomiting, are often present.

Diagnostic approach

The diagnosis is usually made on clinical examination. However, it may be confirmed by US if there is any uncertainty regarding the diagnosis such as when a hydrocele is also present.

> **When attempting to reduce a hernia in a baby, always ensure that they are settled.** Increased intra-abdominal pressure secondary to crying prevents reduction of a hernia. It may then be mistakenly diagnosed as irreducible.

Management

Inguinal herniae in babies are at high risk of incarceration so require surgical repair on an elective basis at the earliest opportunity. An incarcerated hernia warrants urgent surgical reduction to avoid ischaemia of its contents due to pressure on the blood vessels at the tight hernia orifice.

Hydrocele

A hydrocele is a collection of peritoneal fluid in the scrotum (**Figure 7.9**). The fluid enters the scrotum via a patent processus vaginalis, which allows communication between the peritoneum and the scrotum. Hydrocele is present in 5% of newborn boys.

Clinical features and diagnostic approach

A hydrocele appears as a painless fluctuant scrotal swelling. Hydroceles vary in size between individual patients. The condition can be unilateral or bilateral.

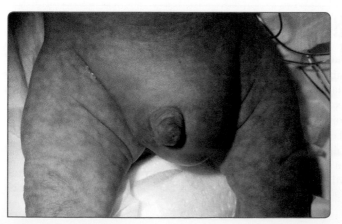

Figure 7.8 A left inguinal hernia in a baby who had been born preterm.

Case 11 *continued*

with the left. His reflexes are more brisk on the right side.

Interpretation of findings

The examination findings are consistent with a right upper motor neurone lesion, which suggests a left-sided cerebral lesion. Jack appears to be developing normally otherwise, playing and interacting socially in a way that is appropriate for his age.

Investigations

A blood sample is obtained for serum creatine kinase concentration, which is normal. A normal creatine kinase excludes a muscular dystrophy. A non-urgent MRI scan of Jack's brain is carried out a few weeks later; the results are normal.

> **Always measure the serum creatine kinase (CK) in boys with delayed walking.**

Diagnosis

A diagnosis of mild hemiplegic cerebral palsy is made. With intensive physiotherapy and the use of splints, Jack's gross motor skills improve significantly. He goes on to attend mainstream school and is progressing well.

Case 12 A seizure at school

Presentation

Ali, a 9-year-old boy, is brought to hospital by his teacher after a collapse at school. He had been his normal self all morning but collapsed in the playground during playtime. A teaching assistant had witnessed what she described as a 'fit'. Ali is now upset and crying, asking for his mother.

Initial interpretation

What is perceived as a 'fit' by a layperson can have many different causes, either epileptic in origin or non-epileptic. For example, it could be:

- a simple faint
- a collapse with a cardiac cause, for example long QT syndrome or another cardiac arrhythmia
- a true epileptic seizure
- a reflex anoxic seizure
- a pseudoseizure or other result of a behavioural problem
- cataplexy

Careful history and examination are essential to clarify the nature of the 'fit' and determine its cause.

History

Ali's teacher was called to the playground by another child. On her arrival, Ali was conscious but confused and disoriented. The teaching assistant explained that she had seen Ali fall to the floor, jerking his arms and legs. The episode lasted about 1 minute. An ambulance was called, and Ali slept all the way to hospital.

Interpretation of history

A good history is the key to distinguishing between epilepsy and non-epileptic causes of an apparent seizure. In Ali's case, features supporting a diagnosis of a generalised tonic–clonic seizure include jerking of all limbs and an apparent postictal phase (the period of recovery after a seizure, during which sleepiness, confusion and emotional upset are common).

Case 12 *continued*

However, generalised tonic–clonic seizure can be caused by both epileptic and non-epileptic conditions. More information is needed regarding the onset of the episode and any other associated features before the cause can by narrowed down to an epileptic seizure.

Further history

Through a phone call to the teaching assistant, it is ascertained that Ali was playing when he suddenly let out a cry, fell to the ground and went completely stiff before both his arms and his legs started jerking rhythmically. He was unresponsive, and his lips turned blue.

Ali's mother arrives. She says that he is normally healthy and doing well at school. There is no family history of epilepsy, seizures or sudden death.

Examination

Reassured by his mother's arrival, Ali is now settled, fully alert and oriented. There is a small bite at the side of his tongue, but no other injuries. Cardiovascular, respiratory and neurological examinations are normal. Ali has recovered fully.

Interpretation of findings

The history is consistent with a first generalised tonic–clonic seizure. There are no other concerning features.

Investigations

The results of 12-lead electrocardiography (ECG) show sinus rhythm with a normal corrected QT interval. No other investigations are indicated at present.

Implications of a diagnosis of epilepsy

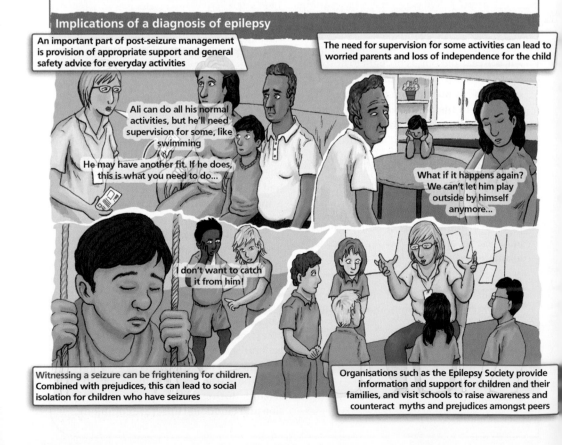

An important part of post-seizure management is provision of appropriate support and general safety advice for everyday activities

The need for supervision for some activities can lead to worried parents and loss of independence for the child

Ali can do all his normal activities, but he'll need supervision for some, like swimming

He may have another fit. If he does, this is what you need to do...

What if it happens again? We can't let him play outside by himself anymore...

I don't want to catch it from him!

Witnessing a seizure can be frightening for children. Combined with prejudices, this can lead to social isolation for children who have seizures

Organisations such as the Epilepsy Society provide information and support for children and their families, and visit schools to raise awareness and counteract myths and prejudices amongst peers

Case 12 *continued*

Diagnosis

One seizure does not constitute epilepsy, and treatment is not indicated at present. Ali's mother is counselled that he could have further episodes, at which point medication would be discussed. She is given first aid advice and advice on general safety measures to take in the event of another seizure before Ali is then discharged home.

Congenital anomalies of the central nervous system

Congenital anomalies of the central nervous system are the result of insults to the fetus occurring at any time up to week 20 of development. The most common are neural tube defects and hydrocephalus. At 0.3–200 per 10,000 births, the prevalence of neural tube defects varies widely across the world, depending on many factors including nutrition; in Europe it averages 9 per 10,000 births. Prevalence is lower in live births, e.g. 2.3 per 10,000 live births versus 16 per 10,000 pregnancies in the UK. For hydrocephalus the corresponding UK figures are 4.5 and 9 per 10,000. Congenital anomalies of the central nervous system are usually detected on antenatal US scans.

> Pregnancies affected by neural tube defects or hydrocephalus can end in spontaneous abortion or be terminated if the anomaly is incompatible with life or there is a risk of severe disability. This is the reason for the discrepancy between the proportion of affected pregnancies and the proportion of affected live births.

Neural tube defects

Neural tube defects are caused by incomplete fusion of the neural folds during formation of the neural tube, the precursor of the spinal cord and brain (see page 7). Therefore neural tube defects can affect either structure:

- the spinal cord is affected in 1.8 per 10,000 live births
- the brain is affected in 0.5 per 10,000 live births

Neural tube defects are the result of herniation of neural tissue through associated defects in the skull or vertebrae.

- A **myelomeningocele** occurs in the spine and involves both meninges and spinal tissue (**Figure 8.1**). It is the most common neural tube defect and is classed as a severe form of spina bifida, comprising 90% of spina bifida cases
- A **meningocele** is herniation of only the meninges through a defect. It is less common than myelomeningocele. It occurs:
  - in the vertebrae (comprising 10% of spina bifida cases)
  - in the skull (cranial meningocele)
- An **encephalocele** is herniation of brain tissue through a skull defect. Posterior encephaloceles are most common in western countries, most being occipital. If below the brain tentorium they are associated with severe cerebellar defects, e.g. Chiari III malformation (see below). In some parts of Asia, anterior encephaloceles are more common and may protrude into the nose, ethmoid or orbit, including olfactory and frontal lobe tissue.
- **Anencephaly** is failure of development of part of the skull and brain; it affects 0.1 per10,000 live births and it is incompatible

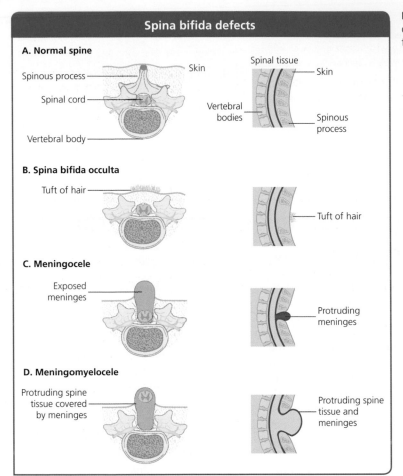

Spina bifida defects

A. Normal spine

Spinous process

Spinal cord

Vertebral body

Skin

Spinal tissue

Skin

Vertebral bodies

Spinous process

B. Spina bifida occulta

Tuft of hair

Tuft of hair

C. Meningocele

Exposed meninges

Protruding meninges

D. Meningomyelocele

Protruding spine tissue covered by meninges

Protruding spine tissue and meninges

Figure 8.1 The defects in different forms of spina bifida.

with life. Up to 75% of the anencephalic fetuses are stillborn with the remainder dying shortly after birth

A major cause of neural tube defects is maternal folic acid deficiency in the first month of pregnancy, when the neural tube is formed. Other risk factors include a family history and the use of antiepileptic medications by the mother (see page 149).

The incidence of neural tube defects has reduced dramatically over the past 50 years in high-economic countries, because of improved maternal nutrition and folic acid supplementation.

Spina bifida is Latin for 'split' spine'.

Clinical features

The clinical outcome depends on the level and type of lesion: the higher (nearer to the brain) the lesion and with nerve tissue involvement, the more significant the morbidity. Most children with a neural tube defect with nerve tissue involvement have some form of difficulty with bowel function (constipation and diarrhoea) and bladder control (frequency, urgency, incontinence or retention).

Myelomeningocele

Myelomeningocele is visible at birth as a cystic swelling (a sac not covered with skin) anywhere along the spinal cord, most commonly in the lumbosacral area (80% of cases). This sac consists of both meninges and spinal cord contents and may leak CSF. Damage to the spinal nerves occurs before delivery, so a neonate with myelomeningocele usually has weakness or total paralysis of the lower limbs with talipes at birth. There is loss of skin sensation in the lower limbs and around the perineum. Frequently, there is increased head circumference because hydrocephalus occurs in approximately 90% of cases of myelomeningocele at birth, although the head circumference may initially be within the normal range. The hydrocephalus usually becomes clinically significant once the spinal lesion is closed, especially if there has been CSF leakage through the defect (thus decompressing the hydrocephalus).

Many children with myelomeningocele have an associated type 2 Chiari malformation, i.e. downward displacement of the cerebellum through the foramen magnum (see page 250). This may lead to hydrocephalus.

Meningocele

A spinal meningocele also presents as a cystic swelling along the spine at birth, most commonly in the lumbosacral area. There is no associated hydrocephalus, and neural examination is usually normal.

Cranial meningocele/encephalocel

This appears as a swelling identified at birth, usually on the posterior midline aspect of the skull or between the forehead and nose. This can be skin which is covered or open. In 80% of encephalocele cases there is hydrocephalus (an increased head circumference).

> **Spina bifida occulta is a defect in the posterior vertebra, but with no herniation of meninges or spinal tissue.** It occurs in about 10% of the population, the incidence varying between populations, for example being higher in Britain than continental Europe and higher in women. It occasionally presents with weakness and lower motor neurone signs in the legs, or difficulties with control of the bladder and anal sphincter.

Diagnostic approach

A neural tube defect is diagnosed on clinical appearance, either antenatally or at birth. Most defects are diagnosed antenatally on fetal US, with fetal MRI used for further assessment. If the defect is first noted at birth on clinical examination, the extent of tissue herniation is determined by MRI, and cranial US is used to assess any associated hydrocephalus (see Figure 3.7).

Management

Neural tube defects require surgical correction. Open defects need to be closed as soon as possible to prevent infection (meningitis).

At birth, the lesion is covered with a sterile dressing, the baby is nursed in a prone position and preventive antibiotics are given. Surgery is carried out within 48 hours of birth.

Ongoing management requires a multidisciplinary team approach. Further surgery may be required to correct complications, for example talipes and hydrocephalus. Regular US monitoring of the renal tract is also essential to identify and manage any neurological bladder outflow obstruction. Intermittent catheterisation several times a day is necessary if there is urinary retention from outflow obstruction.

Prognosis

The prognosis for neural tube defects depends on the site and severity of the lesion, and associated complications. Lower limb paralysis usually leads to the use of a wheelchair. Children with lesser paralysis may walk with crutches or braces, or walk unaided. Children with an encephalocele are more likely to have spastic weakness of all four limbs, uncoordinated muscle movements, delayed developmental milestones, vision problems and seizures.

Hydrocephalus

Hydrocephalus is characterised by excessive accumulation of cerebrospinal fluid in the cerebral ventricles. Cerebrospinal fluid is formed continuously, primarily by the ependymal cells of the choroid plexus in the ventricles. It circulates within the ventricles and subarachnoid space and around the spinal cord. It is reabsorbed by the arachnoid granulations into the dural venous sinuses. Hydrocephalus can be divided into two categories according to the way in which it develops.

- In communicating hydrocephalus, the build-up of cerebrospinal fluid is the consequence of its excessive production or reduced absorption
- In non-communicating hydrocephalus, cerebrospinal fluid accumulates because of obstruction of its outflow from the ventricles

Hydrocephalus is congenital or acquired. Congenital hydrocephalus affects about 0.6 in 1000 live births and is usually non-communicating; the flow of cerebrospinal fluid is obstructed by a structural malformation, for example cerebral aqueduct stenosis or Chiari malformation. Non-communicating hydrocephalus occasionally indicates a congenital infection. Acquired hydrocephalus, such as post-haemorrhagic hydrocephalus in preterm babies or after meningitis in older children, develops as a consequence of impaired absorption of cerebrospinal fluid and is therefore classed as communicating hydrocephalus.

Clinical features

The symptoms of hydrocephalus depend on whether or not the fontanelle has closed and the cranial sutures have fused, and therefore differ in children of different ages.

- In a baby, the first sign may be a rapidly increasing head circumference, with separation of the sutures; later signs (which occur within a couple of weeks if the increased pressure is not relieved) include vomiting, lethargy, dilated scalp veins and 'sunsetting' eyes
- In an older child (> 1 year of age) when the sutures have fused, the signs and symptoms of hydrocephalus are the same as those of increased intracranial pressure (see page 391)

> **The 'sunsetting' sign is a late presenting sign of hydrocephalus.** It is an up-gaze paresis caused by increased intracranial pressure, resulting in both eyes appearing to be driven downwards. The lower portion of the iris and pupil is covered by the lower eyelid, like the sun behind the horizon, and sclera is visible between the upper eyelid and the iris.

Diagnostic approach

Congenital hydrocephalus is usually detected on an antenatal US scan. In a baby, cranial US through the fontanelle is an easy first investigation. In the older child, in whom the fontanelle will have closed, CT or MRI is required.

Management

The aim of hydrocephalus management is to reduce the increased intracranial pressure. For all non-communicating hydrocephalus and communicating hydrocephalus in children outside of the neonatal period, this requires surgical insertion of a ventriculoperitoneal shunt, a catheter and a valve with one end placed in the ventricle and the other end in the peritoneal cavity. The shunt drains cerebrospinal fluid from the ventricle into the peritoneal cavity, where it is reabsorbed into the lymphatics. In cases of post-haemorrhagic hydrocephalus (communicating) in pre-term babies, a temporary 'reservoir' is surgically inserted just under the scalp extending into the ventricle, enabling CSF to be removed by needle and syringe at regular (e.g. daily) intervals while waiting for the blood clots blocking CSF drainage to resolve. If the hydrocephalus continues to increase despite this treatment, a ventriculoperitoneal shunt is inserted.

Prognosis

The outcome primarily depends on any associated abnormalities rather than the hydrocephalus itself, as in a genetic syndrome, and the underlying cause, for example intraventricular haemorrhage and any associated brain parenchymal injury with prematurity. With a straightforward single malformation, such as aqueduct stenosis, outcomes are generally good. Complications of ventriculoperitoneal shunts include infection and blockage.

> **The Chiari (or Arnold–Chiari) malformation is characterised by downward displacement of the cerebellar tonsils through the foramen magnum.** It is graded in terms of increasing severity from type 1 to type 4. Type 1 is reduction or lack of development of the posterior fossa, and type 2 is associated with myelomeningocele. Types 3 and 4 are very rare.

Infections of the central nervous system

Central nervous system infections include meningitis, which affects the meninges, and encephalitis, which affects the brain tissue itself. Such infections can be life-threatening, and meningitis is sometimes associated with generalised sepsis carrying a significant risk of mortality (see page 398).

Epidemiology and aetiology

The causes of meningitis and encephalitis are listed in **Table 8.1**. Many bacteria and viruses cause meningitis, with their prevalence varying according to age group. Encephalitis is usually viral in origin. There is evidence that genetic factors contribute to susceptibility to meningitis and encephalitis and help determine the severity of an infection.

In developed countries the incidence of bacterial meningitis is about half that of viral meningitis. It has fallen in recent years as a result of the introduction of vaccines against some of the causative organisms, i.e. *Haemophilus influenzae* type b, *Pneumococcus* and *Meningococcus*.

Clinical features

Early identification of meningitis is difficult, because the signs and symptoms are vague and in most cases similar to those of a simple viral illness. However, it can quickly progress

Meningitis and encephalitis: causative organisms			
Bacterial meningitis in neonates and infants (0–12 months)	Bacterial meningitis in older children (> 12 months) and adolescents	Viral meningitis (all ages)	Encephalitis (all ages)
Group B *Streptococcus* *	Neisseria *meningitidis* type B*	Enteroviruses*	Herpes simplex*
Streptococcus pneumoniae†	*N. meningitidis* type A†	Herpes simplex	Varicella-zoster
Escherichia coli	*S. pneumoniae*†	Mumps (rare)†	Cytomegalovirus
Listeria	*Mycobacterium tuberculosis* (chronic infection)	Varicella (rare)	Epstein–Barr virus
N. meningitidis		Measles (rare)†	
H. influenzae type B†	*Haemophilus influenzae* type B†		

*The commonest current causes.

†The prevalence of these previously common organisms has been reduced by vaccination programmes in developed countries.

Table 8.1 Bacterial and viral causes of meningitis and encephalitis

to becoming life-threatening over a few hours. **Table 8.2** lists the signs and symptoms of meningitis in children and babies. A tense, bulging fontanelle in a child <1 year old or photophobia with neck stiffness and headache in a child > 1 year old particularly raise the suspicion of meningitis.

Encephalitis may present even more insidiously. Fever, vomiting and headache may be followed by the development of neurological signs, such as abnormal behaviour and confusion, altered consciousness and possibly seizures.

Diagnostic approach

Antibiotic treatment is initiated on clinical suspicion alone – the earlier, the better. Several investigations are used to aid diagnosis and guide management until identification of the causative organism.

Meningitis symptoms	
Babies (< 12 months)	Children and adolescents (1–18 years)
Irritability, with high-pitched cry	Photophobia (intolerance of light)
Tense, bulging fontanelle	Headache
Poor feeding	Neck stiffness
Hypotonia	Spreading rash (classically petechiae or purpuric)
Mottled skin	
Cold hands and feet	Diarrhoea
Fever, vomiting and seizure	Myalgia
	Fever, vomiting and seizure

Table 8.2 Symptoms of meningitis in babies and children

Blood tests

In bacterial meningitis, a full blood count may show neutrophilia. The concentration of C-reactive protein may be increased, but it can be normal in the first 12 h. Coagulation tests are needed in the presence of a purpuric rash or septic shock.

It is vital to obtain a blood sample for culture, ideally before the first dose of antibiotics. A blood sample is also needed for detection of meningococcal DNA by PCR.

In encephalitis, inflammatory markers may not be very high. However, a full blood count usually shows lymphocytosis.

Lumbar puncture

For a definitive diagnosis, a lumbar puncture must be carried out, unless contraindicated. The levels of protein and glucose in the cerebrospinal fluid, and the white cell count, are used to determine whether an infection is present, and if so, whether it is bacterial or viral (**Table 8.3**). Cerebrospinal fluid can also be sent for PCR tests to detect *Meningococcus*, *Pneumococcus*, herpes and enterovirus.

> **Contraindications for a lumbar puncture** are the presence of septic shock, signs of increased intracranial pressure or coagulopathy.

Imaging

If the patient has reduced consciousness, a CT scan is indicated to assess for increased intracranial pressure and to exclude other causes for the clinical picture. In encephalitis, CT may

Cerebrospinal fluid findings in CNS infections			
Feature	Bacterial meningitis	Viral meningitis or encephalitis	Tuberculous meningitis
Appearance	Cloudy or turbid	Clear	Clear or slightly cloudy
Organisms on microscopy?	Sometimes seen (Gram stain)	None	Occasionally seen (acid-fast stain, i.e. Ziehl–Neelsen stain)
White cell count	Increased (predominantly neutrophils)	Increased (predominantly lymphocytes)	Increased (mixed, with greater proportion of lymphocytes)
Glucose concentration	Low	Normal	Low
Protein concentration	High	Normal or high	Very high

Table 8.3 Characteristic features of cerebrospinal fluid in infections of the central nervous system

show signs of cerebral oedema and inflammation, especially in the temporal lobes.

Electroencephalography

This is useful only in suspected encephalitis; it may show abnormalities in the temporal regions.

Management

Prompt recognition and treatment are vital. The latter begins with ABC management and treatment of septic shock (see page 400). Broad-spectrum antibiotics, usually a third-generation cephalosporin (e.g. ceftriaxone) are started as early as possible. If encephalitis is suspected, aciclovir is added. A course of dexamethasone has been shown to decrease the rate of sensorinerual hearing loss in meningitis due to *H. influenzae* in children. Some children with shock or unconsciousness associated with the meningitis or encephalitis need to be nursed in an intensive care unit.

Prognosis

In meningitis, the prognosis depends on the pathogen and the severity of symptoms.

- In bacterial meningitis, mortality can be up to 10%, and potential long-term complications for survivors include deafness and developmental problems
- Most children with viral meningitis recover completely

Survival from encephalitis depends on the child's age (usually a higher death rate in children under 1 year) and the severity of their symptoms. Prompt treatment of herpes simplex encephalitis reduces overall mortality from 70% (untreated) to 10%. Mortality in neonates is up to 30% with disseminated infection. Cognitive, visual or motor neurological deficits may persist, especially if herpes simplex virus was the causative organism.

Collapse and seizures

A collapse is a sudden fall to the ground as a result of loss of consciousness. A seizure (also known as a fit or convulsion) is the consequence of excessive and/or hypersynchronous discharge of neurones in the brain, and is usually brief and self-limiting. Signs and symptoms of the abnormal neuronal activity vary from a momentary loss of awareness or unusual sensation to longer periods of unconsciousness accompanied by rhythmic jerking of the limbs.

In paediatrics, identifying the cause of collapse is not always straightforward, because it can be caused by very different conditions with similar presentations. **Table 8.4** provides information to guide the determination of the cause of collapse in children (see also pages 60 and 188). This section focuses on seizures, the main causes of which in children are epilepsies or fever.

The epilepsies

The epilepsies are a group of conditions characterised by recurrent epileptic seizures. Particular patterns of seizures are recognised and are associated with different prognoses.

Epidemiology and aetiology

About 5% of the population in the developed world will have a seizure at some point in their life; however, this does not mean they have epilepsy especially if there is a trigger for the seizure such as a head injury or hypoglycaemia. Epilepsy is usually idiopathic. A genetic component is likely, although no specific gene has been identified. Symptomatic epilepsies are those for which an underlying cause has been identified, such as a structural brain malformation or damage resulting from hypoxia-ischaemia or infection.

Clinical features

The clinical features of seizures depend on the type.

- In a **generalised seizure,** such as an absence seizure or a tonic–clonic seizure, the

General classification	Sub-classification	Description of episode	Loss of consciousness?	Recovery	Possible associated signs	Investigations
Epileptic: generalised	Generalised tonic–clonic seizure	Sometimes preceded by an 'aura' (unusual perception preceding seizure) Generalised stiffness followed by symmetrical jerking of arms and legs	Yes	Sleepy post-ictal phase	Tongue biting or incontinence	EEG: may be normal between episodes
	Absence (e.g. childhood absence epilepsy)	Suddenly stops mid-task, staring blankly and being non-responsive for a few seconds, then resuming task	Yes	Immediate	Generalised tonic–clonic seizure (minority of cases)	EEG: 3 Hz/s spike and wave pattern
	Myoclonic (e.g. juvenile myoclonic epilepsy)	Brief jerks, usually of an arm; actions are often considered 'clumsiness' if myoclonus is not recognised Often occurs on waking	No	Immediate	Generalised tonic–clonic seizure and absences (up to 60% of cases)	EEG: normal background with polyspike and wave discharges
Epileptic: focal	Motor	Variable (e.g. repetitive movements of one arm, hand or side of face)	Variable	Variable	Todd's paresis; temporary (minutes to hours) weakness of the body part that was involved in the seizure	EEG: may show localised abnormality, involving the frontal lobe (motor cortex)
	Non-motor	Variable symptoms relating to senses (e.g. visions, smells, tastes), cognitive, emotional and autonomic	Variable	Variable	Headache	EEG: may show localised abnormality (e.g. in temporal lobe)
Non-epileptic	Reflex anoxic seizure ('breath holding')	Precipitating unpleasant event, e.g. a fall Cry followed by pallor, stiffening and symmetrical jerks	Yes	Fast	Young children only (start aged 6–18 months, stop by 5 years)	Not indicated
	Daydreaming	Staring blankly, but can be distracted	No	Immediate	None	Not indicated
	Simple faint	Dizziness, nausea, feeling hot before a fall to ground	Yes	Within minutes	May have a few jerks of the limbs	EEG: not indicated ECG: normal
	Cardiac syncope	Sudden collapse	Variable	Fast	May occur during exercise	ECG: may show prolonged QT or arrhythmia (see page 107)

ECG, electrocardiography; EEG, electroencephalography.

Table 8.4 Epilepsy seizure classification and non-epileptic causes of collapse: clinical features and results of investigations

abnormal neuronal activity starts in both cerebral hemispheres simultaneously
- In a **focal seizure**, the activity starts in a distinct part of the brain, even if it later spreads to become generalised; focal seizures can be subdivided according to:
  - whether the symptoms are predominantly motor or sensory
  - the area of the brain that is the focus for the abnormal neuronal activity (e.g. frontal, temporal, parietal or occipital lobe epilepsy)

Table 8.4 lists the clinical features used to distinguish between the different types of epilepsy as well as non-epileptic causes of collapse.

Diagnostic approach

The diagnosis of epilepsy is based mainly on a detailed history. No single test confirms or excludes the diagnosis. However, several investigations are useful to classify seizures and to guide management.

Generally, no investigations are needed for a child presenting with a first seizure and who makes a quick recovery. However, it is prudent to carry out ECG to rule out a cardiac cause, such as a long QT syndrome (see page 107).

Blood tests

These are not indicated unless the clinical situation dictates. For example, glucose and electrolytes are measured if a seizure is ongoing, i.e. in status epilepticus (see page 408).

Imaging

Brain imaging is not routinely carried out unless the seizure is associated with a head injury, in which case an urgent CT scan is indicated. In children who develop epilepsy before the age of 2 years, or whose seizures have a focal onset, an outpatient MRI scan is recommended.

Electroencephalography

This should not be used to confirm or refute the diagnosis of epilepsy. For about 5% of children with a non-epileptic cause for their collapse the results show epileptiform abnormalities; conversely, an interictal electroencephalogram can be normal in children with epilepsy. Nevertheless, when the history strongly suggests epilepsy, electroencephalography can be used to provide information on the type of epilepsy and to assess for precipitating factors, such as photosensitivity.

Management

Drugs are not indicated after a first seizure, because at least 10% of children do not have any more. With recurrent seizures, the aim of medication is to reduce seizure frequency. Various anticonvulsant medications are available, each with its own merit and demerits. Control with a single medication is preferred, but some children require a combination for adequate control of their seizures.

The first-line medications are:

- sodium valproate for generalised seizures. This is contraindicated in sexually active teenage girls because of its teratogenicity. In these situations lamotrigine is prescribed instead
- carbamazepine for focal seizures

The family are given first aid advice and counselled regarding safety when carrying out daily activities, such as bathing.

Prognosis

Between 70 and 80% of children have no more seizures before adulthood. Persistent seizures lead to consideration of adherence to therapy and alternative diagnoses before further medications are started. Withdrawal of medication is considered after a seizure-free period of 2 years.

Epilepsy can be resistant to treatment, especially if there is an underlying brain abnormality. When deciding the appropriate anticonvulsant drug therapy for these patients, it is essential to balance the control of seizures with acceptable levels of adverse effects.

Febrile seizure

A febrile seizure is a seizure associated with fever caused by an infection outside the central nervous system in a 6-month-old to 7-year-old child, who is otherwise neurologically normal. Febrile seizures are not defined as an epilepsy.

Epidemiology and aetiology

Febrile seizures have a genetic component that is likely to be polygenic; siblings of a child who has had a febrile seizure have a 25% chance of having one themselves. They occur in up to 4% of children by the age of 5 years in Western Europe, and are a frequent cause of hospital admission. Febrile seizures occur in all races with the incidence ranging from 0.5–1.5% in China, and 5–10% in India and Japan in children under 5 years of age. Once a child has had a febrile seizure, the risk of a further episode is increased if:

- the first episode occurred at an early age (< 15 months)
- there is a family history of febrile seizure
- the fever had lasted only a short time (< 1 hour) before the seizure occurred
- the fever that precipitated the seizure was mild (<38.5°C)

Clinical features

Febrile seizures are usually generalised tonic–clonic, with stiffening of the body, eye rolling, jerking of the arms and legs, and loss of consciousness. Most are described as simple, but ≥ 30% are complex.

The characteristic features of simple and complex febrile seizures are shown in **Table 8.5**. Knowledge of the differences between the two is essential for guiding investigation and making decisions about hospital admission.

Diagnostic approach

The source of the fever should always be sought. This is usually obvious on examination, for example in children with otitis media or viral upper respiratory tract infection. If there are no clues on clinical examination, investigations for fever, such as analysis of a midstream specimen of urine or chest radiograph, may be helpful (see page 59).

Complex febrile seizures require consideration of:

- a different diagnosis, such as meningitis or encephalitis
- conditions that cause afebrile seizures, such as epilepsy, hypoglycaemia or brain injury

Focal signs may be investigated with a cranial MRI or CT scan.

Management

The underlying cause of the fever requires treatment, if appropriate, for example with antibiotics. Antipyretics help the child feel better but will not prevent further seizures. If the seizure is ongoing on admission, management is as for status epilepticus (see page 408).

Most children with their first febrile seizure are admitted to hospital, primarily to reassure the parents. Admission to hospital is also warranted in children with complex seizures or the possibility of partially treated meningitis, for example if the child is already receiving antibiotics.

Anticonvulsants are not routinely prescribed to prevent further seizures.

Simple and complex febrile seizures: characteristics		
Feature	Simple	Complex*
Type of seizure	Isolated, generalised, tonic–clonic seizures	Focal onset or focal features during the seizure
Duration	< 15 min	> 15 min
Recurrence and recovery	Do not recur within 24 h or within the same febrile illness	Incomplete recovery within 1 h Recurrence within 24 h or within the same febrile illness

*A complex seizure has at least one of the features listed.

Table 8.5 Characteristic features of simple and complex febrile seizures

Prognosis

The prognosis for febrile seizures is excellent. Seizures of short duration are not harmful. About one in three children will have more than one febrile seizure, but only up to the age of 7 years. Their risk of epilepsy is about six times higher than that for the normal population, but most will not develop epilepsy.

> **Parents of a child who has had a febrile seizure are given general advice on managing fever and told what to do if further seizures occur.** Advice includes how to protect their child from injury during a seizure, and when to call for medical help, i.e. in the event of complex features such as duration > 15 min or delayed recovery.

Cerebral palsy

Cerebral palsy is a group of conditions that affect movement, posture and coordination. It results from an insult to the developing brain. Although the insult is static, the signs change and progress as the child grows and develops.

Epidemiology and aetiology

The prevalence of cerebral palsy is 2–3 in 1000 children in developed countries. In most diagnosed children, the exact cause is unknown. Most insults are believed to occur in the antenatal period, for example as a consequence of intrauterine infection, brain malformations, placental insufficiency (i.e. intrauterine growth restriction) and twin pregnancy (even after allowing for increased preterm delivery and growth restriction).

> **There is widespread belief that perinatal hypoxia (birth asphyxia) is the main cause of cerebral palsy.** However, in reality it accounts for only a very small proportion of children diagnosed with cerebral palsy.

> **About 40% of children with cerebral palsy were born prematurely.** In these children, the cause of the cerebral palsy is a combination of antenatal and postnatal complications.

Clinical features

Cerebral palsy is the term for a wide spectrum of clinical presentations, usually including delayed motor skills. Cerebral palsy is classified into three broad categories.

- **Spastic cerebral palsy** (75–80% of cases) is characterised by a persistent increase in muscle tone; patients have upper motor neurone signs with hyper-reflexia
- **Dyskinetic cerebral palsy** (15% of cases) is characterised by involuntary movements and variable tone; there is extrapyramidal tract motor dysfunction
- **Ataxic cerebral palsy** (4% of cases) causes unsteadiness, with poor spatial awareness

These are subcategorised further (**Table 8.6**), and may be 'mixed', with features of more than one type.

The term cerebral palsy describes a motor deficit. However, many children with cerebral palsy, generally those with more severe signs, have other associated problems, such as epilepsy (21%), learning difficulties (31% severe), vision (11%) and hearing (5%) problems and feeding difficulties (up to 60% have oro-motor dysfunction – an inability to control facial and neck muscles – with 6% gastrostomy fed).

Diagnostic approach

The diagnosis of cerebral palsy is clinical. Therefore, although it may be suspected earlier, a confident diagnosis is usually not possible until later infancy or early childhood. Investigations may be carried out to aid management, for example brain MRI to establish the underlying cause and hearing tests and videofluoroscopy swallow test to identify complications.

Cerebral palsy: classification					
Spastic cerebral palsy		**Dyskinetic cerebral palsy**		**Ataxic cerebral palsy**	
Diplegia	Affects lower limbs only	Athetoid	Slow, writhing movements	Unsteady gait, clumsiness and poor balance. Not subclassified further	
Hemiplegia	Affects arm and leg on one side of the body (Figure 8.2)	Chorea	Rapid, unpredictable, jerky movements		
Quadriplegia	Affects all four limbs	Dystonia	Fluctuations of muscle tone, from floppy to stiff, and abnormal posturing		

Table 8.6 Classification of cerebral palsy

In a videofluoroscopic swallow test food or drink containing contrast medium is administered to delineate the swallowing process. In normal swallowing, food and liquid moves from the mouth into the throat, into the oesophagus and then the stomach; the epiglottis and neck muscles prevent aspiration into the lung. When this process is affected, as is the case in cerebral palsy, there is an increased risk of aspiration. If aspiration occurs the child should be fed by a nasogastric or gastrostomy tube.

Management

Management of cerebral palsy is by a multidisciplinary team and coordinated by a community paediatrician. It is tailored to the individual needs of the child and their family.

Children's therapy services

Physiotherapists optimise mobility. Some children require specialised wheelchairs. Speech and language therapists assess coordination of swallowing and work with dieticians to achieve optimum nutrition. Gastrostomy feeds are needed in children with severe cerebral palsy.

Medication

Injections of botulinum toxin or oral baclofen, a skeletal muscle relaxant, reduce spasticity. Medication may be required for

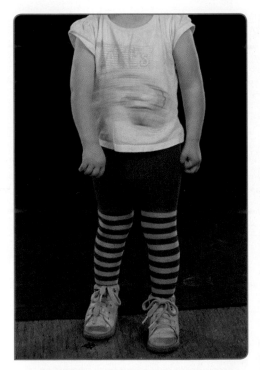

Figure 8.2 The typical hemiplegic posture of a child with a right hemiplegia. Note the pronation of the right arm with flexion at the wrist, and the scuffed toes of the special support shoes, indicating difficulty in walking. The right leg appears shorter because of flexion at the hip and knee.

associated complications, such as melatonin for sleeping difficulties (common in those with associated severe learning difficulties) or anticonvulsant medications for epilepsy.

Surgery

Secondary musculoskeletal disorders are common as a result of spasticity, muscle weakness and immobility. Orthopaedic surgeons regularly screen non-ambulant children with cerebral palsy for evolving scoliosis and hip dislocation. Lengthening the ankle tendon may aid walking, and osteotomy relocates a displaced hip. Selective dorsal rhizotomy surgery followed by intensive rehabilitation is a new procedure that improves spasticity in spastic diplegia if performed on children between 3 and 12 years of age. The surgery involves dividing some of the sensory nerve fibres (at the roots L1 to S2) running from the muscles to the spinal cord, thus reducing spasticity, and leading to improved walking.

Prognosis

This depends entirely on the extent and severity of the cerebral palsy. Children with mild cerebral palsy are able to attend mainstream schools and have a normal life expectancy. Children with severe cerebral palsy depend entirely on carers and often die in childhood from secondary complications such as aspiration pneumonia.

Ataxia

Ataxia is a disorder characterised by uncoordinated movements of the body, with an unsteady gait, clumsiness and poor balance. It may be the result of an insult to the cerebellum and its connecting pathways, the proprioceptive sensory pathways or the vestibular system. The most common cause of ataxia in children is acute cerebellar ataxia (cerebellitis) occurring within 3 weeks of a viral febrile illness, most commonly varicella (chickenpox).

Epidemiology and aetiology

Causes of ataxia are broadly categorised as:

- infectious
- postinfectious
- migraine-related
- toxin-related
- neoplastic
- hereditary

Ataxia in childhood can be acute and self-limiting, or chronic or intermittent. Acute onset ataxia is the most common form (**Table 8.7**). Intermittent or chronic ataxia is more sinister and can be caused by cerebellar tumours and, rarely, hereditary conditions. Cerebral palsy is also associated with ataxia (see page 257).

> **Guillain–Barré syndrome is an acute immune-mediated polyneuropathy usually presenting as an acute paralysing illness, which can start with ataxia triggered by a preceding infection.** An inflammatory demyelinating form is the most common type. Other types include acute axonal degeneration, especially in *Campylobacter*-associated disease.

Clinical features

Symptoms and signs of normal cerebellar function and coordination are outlined in Chapter 2 (see page 80). Associated symptoms for different causes of acute onset ataxia are shown in **Table 8.7** and for hereditary ataxia in **Table 8.8**. Cerebellar tumours are discussed in Chapter 15 (see page 390).

Acute ataxia in children: clinical features of associated conditions		
Condition	Predisposing factor or cause	Clinical features
Acute cerebellar ataxia	Recent viral febrile illness	Mainly gait and coordination problems, but other cerebellar signs (e.g. tremor, nystagmus, dysarthria) may be present No fever or meningism Normal power and deep tendon reflexes
Labyrinthitis	Viral or bacterial otitis media	Otalgia Symptoms of otitis media or upper respiratory tract infection Hearing loss Vomiting Normal tone, power and reflexes
Guillain–Barré syndrome	Preceding viral or bacterial respiratory or gastrointestinal infection	Pain or refusal to walk in younger children Progressive ascending weakness Diminished or absent reflexes Sensation usually preserved
Toxin ingestion or exposure	Possibility of ingestion or exposure to a toxin (e.g. alcohol, some anticonvulsants, lead, carbon monoxide)	Lethargy Confusion Occasionally vomiting Normal tone, power and reflexes

Table 8.7 Characteristics of conditions that present with acute ataxia in children

Diagnostic approach

A detailed history and examination is often sufficient for diagnosis without the need for extensive investigation, for example in labyrinthitis. If a serious underlying is suspected, investigations include:

■ brain MRI (to exclude a brain tumour)
■ lumbar puncture to obtain cerebrospinal fluid for analysis (to exclude meningitis, high white cell count and protein, or Guillain-Barré, high protein with low white cell count)
■ urine toxicology tests (to detect drug ingestion)

Management

Treatment of acute ataxia is supportive. Patients with Guillain–Barré syndrome require intensive care, because the respiratory muscles are affected. Hereditary ataxias require management by a neurologist; cure is seldom possible.

Prognosis

Common causes of acute ataxia are usually self-limiting; full recovery from labyrinthitis and acute cerebellar ataxia can be expected in days to weeks. Most children with Guillain-Barré syndrome also make a full recovery, but this may take months to a year. Hereditary conditions have a poorer prognosis, usually with progressive deterioration over time and significant morbidity and mortality.

Childhood inherited ataxias: characteristics				
Type	Inheritance	Incidence	Typical age of presentation	Clinical features and associations
Friedreich's ataxia	Autosomal recessive	1 in 50,000	8–15 years	Pes cavus* Clumsy gait Loss of postural and vibratory sensation Impaired tendon reflexes May have optic atrophy Associated with cardiomyopathy
Ataxia-telangiectasia	Autosomal recessive	1 in 100,000	< 5 years	Increasing cerebellar ataxia Telangiectasiae† over the bulbar conjunctiva and face Associated with impaired cellular immunity Predisposition to malignancy

*Pes cavus (claw foot) is a foot deformity with a very high fixed arch and stiffness of the foot.

†Telangiectasiae (spider veins) are small clusters of dilated blood vessels near the surface of the skin or mucous membranes.

Table 8.8 Characteristics of childhood inherited ataxias

Neuromuscular disorders

Neuromuscular disorders affect the lower motor neurones and muscles, and are classified according to site within the peripheral nervous system. Figure 8.5 Children present with floppy weakness and delayed motor milestones, most commonly with:

- a muscular dystrophy
- spinal muscular atrophy, or
- myasthenia gravis

Rarer disorders are the myopathies, which affect the muscle cells, and inborn errors of metabolism that impair production of cellular energy.

Muscular dystrophy

In the muscular dystrophies, muscle weakness results from abnormalities in muscle fibre structure. They are genetic conditions inherited in an X-linked recessive manner, so affect only boys. The defect impairs formation of dystrophin, a protein which, as part of a protein complex, strengthens the muscle cell's structural framework (cytoskeleton), reducing injury during muscle contraction and relaxation, by acting as a structural link with the extracellular matrix. There are two common types:

- Duchenne's muscular dystrophy, in which little or no dystrophin is produced; it affects 1 in 3500 males
- Becker's muscular dystrophy, in which dystrophin is produced but is faulty; it affects 1 in 17,000 males

Clinical features

Typical clinical features are listed in the comparison of Duchenne's and Becker's muscular dystrophy in **Table 8.9**.

Pseudohypertrophy of the calf muscles in muscular dystrophy is caused by muscle atrophy with overgrowth of fatty and fibrous tissues.

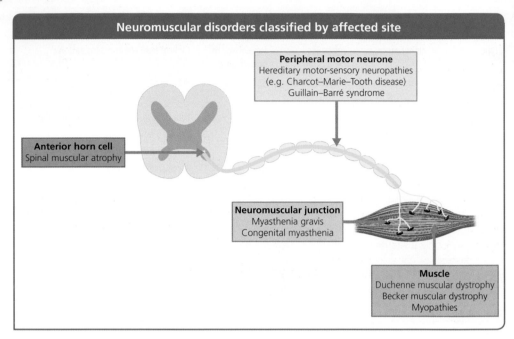

Figure 8.3 Classification of neuromuscular disorders by affected site.

Duchenne's and Becker's muscular dystrophy: characteristics		
	Duchenne's muscular dystrophy	Becker's muscular dystrophy
Age of onset	2–3 years	Teenage years
Initial symptoms	Delayed motor milestones of lower limbs: 'waddling' gait, Gower's sign (see page 84)	Proximal weakness: ■ difficulty climbing stairs ■ difficulty running
Limbs	Pseudohypertrophy of calf muscles	Proximal muscle wasting Pseudohypertrophy of calf muscles
Respiratory	Respiratory failure (resulting from respiratory muscle weakness and scoliosis)	Less marked symptoms than in Duchenne's muscular dystrophy
Cardiac	Cardiomyopathy from late teenage years	Symptomatic cardiomyopathy early in diagnosis
Orthopaedic	Progressive scoliosis	Lesser degree of scoliosis Joint contractures
Cognitive	Usually have a mild impairment (average IQ 85; 30% IQ<70)	Higher incidence of learning difficulties than in the general population (25%)

Table 8.9 Characteristic clinical features of Duchenne's and Becker's muscular dystrophy

Diagnostic approach

Initial tests include measurement of the serum concentration of creatine kinase, which is markedly increased in muscular dystrophy. Myopathic changes are visible on electromyography. In most cases, the diagnosis is confirmed on genetic testing. Muscle biopsy is useful if the exact gene responsible for the muscular dystrophy cannot be determined.

Management

There is no cure for muscular dystrophy. Management is supportive, with physiotherapy. Steroids can be useful in delaying the need for a wheelchair. Care in later life focuses on treatment of respiratory complications (see Figure 4.8). Cardiac monitoring is needed to detect cardiomyopathy.

Prognosis

Most patients with Duchenne's muscular dystrophy require a wheelchair by their early teens, and die from respiratory complications in their mid-twenties. The prognosis is much better for patients with Becker's muscular dystrophy; most are able to walk independently until 16 years of age and are still able to walk with aids into their twenties and survive into their forties. Death is usually from cardiac complications.

Spinal muscular atrophy

In spinal muscular atrophy, the muscle weakness is the result of a peripheral motor neurone disease affecting the anterior horn cells. It is an autosomal recessive condition usually caused by deletion of a gene on chromosome 5 or more rarely inherited in an X-linked manner with a mutation on the X chromosome. The condition affects fewer than 1 in 10,000 births.

Clinical features

There are four types of the most common autosomal recessive spinal muscular atrophy, three of which present in childhood:

- **Type 1** (Werdnig–Hoffmann disease) is the commonest; it presents with marked hypotonia and muscle weakness from birth or up to 6 months, (**Figure 8.4**), and a poor suck and swallow

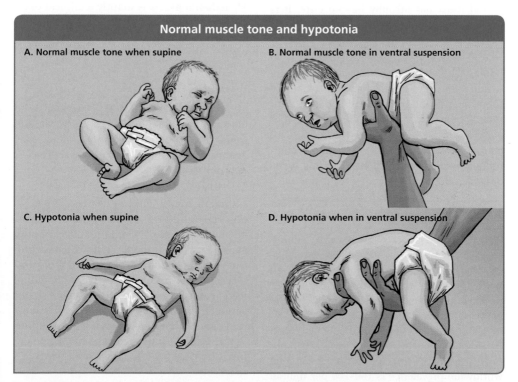

Normal muscle tone and hypotonia

A. Normal muscle tone when supine

B. Normal muscle tone in ventral suspension

C. Hypotonia when supine

D. Hypotonia when in ventral suspension

Figure 8.4 Normal muscle tone and hypotonia in a newborn baby when placed supine or held in ventral suspension. A baby with normal muscle tone has a flexed posture when supine. Head lag is minimal when they are pulled to the sitting position. Their posture is flexed in the prone position, and they are able to lift their head. In a baby with hypotonia, head lag is marked when the baby is pulled to sit. When held prone, they are unable to lift their head, and their limbs are floppy.

- **Type 2** presents at 7–18 months with delayed motor development or increasing proximal weakness
- **Type 3** presents after 18 months with the same characteristics as type 2

> **In spinal muscular atrophy type 1**, despite extreme muscle weakness, the baby has an alert facial expression. Tongue fasciculation, muscular twitching giving the tongue a 'bag of worms' appearance, may be seen.

Diagnostic approach

In spinal muscular atrophy, creatine kinase concentration is normal or only slightly increased. Electromyography shows diminished signals, and muscle biopsy finds muscle atrophy.

Management

Spinal muscular atrophy has no cure. It is managed with supportive therapies.

Prognosis

Babies with spinal muscular atrophy type 1 usually die from respiratory failure before their first birthday. Those diagnosed with type 2 spinal muscular atrophy survive into early adulthood, and those with type 3 can usually have a normal lifespan although many are unable to walk past their late-teens or early adulthood.

Myasthenia gravis

In myasthenia gravis, there is variable muscle weakness characterised by fatigability. It is an autoimmune condition caused by circulating antibodies that block, alter or destroy postsynaptic acetylcholine receptors at the neuromuscular junction.

The prevalence of myasthenia gravis in developed countries is 15–20 per 100,000 but only 10% of cases are children. The estimated worldwide prevalence is 100–200 per million population, the incidence being significantly higher in Afro-Carribean women. In adults, it is more common in females, but it affects both genders equally pre-puberty. A genetic link has yet to be established, but familial patterns are occasionally seen. Transient neonatal myasthenia can be encountered if mothers are affected, because the antibodies cross the placenta (see Table 3.10).

Clinical features

The muscle fatigability and weakness are more marked around the eye and eyelids, manifesting as ptosis and squint. There is facial weakness, and the proximal limb muscles and trunk are also affected. The child becomes weaker over the course of the day and subsides after a period of rest. Muscle bulk, tone and reflexes are normal.

Diagnostic approach

Myasthenia gravis is mainly a clinical diagnosis. However, blood tests for anticholinesterase antibodies usually give a positive result.

Management

Myasthenia gravis is initially treated with anticholinesterase inhibitors. However, steroids or other immunosuppressants may eventually be required in a minority of cases.

Prognosis

Although myasthenia gravis has a relapsing and remitting course, symptoms usually becoming more sporadic, and a minority experience a myasthenic crisis which is a life-threatening condition in which the respiratory muscles become very weak. Potential triggers for myasthenic crisis include stress, acute illness, surgery or certain medications such as aminoglycosides and fluoroquinolones. Despite intensive care management, myasthenic crisis is associated with 5% mortality.

Neurodegenerative disorders

Neurodegenerative disorders are characterised by progressive deterioration of the structure or function of the nervous system as a result of neuronal death. The term encompasses a large, heterogeneous group of diseases resulting from specific genetic or biochemical defects, and many unknown causes. They include inborn errors of metabolism (storage disorders; see page 347) and rare genetic disorders. The likelihood of developing a neurodegenerative disease increases with age; children are rarely affected.

Clinical features

The key feature is progressive decline in nervous system function, usually with loss of previously acquired skills (developmental regression) and intellectual impairment. There may be other features characteristic of any individual underlying disease, such as hepatosplenomegaly or coarse facial features in storage disorders.

Diagnostic approach

Determination of the exact cause for the regression is guided by the age of onset and certain physical findings, supported by the result of targeted investigations, such as a brain MRI and a urine metabolic screen (looking for the presence of excessive amounts of certain metabolites, compared with normal, in the urine).

Prognosis

Neurodegenerative diseases have a generally poor prognosis, with increasing impairment of nervous system function as the disease progresses. However, a minority of metabolic conditions can have their progression halted with enzyme replacement therapy or bone marrow transplantation, if the disease is expressed in stem cells (such as lysosomal storage diseases and mucopolysaccharidoses), as the haematopoietic stem cell transplantation provides a continuous source of enzyme replacement.

Neurocutaneous syndromes

Neurocutaneous syndromes are disorders of the central nervous system associated with typical skin lesions and the growth of tumours. The neurocutaneous syndromes most commonly encountered in children are:

- neurofibromatosis types 1 and 2
- tuberous sclerosis
- encephalotrigeminal angiomatosis (Sturge-Weber syndrome) (see page 353)
- ataxia telangiectasia

Some neurocutaneous syndromes are inherited; neurofibromatosis and tuberous sclerosis have autosomal dominant inheritance (although a significant number arise from new mutations), and ataxia telangiectasia is autosomal recessive. Encephalotrigeminal angiomatosis occurs sporadically.

The manifestations of the neurocutaneous syndromes are related to the common ectodermal origin (neural crest) of the affected organs. The diverse features result from abnormal neural crest differentiation in the embryo with abnormal angiogenesis, nerve sheath proliferations, abnormal pigmentation and benign or malignant tumours.

Neurofibromatosis

Neurofibromatosis is characterised by the growth of neurofibromas (tumours on neurons). It is the most common neurocutaneous syndrome, affecting 1 in 3000 live births in northern Europe. There are two different forms: type 1 and type 2.

Clinical features

Neurofibromatosis type 1 accounts for 90% of cases of neurofibromatosis. The diagnosis of type 1 requires the presence of at least two of the following:

- history of neurofibromatosis type 1 in a first-degree relative
- six or more café au lait spots (**Figure 8.5**)
- two or more typical neurofibromas or one plexiform neurofibroma
- axillary or inguinal freckling
- two or more iris hamartomas (Lisch nodules) on slit lamp examination
- optic nerve glioma (rarely malignant)
- bony lesions, for example dysplasia or pseudoarthrosis

Typical neurofibromas are nerve sheath tumours, usually in the skin, affecting a single peripheral nerve. **Plexiform neurofibromas** affect a nerve bundle and can be deep.

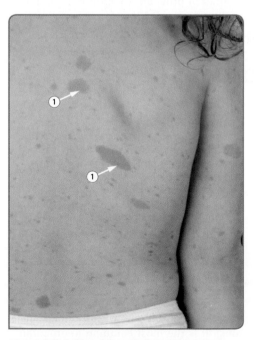

Figure 8.5 Café au lait spots (hyperpigmented macules) ①. This child also had axillary freckling, typical of neurofibromatosis.

The neurofibromas are benign but may cause serious damage by compressing nerves and other tissues. There is an associated increased risk of epilepsy, learning difficulties, scoliosis, osteoporosis and hypertension.

Neurofibromatosis type 2 is a completely separate condition characterised by acoustic neuromas.

The most common cause of hypertension in children with neurofibromatosis type 1 is renal artery stenosis. Other causes are phaeochromocytoma and coarctation of the aorta.

Management

The management of neurofibromatosis type 1 is largely surveillance, based on monitoring of growth, blood pressure and visual acuity. Complications may require surgery, for example excision of disfiguring neurofibromas.

Tuberous sclerosis

Tuberous sclerosis is characterised by formation of 'tubers' (hamartomas) in many organs, including the brain. It affects 1 in 6000 live births in northern Europe and the USA.

Clinical features

Typical skin lesions include depigmented ash leaf macules (so called as they are the shape of leaves from an ash tree), and adenoma sebaceum, which resembles acne in a prepubertal child. Other symptoms are caused by tumours in other organs, typically the brain, kidneys, heart, eyes and lungs. More than half of children with tuberous sclerosis will have learning difficulties and epilepsy.

Management

The management of tuberous sclerosis consists of surveillance, control of epilepsy and treatment of tumour complications, including bleeding from renal angiomyolipomas and hydrocephalus caused by brain astrocytomas.

Headache

A headache is pain in the region of the head or neck. Headaches are common in children, and tend to run in families. The commonest types in children are tension headache and headache associated with a viral illness, e.g. meningitis.

Clinical features

Table 8.10 lists the characteristic features of different types of headache. Always be alert for 'red flag' symptoms or signs suggesting increased intracranial pressure or other serious underlying pathology.

> **Headache 'red flags'** include early morning headache, nausea and vomiting, visual changes and an abnormal neurological examination.

Diagnostic approach

A brain imaging study, either CT or MRI, is carried out only when 'red flag' signs or symptoms are present. If meningitis is suspected, a lumbar puncture is carried out unless there are contraindications such as signs of increased intracranial pressure.

Management

Benign types of headache require only simple analgesia together with child and parental reassurance. For migraines, simple analgesia is advised, as well as avoidance of precipitating factors, for example dehydration, dietary triggers and exhaustion. If migraines are severe, preventive medication, for example pizotifen, can be considered. Brain tumours and intracranial bleeds require specialist referral.

Types of headaches in children	
Headache	Features
Migraine	Acute, recurrent
	Bifrontal, bitemporal
	Symptoms of nausea, photophobia
	Improves with sleep in dark room
Tension headache	Chronic, recurrent
	Frontal, 'band-like'
	Caused by stress
Idiopathic intracranial hypertension	Recurrent, variable characteristics
	Visual symptoms (may lead to loss of vision), papilloedema
	Tinnitus
Meningitis	Acute
	Symptoms of fever, photophobia, neck stiffness, vomiting
Space-occupying lesion	Chronic, recurrent
	Focal or diffuse early morning headache
	Associated symptoms of nausea, vomiting, visual disturbance
	Papilloedema on fundoscopy
Cluster headaches	Severe unilateral orbital and/or supraorbital pain
	Several short-lived episodes during attack
	Associated with restlessness and autonomic symptoms, e.g. miosis, lacrimation

Table 8.10 Types of headaches in children and their features

Answers to starter questions

1. Seizures in a young child are the first sign of a neurocutaneous syndrome; if the skin is not examined this diagnosis will be missed. Some lesions, such as hypopigmented lesions or café au lait spots, are difficult to see with the naked eye; examination under UV light makes them more obvious.

2. Ten per cent of children carry *Neisseria meningitidis* with no symptoms; it can persist for months and induces immunity. It is not known why it enters the bloodstream and causes invasive infection in some cases.

3. Examining the eyes reveal crucial information in relation to recurrent headache. This includes strain from short or long sightedness, or more serious pathology in the presence of a VIth nerve palsy or papilloedema, as signs of raised intracranial pressure secondary to tumour or hydrocephalus.

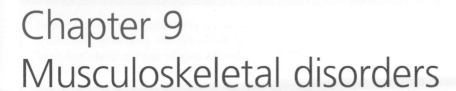

Chapter 9
Musculoskeletal disorders

Starter questions

Answers to the following questions are on page 286.

1. Why should the hip be examined in children with knee pain?
2. Why is uveitis screened for in children with arthritis?
3. Why might osteogenesis imperfecta be confused with a non-accidental injury?
4. Why is it crucial to screen for developmental dysplasia of the hip early in life?

Introduction

In children, most musculoskeletal problems are benign and self-limiting. However, some can cause lifelong disability if not treated promptly and appropriately, for example, septic arthritis and developmental dysplasia of the hip. Diagnosis requires a sound knowledge of the common presenting features of these conditions, and the ages at which they tend to present.

Chronic musculoskeletal disorders are managed by a multidisciplinary team of physicians, specialist nurses, physiotherapists, occupational therapists and pain specialists. The disorders requiring this approach are chronic arthritis, osteogenesis imperfecta, and scoliosis.

Case 13 Sudden limp in a 6-year-old boy

Presentation

Thomas, aged 6 years, presents with a 24-hour history of limp. He has been unwell with fever, sore throat and 'common cold' symptoms for a couple of days. His mother says he fell over in school yesterday but appeared unharmed.

Initial interpretation

Most children of school age are able to localise pain, but Thomas is still young and his limp could indicate pathology in the hip, knee or foot (or even the groin or lower abdomen). All these sites should be examined carefully. In practice, the most likely diagnosis in a child of school age is transient synovitis ('irritable hip'), but a traumatic cause should be considered in view of the history of a fall. Septic arthritis must always be considered in a child of any age presenting with fever and limp, and osteomyelitis is also a possibility. **Table 9.1** lists by age the likely causes of limp in a child.

History

Thomas's mother reports that he initially became unwell a couple of days earlier, with a runny nose and sore throat. His temperature at home had been up to 38°C. Yesterday evening, he was intermittently complaining of pain in his right hip, and he was limping when he got up this morning. Thomas is adamant that although he fell over while playing football yesterday, he got straight up and carried on playing. He is normally fit and well, and there are no concerns about his growth. Thomas has never complained of joint pains before.

Causes of limp in children				
Acute or chronic?	Any age	3–5 years (preschool in the UK)	5–11 years (primary school in the UK)	12–17 years (adolescence)
Acute	Fracture	Non-accidental injury	Myositis	Sprain
	Septic arthritis	Transient synovitis	Transient synovitis	Tendonitis
	Reactive arthritis	Henoch–Schönlein purpura		
	Rheumatic fever	Toddler's fracture		
	Haemarthrosis (common in haemophilia)			
Acute or chronic	Osteomyelitis	No specific cause	No specific cause	Slipped upper femoral epiphysis
Chronic	Poorly fitting shoes	Developmental dysplasia of the hip	Perthes' disease	Osgood–Schlatter disease
	Tuberculosis arthritis	Juvenile idiopathic arthritis (systemic onset or oligoarticular)	Leukaemia	Scoliosis
		Cerebral palsy	Juvenile idiopathic arthritis (oligoarthritis or polyarthritis)	Inflammatory bowel disease (enthesis-related juvenile idiopathic arthritis) or polyarthritis juvenile idiopathic arthritis
		Leg length asymmetry	Dermatomyositis	Systemic lupus erythematosus
			Rheumatic fever	Tumour

Table 9.1 Causes of limp in different age groups

Case 13 *continued*

Interpretation of history

A fracture seems less likely, considering Thomas's recovery after his fall. If Thomas were older (over 10 years), even mild trauma would prompt investigations to exclude a slipped upper femoral epiphysis. His mother has described a short history of symptoms of a viral illness. The pain is intermittent and difficult to localise, making transient synovitis more likely. However, the symptoms are also consistent with septic arthritis or osteomyelitis, especially in view of the fever. A neoplastic cause is extremely unlikely given such a short history.

Examination

Thomas looks well but has a low-grade fever (temperature, 38.2°C). His observations are otherwise normal. He is able to bear weight on his right leg, but his walking gait is antalgic (adjusted to avoid pain). While lying on the bed, he is holding his right hip slightly abducted and externally rotated. Inspection of the hips and legs is otherwise normal, apart from some superficial grazes on the right knee.

There is full range of active and passive movement of the hip, but pain at the extremes of rotation. Thomas's abdomen is soft. The rest of the systems examination is normal, except for the finding of slightly inflamed tonsils.

When examining a child with a limp:

- check the soles of the feet for any local causes of limp, such as a painful verruca or blisters from poorly fitting shoes
- examine the joints above and below a painful joint to assess whether the pain is referred from these structures

Interpretation of findings

Rotation produces pain in traumatic, infectious or inflammatory conditions of the hip. Septic arthritis produces pain with minimal movement, whereas transient synovitis may produce pain only at extremes of rotation. Considering this latter finding, combined with the symptoms of viral tonsillitis and the absence of swelling, erythema or tenderness of the joint, the most likely diagnosis is transient synovitis. However, children with septic arthritis are not always 'unwell', so this alternative diagnosis cannot be completely ruled out.

Investigations

Because of its potentially serious consequences, septic arthritis must be excluded by further investigations. Appropriate blood tests are full blood count, measurement of C-reactive protein (CRP) and determination of erythrocyte sedimentation rate (ESR). A hip US scan is also indicated. A plain radiograph is useful only when a fracture, Perthes' disease (avascular necrosis of the femoral head) or slipped upper femoral epiphysis is suspected. An effusion may be caused by septic arthritis or transient synovitis. In transient synovitis a bilateral effusion is present in a quarter of cases even when the symptoms are unilateral. A useful approach to diagnosing acute limp in a child is shown in **Figure 9.1**.

Thomas's blood test results show:

- white cell count $11.2 \times 10^9/L$
- CRP 18 mg/L
- ESR of 12 mm/h

A small effusion of the right hip is seen on US.

Diagnosis

A diagnosis of transient synovitis is made. Thomas is discharged home, and his parents are advised to give him ibuprofen for symptomatic relief. He recovers fully within a week.

Case 13 *continued*

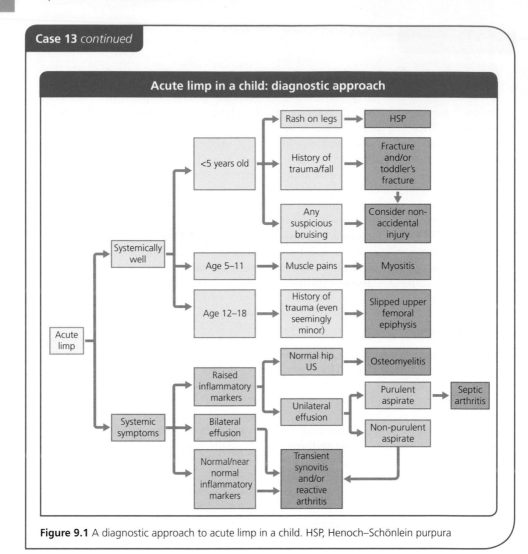

Figure 9.1 A diagnostic approach to acute limp in a child. HSP, Henoch–Schönlein purpura

Congenital anomalies

Congenital musculoskeletal anomalies are detected on antenatal US or identified at the newborn examination. The cause is usually multifactorial, and includes genetic and environmental factors such as restricted movement in utero or amniotic bands. The foot and the hip (**Figure 9.2**) are the structures most commonly affected. They can be minor, for example extra digits (polydactyly) or fused digits (syndactyly), or more significant, for example an absent limb.

The cause is often multifactorial, and includes genetic and environmental factors such as restricted movement in utero or amniotic bands.

> **Amniotic band syndrome** is a congenital abnormality caused by fibrous strands of the amniotic sac encircling a limb or digit, thereby constricting its blood supply and causing amputation or a deep indentation.

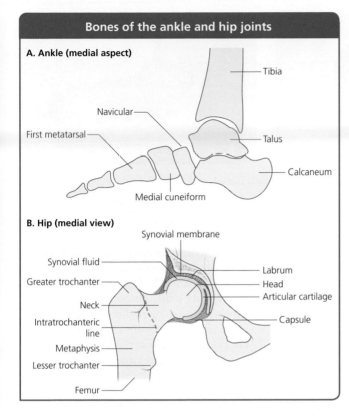

Bones of the ankle and hip joints

A. Ankle (medial aspect)

- Tibia
- Navicular
- First metatarsal
- Talus
- Calcaneum
- Medial cuneiform

B. Hip (medial view)

- Synovial membrane
- Synovial fluid
- Greater trochanter
- Neck
- Intratrochanteric line
- Metaphysis
- Lesser trochanter
- Femur
- Labrum
- Head
- Articular cartilage
- Capsule

Figure 9.2 Normal bony anatomy of the ankle and hip joint. The cavity of the hip joint is lined by synovial membrane, which extends from the margins of one articular surface to the other. The synovial membrane is protected by a tough fibrous membrane, the capsule of the joint, which extends past the growth plate.

Talipes

Talipes are abnormalities of the ankle and foot that are present at birth. The two most common types are:

- **talipes equinovarus** ('fixed talipes'), a fixed abnormality that restricts active and passive movement at the ankle
- **positional talipes,** which resembles talipes equinovarus but passive movement at the ankle joint is normal

> The word **talipes** comes from the Latin words talus ('ankle') and pes ('foot'). **Equino** refers to the heel in an elevated position, like that of a horse. **Varus** means that the distal foot is turned inwards and **valgus** describes the distal foot turned outwards.

Talipes equinovarus

This structural deformity of the foot, also known as clubfoot, affects about 1 in 1000 births. The male to female incidence ratio is 2:1. Half of cases are bilateral.

In talipes equinovarus, fixed adduction at the talonavicular joint and inversion at the subtalar joint prevent normal movement at the ankle. The cause is not completely understood, but it is associated with:

- oligohydramnios
- developmental dysplasia of the hip
- spina bifida
- genetic conditions

Diagnosis is made on examination, when the foot is found to be fixed in plantar flexion, with the forefoot turned medially and the sole facing inwards (**Figure 9.3**), and both active and passive movement are restricted.

Management of talipes equinovarus is guided by an orthopaedic surgeon. The condition is usually managed by manipulation and the use of serial plaster casts (Ponseti's method) to try to achieve a satisfactory foot position. Surgery to the Achilles tendon, ligaments and bones may occasionally be required.

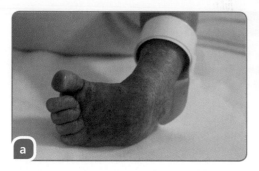
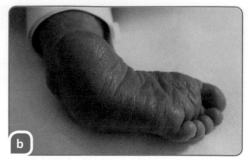

Figure 9.3 Talipes equinovarus: (a) plantar flexed, medially placed forefoot and (b) sole facing inwards.

Positional talipes

This deformity has the appearance of talipes equinovarus but the position of the foot is not fixed; it is easily moved into the neutral and dorsiflexed positions. The condition affects 15 in 1000 neonates and is caused by lack of space in utero. It is self-correcting but regular stretching exercises are helpful.

Developmental dysplasia of the hip

Developmental dysplasia of the hip, also known as congenital dysplasia of the hip, is abnormal development of the hip joint in utero. Its severity ranges from mild dysplasia of the acetabulum to frank hip dislocation. Risk factors for its development include:

- developmental dysplasia of the hip in a first-degree relative
- breech presentation (all babies in a multiple pregnancy are at risk if one is breech)
- abnormalities suggesting restricted fetal movement in utero, for example torticollis, arthogryposis and fixed foot deformities (e.g. talipes equinovarus)

About 1% of newborns are affected. It is more common in firstborn children. Most affected children (80%) are female. Developmental dysplasia of the hip is unilateral in 80% of cases; the left hip is more commonly affected (possibly due to the usual in utero positioning of the fetal left hip against the mother's sacrum, keeping it in an adducted position).

Clinical features

Clinical features of developmental dysplasia of the hip in the neonatal period a click or clunk of the hips, the feeling felt by the examiner's hands when Ortolani's and Barlow's manoeuvres are carried out at the newborn examination (see Figure 2.28). Asymmetrical skin creases such as at the inner upper thigh are suggestive but not diagnostic of developmental dysplasia of the hip. If the condition is not identified at birth, the child presents with other features, as listed in **Table 9.2**.

Diagnostic approach

In the newborn period, US of the hip is carried out to confirm the diagnosis when suspected

Developmental dysplasia of the hip: clinical signs	
Age	Findings
Birth to 3 months	Positive finding on clinical examination (Ortolani's or Barlow's test)
	Asymmetry of leg creases (inguinal, gluteal or thigh)
3 months to 1 year	Limited hip adduction
	Leg length discrepancy
	Asymmetry of leg creases
Mobile child	Limp
	Excessive lumbar lordosis (especially in bilateral cases)
	Waddling gait (bilateral cases)

Table 9.2 Clinical signs suggesting developmental dysplasia of the hip

on clinical examination. US scans are also required for babies with risk factors, even if clinical examination is normal. If there is suspicion of developmental dysplasia of the hip in a child older than 6 months, a hip radiograph is carried out, because ossification of the epiphysis of the femoral head should have occurred by this age, making the dysplasia easier to see. Shenton's line is disrupted in developmental dysplasia of the hip (**Figure 9.4**).

> **Hip screening by clinical examination is carried out during the newborn examination and at the 6-week check to diagnose developmental dysplasia of the hip early.** Treatment can then start immediately after diagnosis, thereby avoiding permanent structural damage to the child's hips and associated functional limitations.

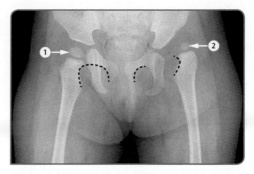

Figure 9.4 Radiograph showing developmental dysplasia of the left hip in an 18-month-old child. The femoral head is displaced upwards and laterally, with interruption of Shenton's lines (dotted line). There is less ossification of the left femoral head epiphysis ② compared with the normal right hip ①.

Management

A neonate with developmental dysplasia of the hip is placed in a Pavlik harness (**Figure 9.5**). This prevents hip extension and adduction while allowing flexion and abduction, thereby enabling the hip to develop normally. Surgery is required if the harness does not help or if the condition presents late (> 6 months of age).

With early diagnosis and appropriate treatment, prognosis is excellent. Prognosis is worse if the condition is diagnosed after the newborn period, (estimated 1 in 50 cases of DDH), by which time the femoral head is usually out of the acetabulum. In these babies, complex orthopaedic surgery, including open reduction and femoral osteotomy, is needed.

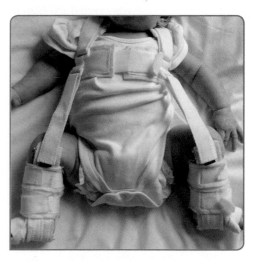

Figure 9.5 A baby in a Pavlik harness for management of developmental dysplasia of the hip.

Osteodysplasias and chondrodysplasias

The osteodysplasias and chondrodysplasias are a group of conditions in which there is abnormal development of bone and cartilage, respectively. They are caused by genetic mutations. The commonest osteodysplasia is osteogenesis imperfecta, and the commonest chondrodysplasia is achondrodysplasia.

Achondroplasia

In achondroplasia, the formation of abnormal cartilage results in short stature and other skeletal abnormalities. About 1 in 25,000 live births are affected. It is caused by a mutation in a fibroblast growth factor receptor gene (*FGFR3*) and is inherited in an autosomal dominant fashion. About 75% of cases are caused by a sporadic mutation.

Clinical features

The clinical features of achondroplasia are listed in **Table 9.3**. The final average adult height is 125 cm (4 ft, 1 in).

Diagnostic approach

Achondroplasia may be suspected if short limbs, particularly short femur length, are seen on an antenatal US scan relative to the abdominal and head circumference measurements. Genetic testing confirms the diagnosis. Skeletal survey can also be carried out to determine the exact type of dwarfism, as less common causes can present with typical vertebral or other, e.g. rib characteristics.

> There are special growth charts for children with achondroplasia as these children do not follow standard height centile charts, due to their shortened limbs.

Management

Children with achondroplasia undergo regular monitoring for common complications associated with the condition. These include

Achondroplasia: clinical features	
Head and face	Body and limbs
Large head with midfacial hypoplasia	Short arms and legs, primarily as a consequence of humeral and femoral shortening, i.e. rhizomelic (proximal) limb shortening
Frontal bossing (large forehead)	
Occipital bossing	Short fingers and space between the middle and ring fingers (trident hands)
Flat, wide nasal bridge	
Prominent (protruding) jaw	Short stature (normal trunk length)
Crowded teeth	Lumbar lordosis and kyphosis
	Bowing of legs
	Flexible joints
	Decreased muscle tone
	Bulky arms and legs

Table 9.3 Clinical features of achondroplasia

joint pain, otitis media (hearing loss), spinal cord compression and hydrocephalus. Individuals with achondroplasia have twice the risk of death to the normal population for all age groups. In children this is due to central nervous system (respiratory insufficiency and sudden death due to brain stem compression) and respiratory abnormalities (upper airway obstruction, pneumonia, apnoea). In adults death is most frequently due to cardiovascular problems.

> **Mild achondroplasia may present as apparent delayed development** because the large size of the child's head makes head control difficult.

Osteogenesis imperfecta

Osteogenesis imperfecta is a skeletal dysplasia in which there are abnormalities in type I collagen, a component of bone, ligament and sclera. There are eight different types of osteogenesis imperfecta, the most common being types I–IV (**Table 9.4**). The disorder is usually inherited, but 35% of cases result from sporadic mutations. It affects 1 in 20,000 live births. Type I is the most common form.

Clinical features

Table 9.5 shows the clinical features of osteogenesis imperfecta in children; these features are typically apparent after multiple fractures lead to skeletal deformities. Severe types of osteogenesis imperfecta, i.e. type II is suspected in utero or soon after birth because of the presence of major limb deformities due to fractures that have occurred in utero. The less severe types of osteogenesis imperfecta are detected during investigation of fractures sustained by minimal trauma or a history of multiple fractures.

> **Blue sclera does not always indicate osteogenesis imperfecta**, and it is not present in all types of osteogenesis imperfecta. Many healthy newborn babies have the appearance of blue sclera but the colour disappears over time. Blue sclera is not typical of any other disorders.

Osteogenesis imperfecta: classification				
Type	Pathogenesis	Severity	Inheritance	Characteristics
I	Normal collagen but inadequate amount	Mild	AD	Fewer fractures than other types, minimal deformity Often develop hearing loss Blue sclera
II	Abnormal collagen and inadequate amount	Lethal	AD	Most die in antenatal or newborn period Blue sclera, can be very dark
III	Defective collagen, adequate amount	Severe	AD	Fractures from birth Severe bone deformity Blue sclera at birth, becoming white with age Dentinogenesis imperfecta Often hearing loss
IV	Defective collagen, adequate amount	Moderate or mild	AD	Age of fractures varies – worse before puberty May have dentinogenesis imperfecta White or grey sclera

Table 9.4 Classification and characteristics of osteogenesis imperfecta

Osteogenesis imperfecta: clinical features	
Head and face	Body and limbs
Basilar skull deformities†	Short stature
Wormian bones (**Figure 9.6**)	Scoliosis
Blue sclera	Increased laxity of ligaments and skin
Dentinogenesis imperfecta: discoloured (blue-grey or yellow-brown) and translucent teeth, weaker than normal teeth	Bowing and deformities of long bones*

*Bone deformities are the result of healed fractures.
†Basilar skull deformities compress nerves and cause deafness.

Table 9.5 Clinical features of osteogenesis imperfecta

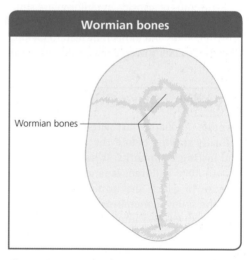

Wormian bones

Wormian bones

Figure 9.6 Wormian bones: pieces of bone that occur within a suture of the cranium in conditions such as osteogenesis imperfecta.

Diagnostic approach

Diagnosis is based on clinical findings and confirmed by genetic investigations.

Osteogenesis imperfecta can be mistaken for non-accidental injury if a child presents with multiple fractures of different ages and no history, or minimal history, of trauma (see page 432).

Management

The aims of management are to prevent deformities caused by fractures with splinting and to correct any that do occur. Families are given advice and practical support on avoiding injury and consequent fractures. Low impact exercise such as swimming is encouraged to strengthen muscles and bones.

Oral biphosphonate such as pamidronate is used for the severe forms of osteogenesis imperfecta, under specialist advice, to reduce fracture rates.

Prognosis depends on the type of osteogenesis imperfecta. Hearing loss is common in types I and III. Patients with type 1 osteogenesis imperfecta have a normal life expectancy and those with type IV only have a modest reduction in life expectancy. Type II are either stillborn or die soon after birth and type III have a shortened life expectancy, many dying in childhood.

Arthritis

Arthritis is inflammation of a joint (or joints), which presents as pain and swelling. The types of arthritis encountered in children differ significantly from those in adults; for example, very few children develop rheumatoid factor-positive arthritis. Reactive arthritis is the commonest type of arthritis in children, and juvenile idiopathic arthritis is the most common chronic form.

Symptoms of arthritis in children are similar to those in adults. However, its effects on growing bones and joints may lead to lifelong physical disability even after remission of the active disease.

Juvenile idiopathic arthritis

Juvenile idiopathic arthritis is defined as arthritis starting before the age of 16 years and lasting $\geq$ 3 months. It has a prevalence of 1 in 1000 children. It is an autoimmune disease in which the immune system targets the synovial membrane lining the joint. The cause of the autoimmune reaction is unknown.

The condition is classified according to the number of joints affected. The three main types are:

- systemic onset juvenile idiopathic arthritis, in which systemic symptoms are present and joint involvement may be minimal
- oligoarthritis, in which up to four joints are affected
- polyarthritis, in which five or more joints are involved

Additional types include enthesitis-related arthritis, in which there is inflammation at the attachments of tendons or ligaments to bone, and psoriasic arthritis, in which there is psoriatic rash and nail involvement. Enthesitis-related arthritis is associated with the HLA-B27 surface antigen. HLA-B27 is present in about 8% of Caucasians, higher in Scandinavians and lower in North Africa (4%) China (4%) and Japan (0.5%). The chance that an HLA-B27 patient will develop arthritis or eye disease is 1 in 4.

> **Human leukocyte antigen (HLA) B27 found on the surface of cells is encoded on chromosome 6.** It plays a role in immunity and self-recognition presenting peptides to T cells. It is strongly associated with inflammatory disease such as enthesitis-related arthritis, inflammatory bowel disease and many systemic diseases with ocular manifestations (uveitis).

Clinical features

Juvenile idiopathic arthritis presents with pain, redness, swelling and restricted movements of one or more joints. The affected joint or joints feel warm, and morning stiffness is typical. Systemic onset juvenile idiopathic arthritis may initially present with predominantly systemic features, such as swinging fever, salmon pink macular rash, organomegaly and pericarditis, before arthritis occurs (**Table 9.6**).

Juvenile idiopathic arthritis: clinical features

Type	Epidemiology	Joint involvement and other clinical features
Systemic onset (formerly called Still's disease)	10–15% of cases of JIA Typically affects children < 5 years of age, but may occur at any age Equal sex distribution before the age of 5 years, after which girls are predominantly affected	Usually symmetrical Mainly affects knees, wrists, hands and feet Joint involvement usually preceded by swinging fever, tiredness, rash, enlarged glands; sometimes also enlarged liver and spleen and/or pericarditis
Oligoarticular (pauciarticular)	Commonest type: 50% of children with JIA Girls more likely to be affected than boys Young age (< 6 years)	Asymmetrical Knee, ankle and elbow most commonly affected
Polyarticular	30–40% of children with JIA Girls more likely to be affected than boys Usually occurs in children > 8 years of age	Symmetrical Affects large and small joints Later involvement of temporomandibular joints and cervical spine
Enthesitis-related arthritis	Juvenile anklyosing spondylitis Primarily affects boys > 8 years old	Initially oligoarticular Sacroiliac involvement develops gradually during adolescence
	Psoriatic arthritis Children typically > 10 years of age at presentation	Monoarthritis or asymmetrical polyarthritis, usually involving the fingers Nail pitting Psoriatic rash

JIA, juvenile idiopathic arthritis.

Table 9.6 Clinical features of the most common types of juvenile idiopathic arthritis

> It is often difficult to elicit whether a young child has morning stiffness. Therefore it is helpful to ask parents if the child finds the first nappy change of the day particularly uncomfortable. If the answer is 'yes', this may indicate morning stiffness.

Diagnostic approach

Juvenile idiopathic arthritis is primarily a clinical diagnosis and requires exclusion of other causes of polyarthritis (**Table 9.7**). A detailed history is needed to explore serious disorders, such as septic arthritis and malignancy, that can present similarly. Radiographs are not indicated unless there is a history of trauma. Genetic testing may be appropriate in enthesitis-related arthritis, because it is associated with the HLA-B27 surface antigen.

Childhood polyarthritis: causes

Category	Causes
Mechanical or degenerative disorders	Overuse
	Trauma
	Non-accidental injury
Inflammatory or infective disorders	Reactive arthritis
	Rheumatic fever
	Henoch–Schönlein purpura
	Juvenile idiopathic arthritis
	Connective tissue diseases: systemic lupus erythematosus, dermatomyositis
Haematological or neoplastic	Haemoglobinopathies (e.g. sickle cell disease)
	Leukaemia
	Lymphoma
	Neuroblastoma (metastases)
	Bone or cartilage tumours
	Bleeding disorders (e.g. haemophilia A)

Table 9.7 Causes of childhood polyarthritis

About one in five children with juvenile idiopathic arthritis develop chronic anterior uveitis, i.e. inflammation of the uvea (the iris, ciliary body and choroid). Untreated, it can lead to glaucoma, cataracts and blindness. It is often asymptomatic, so regular slit lamp eye examinations are essential for all children with juvenile idiopathic arthritis.

Management

The aims of management are to maintain joint function and to reduce joint inflammation, pain and the potential for joint deformity. Many children with juvenile idiopathic arthritis go into remission. A small minority of patients have longer term problems, including joint damage, osteoporosis and altered growth at affected joints.

Good pain management facilitates exercise and physiotherapy. Regular exercise is fundamental to a good outcome and includes passive exercises, weight-bearing exercises and hydrotherapy. Night splints keep joints in a comfortable position to prevent contractures or deformity.

Medication

The medications used to treat juvenile idiopathic arthritis are primarily analgesic nonsteroidal anti-inflammatory drugs, to ease pain. Drugs to suppress the immune system are also used early, under specialist supervision, to induce remission and minimise joint damage:

- disease-modifying antirheumatic drugs (methotrexate)
- corticosteroid injections into the joint
- systemic steroid tablets (oral or pulsed intravenous methylprednisolone)
- Cytokine modulators ('biologics') and other immunotherapies such as tumour necrosis factor alpha (TNF-A) inhibitors, interleukin inhibitors and T-cell activation inhibitors

Uveitis is treated with antimuscarinic eye drops.

Prognosis

At least 30% of affected children will continue to have active disease into adulthood. Even with disease remission, joint damage that has already occurred frequently leads to joint replacement surgery in young adulthood being necessary.

Reactive arthritis

Reactive arthritis is transient (< 6 weeks). It develops in response to an infection in another part of the body, typically an upper respiratory tract infection. It is caused by an autoimmune 'cross-reactivity', between viral and self-antigens. The condition occurs most frequently between 2 and 10 years of age. Boys are affected more often than girls.

Clinical features

There is typically pain, redness or swelling of the affected joint. The pain may reduce the range of movement of the joint. The child is not systemically unwell, and has a mild or no fever.

Diagnostic approach

The diagnosis can usually be made clinically. Blood tests may show normal or mildly increased levels of inflammatory markers (e.g. CRP and ESR).

Transient synovitis of the hip is a type of reactive arthritis specifically affecting the hip. The child typically presents with a limp but is generally well. The diagnostic approach and management are the same as for reactive arthritis.

Management

Treatment is with rest and simple analgesia until the symptoms have fully resolved. Normally this takes a few days.

Bone and joint infections

Bone and joint infections are uncommon, with about 12 cases per 100,000 children diagnosed per year in high-income countries. At least 50% occur in children under 5 years old. Prompt recognition and treatment of these infections are vital to prevent lifelong damage to the bone or joint.

> **Always consider septic arthritis in a child newly presenting with a limp, especially a toddler.** Septic arthritis of the hip (a deep joint) may not manifest with the classic presentation of a hot, swollen joint. The depth of the joint and subcutaneous fat mask this.

Septic arthritis

Septic arthritis is an infection of the joint space. It is caused by bacteria, which have reached the joint by haematogenous spread, for example *Staphylococcus aureus* (in 75% of cases). Septic arthritis commonly affects the hip and knee.

Clinical features

A child with septic arthritis is usually systemically unwell, with a high temperature. The affected joint is usually red, hot and swollen, and is particularly painful, even with the slightest of movements.

> **A child with sickle cell anaemia is especially at risk of contracting septic arthritis by encapsulated Gram-negative bacteria such as salmonella.** This is due to the functional asplenia seen with sickle cell disease, caused by microinfarcts in the spleen.

> **In any child with a high temperature and a swollen, painful joint** assume septic arthritis is the cause until proven otherwise.

Diagnostic approach

Blood tests show increased levels of inflammatory markers. Blood culture may give positive results for the causative organism. US shows a joint effusion.

Management

Septic arthritis is an orthopaedic emergency. It requires urgent aspiration of the joint effusion followed by irrigation of the joint and IV antibiotics. The aspirated fluid is sent for microscopy, culture and sensitivity. Administration of IV antibiotics guided by sensitivities of the pathogen identified is then continued for ≥ 3 weeks.

Prognosis

With prompt treatment, the prognosis is excellent. However, if there is a delay in the diagnosis of septic arthritis, the articular cartilage, and therefore the joint, will be permanently damaged.

Osteomyelitis

Osteomyelitis is an infection of the bone, typically occurring at the metaphysis of long bones (femur, tibia and humerus). It is the consequence of bacteria reaching the bone, either through haematogenous spread or direct inoculation, for example after trauma. The epiphyseal plate normally prevents spread of infection from the bone into the adjacent joint space. However, in children under 2 years of age the hip capsule is inserted below the metaphysis and the growth plate is immature. This allows bacteria causing osteomyelitis to spread to the joint to cause septic arthritis, and bacteria causing septic arthritis to spread to the bone to cause osteomyelitis.

Clinical features

Osteomyelitis presents with systemic features of malaise and fever, or its onset can be more insidious. There may be localised swelling and erythema of the skin, and extreme tenderness over the area of long bone affected.

> **Osteomyelitis is an essential diagnosis to consider in young children with 'pyrexia of unknown origin',** because they cannot localise the pain, and the swelling may not be obvious.

Diagnostic approach

Blood tests show increased levels of inflammatory markers. Blood cultures may give positive results for the causative organism (e.g. *Staphylococcus aureus*). Radiographs can be helpful if they show abnormality of the bone, but they are often normal in the early stages of infection. Radionuclide bone scans detect infection earlier than radiographs.

Management

The child is started on IV antibiotics. If there is no improvement within 48 h, surgical debridement is indicated. Antibiotics are continued for ≥ 4 weeks to ensure adequate treatment and prevent chronic osteomyelitis.

Prognosis

The prognosis is good if osteomyelitis is treated promptly. However, there is a risk of pathological fractures, and if the epiphyseal growth plate is involved, growth arrest of the limb.

Disorders of the hip and knee

Disorders of the hip and knee usually present with limp, which is painful or painless. Several of the causes are peculiar to children, secondary to the effects of growth, hormones and exercise on the growing bones and joints. The child's age and sex, and the duration of onset of symptoms, give clues to the diagnosis, but radiographs are the most useful diagnostic tool. Knowledge of normal bone and joint anatomy (**Figures 9.2** and **9.7**) is helpful for understanding these conditions.

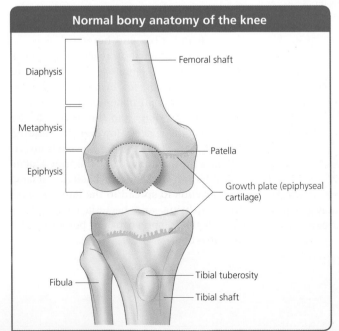

Normal bony anatomy of the knee

Diaphysis — Femoral shaft
Metaphysis
Epiphysis — Patella
Growth plate (epiphyseal cartilage)
Fibula — Tibial tuberosity
Tibial shaft

Figure 9.7 Bony anatomy of the normal knee (the joint space is exaggerated in this view). The patella is attached by ligaments to the tibia at the tibial tuberosity, and to the femur. The tuberosity is subject to a great deal of stress during physical activity, which makes it vulnerable to microfractures and inflammation. Growth plates are visible on imaging at the distal and proximal ends of long bones and are also vulnerable to injury.

Perthes' disease

Perthes' disease occurs when there is a lack of blood supply to the epiphysis of the femoral head; the consequent avascular necrosis results in loss of bone mass and deformity of the femoral head. The exact cause of the avascular necrosis is unknown.

The disease is uncommon, affecting 1 child in 100,000. It typically presents in children aged about 4–10 years, and is usually unilateral (bilateral in 10–15% of cases). Boys are preferentially affected (male to female ratio, 5:1).

Clinical features

Perthes' disease presents with a painless limp or mild and often intermittent hip or referred knee pain, described as 'sore' by the child. The affected hip has reduced abduction or internal rotation. There may also be quadriceps muscle wasting.

Diagnostic approach

Radiography shows a flattened femoral head with increased bone density (**Figure 9.8**).

Management

The aim of treatment is to enable revascularisation and reossification of the femoral head. To achieve this, the femoral head needs to be kept in the acetabulum, with the use of either mechanical appliances or surgical osteotomy. The outcome is good if Perthes' disease is identified and treated early.

Slipped upper femoral epiphysis

Slipped upper femoral epiphysis is diagnosed when the femoral epiphysis slips posteroinferiorly at the level of the growth plate, thereby separating from the metaphysis. Its cause is unknown, but there is thought to be an endocrine link because it usually occurs around adolescence and is associated with hypothyroidism and obesity. Boys are affected more often than girls. The condition predominantly affects children aged 10–15 years. It is bilateral in 20% of cases.

Clinical features

Slipped upper femoral epiphysis presents with sudden onset of a painful limp. The affected leg can appear externally rotated. There is limited abduction and internal rotation of the hip joint.

Diagnostic approach

Radiography confirms the diagnosis by showing displacement of the epiphysis (**Figure 9.9**).

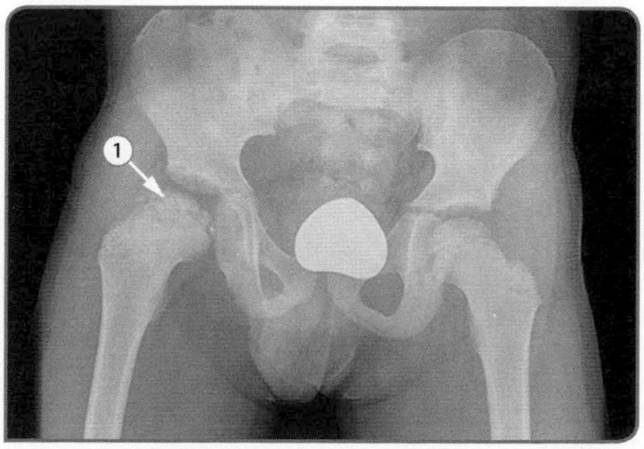

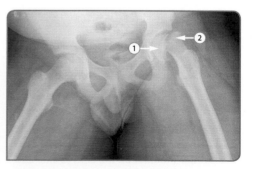

Figure 9.8 Radiograph showing Perthes' disease of the right hip in a 7-year-old child. The femoral head ① is flattened, with increased bone density (whiter, brighter bone) compared with the bone in the opposite, normal hip.

Figure 9.9 Radiograph showing slipped upper femoral epiphysis of the left hip in a 14-year-old boy. The capital epiphysis ① has slipped off the femoral head ②, an appearance that has been likened to 'ice cream slipping off a cone'.

Management

Slipped upper femoral epiphysis requires early surgery to correct the abnormality and to prevent serious complications, which include avascular necrosis and osteoarthritis. Treatment is with screw fixation of the epiphysis, along with analgesia and bed rest. There is a 20% risk of the opposite side being affected within 18 months of the initial slipped upper femoral epiphysis.

Osgood–Schlatter disease

Osgood–Schlatter disease is characterised by pain and swelling of the tibial tuberosity at the site of insertion of the patellar ligament. It is thought to be the result of multiple subacute microavulsion fractures of the tuberosity before fusion of the tibial growth plate and the ossification centre of the tibial tuberosity. It is more common in active children aged 10–16 years, particularly boys (male to female ratio, 3:1), associated with repetitive use of the quadriceps muscles during the rapid adolescence growth spurt. It affects 10–15% of athletic, and up to 4% of non-athletic, adolescents. It is bilateral in 20–50% of patients.

Clinical features

The disease presents with knee pain , particularly after repetitive running or jumping activities, localised point tenderness and frequently a lump (callus formation) over the tibial tuberosity due to new bone laid down in the avulsion space during the repair of the stress fracture. There is a full range of movement of the knee.

Diagnostic approach

The diagnosis is clinical but a plain radiograph of the knee is usually undertaken to exclude other pathologies such as neoplasm and acute tibial apophyseal fracture. Best seen on the lateral view, a radiograph usually shows irregular ossification of the tibial tubercle and soft tissue swelling.

Management

Osgood–Schlatter disease is a self-limiting condition, treated with rest, analgesia, stretching exercises and occasionally orthopaedic bracing. In 10% of cases the symptoms continue into adulthood.

Growing pains

Growing pains are common in children aged 3–12 years. The cause is unknown. The child has leg pain that occurs only at night, often waking the child. Physical examination is normal. There is no specific treatment, but massage is thought to help.

Scoliosis

Scoliosis is lateral curvature of the spine (**Figure 9.10**). It is either structural or postural.

- In structural scoliosis, there is apparent curvature of the spine on standing, and a 'rib hump' on bending forwards (**Figure 9.11**); other findings include elevated shoulder on the convex side and apparent unequal leg length
- Postural scoliosis appears as curvature on standing, but there is no rib hump on bending forwards

The cause is unknown in most (85%) children diagnosed with structural scoliosis; it is then termed idiopathic scoliosis. Idiopathic scoliosis affects about 3% of children, most of whom are girls, during their pubertal growth spurt. There is a family history in 30% of cases.

Non-idiopathic scoliosis is secondary to an underlying problem, usually neuromuscular disease (**Table 9.8**).

Diagnosis is confirmed by spinal radiographs (see **Figure 9.10**).

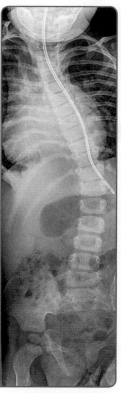

Figure 9.10
Radiograph showing a scoliotic spine in a 1-year-old child.

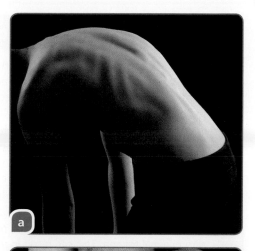

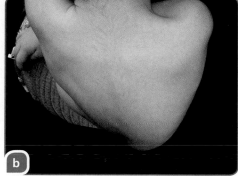

Figure 9.11 Scoliosis is most easily seen on the forward-bending test. It is evident as a 'rib hump', seen here on the right side of the chest. (a) Idiopathic scoliosis. (b) Scoliosis secondary to muscle disease (seen from above).

Scoliosis: associated conditions	
Category	Condition
Connective tissue disorders	Marfan's syndrome
	Ehlers-Danlos syndrome
Neuromuscular conditions	Neurofibromatosis
	Muscular dystrophies
	Spinal muscular atrophy
	Spina bifida
	Cerebral palsy
	Vertebral or intraspinal tumours
Skeletal conditions	Leg length discrepancy
	Developmental dysplasia of the hip

Table 9.8 Conditions associated with scoliosis

Management

All children with scoliosis, unless very mild, are monitored regularly with radiographs 6–12-monthly to check the angle of the curve and whether the condition is progressing.

Treatment consists of bracing or casting. In severe scoliosis, surgery to insert spinal rods or to carry out vertebral fusion may be required. About 10% of teenagers with idiopathic scoliosis require intervention.

Answers to starter questions

1. As with adults, children can present with referred pain from the joint above or below the painful one. Young children sometimes have difficulty localising pain: they will point vaguely at a large section of the leg or not complain of pain at all despite limping.

2. Juvenile idiopathic arthritis (JIA) is an autoimmune condition that affects multiple systems in the body. Anterior uveitis is associated with JIA and is actively sought for with regular screening because it can be asymptomatic and lead to blindness if untreated. Oligoarticular arthritis is associated with a high risk of uveitis, a medium risk of polyarticular and a low risk of systemic onset. All children with JIA are screened regardless of their type.

3. Children with osteogenesis imperfecta have fragile bones that easily fracture, often with minimal trauma. This can result in multiple fractures of different ages being seen on an X-ray; with little history of trauma, this is also a red flag non-accidental injury (see page 432).

4. If developmental dysplasia of the hip is detected within the first few months of birth its management is straightforward: the vast majority of patient only requiring splinting. If the abnormality is not noted in this early period the child will usually not then present until they have started walking, by which time the femoral head is usually out of the underdeveloped acetabulum and significant surgery is required.

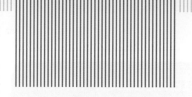

Chapter 10
Allergy, immunodeficiency and infections

Starter questions

Answers to the following questions are on page 301.

1. How does measles cause personality changes later in life?
2. Why should a child on regular oral steroids for asthma avoid contracting chickenpox?

Introduction

The normal function of the immune system is to defend the body from disease-causing organisms. Disorders of the immune system result from its over- or underactivity.

Illness results when the immune system cannot produce an adequate defence against an infectious organism, or is over- or underactive. In the latter two categories:

- Allergy develops when the immune system starts to recognise normally harmless substances as a threat; the resulting inappropriate immune response causes the symptoms of allergic disease
- In immunodeficiency, the immune system is unable to produce an adequate immune

response against disease-causing organisms; it is an uncommon but serious condition

Infection occurs when the immune system is unable to prevent a disease-causing organism becoming established. With their immature immune systems that have not yet been primed by exposure to infectious organisms, or to many strains of the more common ones, children are especially susceptible to many infectious diseases. However, since the introduction of vaccines conferring immunity to many diseases, formerly common childhood diseases with serious complications are now relatively rare in developed countries.

Case 14 Rash after eating a takeaway meal

Presentation

Joshua, aged 3 years, is referred to the allergy clinic after an episode of urticarial rash appearing immediately after eating a Chinese takeaway meal.

Initial interpretation

Urticarial rashes have several causes, viral or bacterial infections being the most common cause in children (see page 358), but are also commonly associated with an allergic reaction. Joshua showed no viral or bacterial symptoms, and was well before the rash appeared. If a food allergy is suspected, a detailed history is essential, focusing on what the child was doing, what they were eating and what they were exposed to shortly before the rash appeared. In this case, the timing of the reaction suggests that a food in the takeaway meal is the cause of the rash.

Further history

Joshua had eaten prawn toast and chicken with peanuts. His mother describes the rash as itchy and 'like nettle stings' all over his body, and says that they appeared within 10 minutes of eating. There was no swelling of his lips, or any difficulty in swallowing or breathing. Joshua has never had a similar reaction before, but to his mother's knowledge he has never previously eaten nuts or prawns.

He had mild eczema as a baby. He now has asthma, for which he needs to regularly use a preventer inhaler delivering a low dose of steroid.

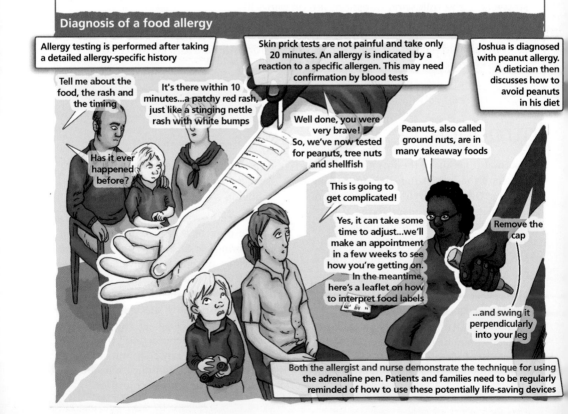

Diagnosis of a food allergy

Allergy testing is performed after taking a detailed allergy-specific history

Skin prick tests are not painful and take only 20 minutes. An allergy is indicated by a reaction to a specific allergen. This may need confirmation by blood tests

Joshua is diagnosed with peanut allergy. A dietician then discusses how to avoid peanuts in his diet

Tell me about the food, the rash and the timing

It's there within 10 minutes...a patchy red rash, just like a stinging nettle rash with white bumps

Well done, you were very brave!
So, we've now tested for peanuts, tree nuts and shellfish

Peanuts, also called ground nuts, are in many takeaway foods

Has it ever happened before?

This is going to get complicated!

Yes, it can take some time to adjust...we'll make an appointment in a few weeks to see how you're getting on.
In the meantime, here's a leaflet on how to interpret food labels

Remove the cap

...and swing it perpendicularly into your leg

Both the allergist and nurse demonstrate the technique for using the adrenaline pen. Patients and families need to be regularly reminded of how to use these potentially life-saving devices

Case 14 *continued*

Examination

The rash has now gone, but Joshua's mother had taken a photograph of it. Its appearance matches the raised wheals of urticaria. The rash's transient and pruritic nature are also consistent with a diagnosis of urticaria. The examination is normal.

Interpretation of findings

The short time between eating and the appearance of the rash strongly suggests food allergy. Common food allergens include nuts (peanuts and groundnut oil, which is derived from peanuts; and tree nuts) and seafood, both of which were in the takeaway meal.

Investigations

Skin prick tests are carried out in the clinic to determine Joshua's response to allergens from various nuts (including peanuts) as well as from prawns and other seafood. He has a moderately positive skin reaction to peanuts, but no reaction to any of the other allergens tested.

Diagnosis

Peanut allergy is diagnosed. Joshua requires an adrenaline (epinephrine) auto-injection device for self-administration, as he is at risk of a severe allergic reaction (anaphylaxis) in the future. Most developed countries now give an adrenaline pen to all children with nut allergy. In Joshua's case his asthma and his requirement for inhaled steroids indicates a high degree of atopy and therefore he has a high risk of anaphylaxis. It is explained to Joshua's mother when the auto-injection device would be needed and they are both shown how it is used. They will be seen annually for regular refresher sessions on its use.

Joshua and his mother see the dietician to learn what foods may contain peanuts and therefore what to avoid. The staff at Joshua's nursery, and later his school, will need to be made aware of his allergy and how to use the auto-injector, because he may inadvertently be exposed to nuts in the preschool or school environment. Peanut allergy is typically a lifelong problem.

Allergy

Allergy is the term for a number of diseases in which the immune system has become hypersensitive to a normally harmless substance commonly found in the environment, for example pollen. The immune system reacts to this substance as a threat. Exposure to the substance, i.e. the allergen, triggers a complex reaction at a cellular level that results in the typical symptoms of allergy.

Epidemiology

Allergy is very common: half of children have at least one type of allergy. It affects boys more commonly than girls.

Aetiology

Children who have a parent with an allergy are more likely to have an allergy themselves. Interestingly, they may not be allergic to the same substances as their parent.

According to the 'hygiene hypothesis', children exposed to fewer allergens are more likely to become sensitised to common environmental substances and develop allergies in consequence.

Pathogenesis

There are two types of allergic reaction: those mediated by immunoglobulin (Ig) E antibodies and those not mediated by IgE antibodies.

Immunoglobulin E-mediated allergic reactions occur immediately on the body's recognition of an allergen. In response, the immune system produces large numbers of IgE antibodies which act against the specific allergen. The antibodies bind to the allergen and to mast cells; this latter action causes the mast cells to release histamine (**Figure 10.1**). Histamine causes immediate symptoms, including rhinorrhoea (runny nose), sneezing and urticarial rash. Severe reactions can result in anaphylaxis.

Non-immunoglobulin E-mediated reactions are not immediate, so it is difficult to associate the associated symptoms with exposure to a specific allergen. The exact pathophysiology of non-IgE-mediated allergic reactions is unclear.

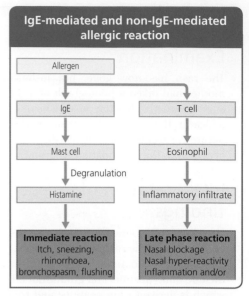

IgE-mediated and non-IgE-mediated allergic reaction

Figure 10.1 Immunoglobulin (Ig) E-mediated and non-IgE-mediated allergic reaction. When IgE-mediated there is an immediate reaction. When non-IgE mediated there is a late phase reaction.

Anaphylaxis is a severe, life-threatening condition caused by an overwhelming allergic reaction. Symptoms include stridor, bronchoconstriction (wheeze), urticarial rash, vomiting and hypotension. Urgent treatment with adrenaline (epinephrine) injected into the muscle is needed. Susceptible children must carry an adrenaline pen with them at all times in case such a reaction occurs.

Clinical features

Clinical features of IgE-mediated reactions include immediate sneezing, rhinorrhoea, red and itchy eyes, wheeze, cough or urticarial rash on contact with the allergen.

Always consider the possibility of fabricated or induced illness in unexplained allergy, particularly if the history and clinical picture are inconsistent. Parents may report exaggerated allergic reactions or place a child on an inappropriately restricted diet. It can be helpful to admit these children to hospital to obtain more objective information such as by challenging the child with the alleged allergen.

Symptoms of non-IgE-mediated allergic reactions are non-specific and do not occur immediately after exposure to the allergen, rather 24–48 hours later. Symptoms may include diarrhoea, dry and itchy skin or chronically blocked nose.

Diagnostic approach

An allergy can usually be diagnosed clinically, without the need for invasive tests, if the typical symptoms occur after exposure. Where there is uncertainty, a diary to document exposure to potential allergens and the symptoms experienced may be helpful to identify the specific one.

Skin prick testing is commonly used to identify allergens. The allergens tested against are those directed by the history, and the allergens commonly seen. Allergens in liquid form are applied to the skin, and the skin below the liquid is superficially scratched. An allergy is confirmed if the skin develops an urticarial reaction within 15 min of exposure.

Antihistamines should not be taken for a few days before the skin prick test, because their use could affect the results by preventing a reaction.

Total levels of IgE antibody in the blood are unhelpful, because they can be increased in conditions associated with allergy, such as asthma, but not the allergy itself.

Levels of a specific IgE antibody may be increased in children with 'sensitisation' to a particular allergen. This means that antibodies are formed against the allergen and can be detected in the blood, but the child does not have symptoms of allergy when exposed to the allergen. Therefore results of increased IgE are interpreted in the context of the clinical history and symptoms.

Blood tests can be carried out to measure the number of specific IgE antibodies present for a particular antigen, for example IgE antibodies specific to peanuts or to tree pollen, which is useful when skin prick testing is not available, although this is less sensitive (particularly for inhaled allergens) than skin prick testing.

Management

Management consists of avoiding the allergen. Symptomatic relief can be obtained from antihistamine medications available as tablets, eye drops or skin creams. Adrenaline (epinephrine) auto-injection devices are given to all children with nut allergies (peanut and tree nut), and to those who presented with anaphylaxis symptoms, or children on inhaled steroids for asthma who also have other food allergies.

Allergic diseases

The common allergic diseases are allergic rhinitis, asthma, eczema, food allergy, venom allergy (e.g. against bee stings) and drug allergy. The most common of these are allergic rhinitis and food allergy. Eczema is discussed on page 362 and asthma on page 160. The most severe allergic reaction – anaphylaxis – is discussed on page 403.

Allergic rhinitis

Allergic rhinitis is inflammation of the inside of the nose as a result of the immune reaction to an allergen, usually an allergen circulating in the air, i.e. an aeroallergen. Aeroallergens are divided into seasonal allergens and perennial allergens (**Table 10.1**).

Clinical features

In addition to sneezing and rhinorrhoea, secondary to nasal inflammation, the child may have red, itchy, watery eyes (allergic conjunctivitis) and other clinical features of atopy

Allergic rhinitis: common sources of aeroallergens	
Type of allergic rhinitis	Allergens
Seasonal allergic rhinitis (hay fever)	Grass pollens
	Tree pollens
	Weeds
	Fungal spores
Perennial allergic rhinitis	House dust mite faeces
	Animal hair (from cats, dogs, horses, mice, rats)
	Moulds

Table 10.1 Common allergens causing allergic rhinitis

(**Table 10.2**). Allergic rhinitis is associated with sinusitis, otitis media, eczema and asthma.

Nasal speculum examination shows:

- pale blue, enlarged nasal turbinates with a clear watery discharge

Atopy: clinical features	
Head and face	Body and limbs
Itchy eyes and nose	Patches of eczema on flexures (e.g. elbows and knees)
Runny nose	
Allergic shiners (dark circles under the eyes associated with itchy eyes and caused by rubbing)	Scratch marks on the skin (from the child's own finger-nails)
Red conjunctiva	
Crease across the nose (from the 'allergic salute')	
Mouth open for breathing (to compensate for chronically blocked nose)	

Table 10.2 Clinical features of atopy

- inflamed mucosa
- nasal polyps (occasionally)

> Many children with allergic rhinitis also have eczema and asthma. If the child has these three conditions, they are said to have atopy and may be described as being 'atopic'.

> The **'allergic salute'** is the habitual gesture in children with allergic rhinitis of using a hand to push the tip of their nose upwards to relieve nasal itch. This produces a horizontal skin crease at the distal end of the nose.

> The presence of **nasal polyps** in a child prompts consideration of cystic fibrosis. Nasal polyps are associated with cystic fibrosis as well as allergy.

Management

Treatment for allergic rhinitis includes allergen avoidance, although aeroallergens, especially those from house dust mite faeces, are difficult to avoid. Topical nasal corticosteroids, antihistamines and decongestants are used. For severe allergic rhinitis, regular use of oral steroids or allergen immunotherapy is tried to suppress the immune system.

> Severe allergic rhinitis can significantly reduce a child's quality of life, diminishing their enjoyment of outdoor activities and even reducing school attendance. Oral steroid therapy is only a short-term treatment due to the adverse effects of long-term steroid use. It is usually used at times when relief of symptoms is particularly important, for example when the child is taking examinations at school.

Food allergy

In food allergy, a certain food causes an allergic reaction: the allergy is usually either IgE-mediated or non-IgE-mediated, cows' milk protein allergy being the exception (**Table 10.3**). Common food allergens include milk and eggs. Peanut, tree nuts, soy, wheat, fish and shellfish are also known food allergens. Food allergy affects about 1 in 14 children. Most children affected are younger than 3 years.

IgE-mediated food allergy and non-IgE-mediated food sensitivity		
Type	Timing	Symptoms
IgE-mediated (e.g. peanut allergy)	Occurs within 60 min of ingesting the food	Swelling (angio-oedema), especially of the face
		Urticaria
		Vomiting
		Wheezing and coughing
		Anaphylaxis
Non-IgE-mediated, (e.g. 40% of cows' milk protein allergy)	Occurs 24 hours to days after ingestion	Vomiting
		Diarrhoea (bloody if severe)
		Abdominal cramps (colic)
		Malabsorption or slow weight gain
		Eczema

Table 10.3 Characteristics of immunoglobulin (Ig) E-mediated food allergy and non-IgE-mediated food hypersensitivity

> **Children with egg allergy cannot receive the standard flu vaccine.** The vaccine virus is grown in fertilised hens' eggs, so there is a risk of allergic reaction. Instead, they are given special egg-free flu vaccine. They can receive all other vaccines as normal.

Nut allergy

This is an IgE-mediated food allergy with symptoms occurring immediately after ingestion of a nut, either a peanut (a ground nut; legume) or a tree nut (most other types of nut; hard-shelled fruit). Nut allergy is estimated to occur in about 1 in 50 children, mainly peanut allergy. Typical symptoms are:

- rash
- swelling of the lips, eyes and/or face
- itchy throat
- vomiting
- diarrhoea

> **A food challenge consists of giving the child small amounts of the food to which they are allergic in a stepwise manner.** The food is first placed on the lips, then the tongue; the food is then ingested in gradually increasing amounts. If a reaction occurs, the child should continue to avoid the offending food. If no reaction occurs, the food can be reintroduced into their diet.

Anaphylaxis can occur if the reaction is severe. Diagnosis is based on clinical history. Management includes avoidance of ingestion and sometimes other types of exposure to nuts, or if symptoms develop, use of antihistamines. The child needs to have an adrenaline pen at all times. Peanut allergies tend to be lifelong; about 10% of children with tree nut allergy grow out of the allergy.

Cows' milk protein allergy

Non IgE-mediated food allergy is more difficult to detect. Cows' milk protein allergy is an allergy to one or more proteins in cows' milk. It can be an IgE-mediated reaction (in up to 60% of cows milk allergy) or non-IgE mediated (the most common recognised non-IgE mediated food allergy).

Cows' milk protein allergy affects up to 5% of neonates and infants in developed countries. Ingestion of milk, either breast or formula, causes either an immediate IgE allergic reaction (see above) or delayed non-specific symptoms (non-IgE mediated), including colic, diarrhoea or mucus-containing stools, eczema and in severe cases failure to thrive.

Diagnosis of the Ig-E mediated allergy is skin prick testing for milk protein or serum milk IgE levels. Diagnosis of the non-IgE mediated milk allergy is clinically based; there is no test for this type of allergy. A trial of hypoallergenic formula milk, or a dairy-free diet for the mother if the baby is breastfed, is given. If symptoms improve as a result, this confirms the diagnosis and the avoidance of cows' milk should continue, even when the child is weaned.

Dairy products are gradually reintroduced from the age of 9–12 months, under the supervision of a dietician, but stopped if symptoms occur again. In children with non-IgE mediated cows' milk allergy symptoms resolve in 50% of children by the age of 1 year, and in nearly all (90%) children by the age of 3 years. With IgE-mediated cows' milk allergy 50–60% outgrow the allergy by 5 years of age.

Immunodeficiency

In immunodeficiency, a child is at risk of infection because their immune system is functioning inadequately. Immunodeficiency is either primary or secondary (**Table 10.4**).

- In primary immunodeficiency, a genetic problem with the immune system underlies the increased susceptibility to infection
- In secondary immunodeficiency, immune system function is impaired secondary to causes other than a genetic problem with the immune system

It can be difficult to recognise immunodeficiency among the many minor, often viral, infections that children contract each year.

> **The use of live vaccines is avoided in children with immunodeficiency.** Unlike other types of vaccine, live vaccines consist of a viable pathogen, so they have the rare potential to cause disease. Therefore there is a risk of overwhelming infection in immunocompromised individuals.

Primary immunodeficiency

Primary immunodeficiencies are caused by various genetic abnormalities that can affect

any part of the immune system, thereby impairing its normal function. This results in an increased susceptibility to infections.

> **Immunodeficiency is suspected when there is a history of 'SPUR':** Severe, Persistent, Unusual or Recurrent infections.

Epidemiology and aetiology

Although there are more than 200 known primary immunodeficiencies, they are uncommon. They are estimated to affect 1 in 10,000 of the population, although the incidence could be higher because many people with minor deficiency go undiagnosed. In 80% of cases, the condition is diagnosed before the age of 20 years.

> **Primary immunodeficiencies do not present until the age of 6 months,** because up to this age maternal antibodies are still circulating in the child's body and helping to fight infection.

Specific primary immunodeficiencies are associated with specific syndromes, including DiGeorge's syndrome (chromosome 22q11 deletion syndrome), Job's syndrome and Wiskott-Aldrich syndrome.

Clinical features

It is normal for children to have frequent and recurrent mild infections, with up to 12 viral infections a year. A primary immunodeficiency is suspected when a child presents with multiple infections in close succession that are more severe than normal childhood infections; for example, children with primary immunodeficiency may contract septicaemia, meningitis or infections with unusual organisms. The infections are usually severe enough to require treatment with intravenous antibiotics.

Primary and secondary immunodeficiency: causes	
Primary immunodeficiency*	Secondary immunodeficiency
Severe combined immunodeficiency	Chemotherapy
X-linked hypogammaglobulinaemia	Leukaemia or lymphoma
	HIV
Common variable hypogammaglobulinaemia	Malnutrition
	Nephrotic syndrome (protein-losing conditions)
Immunoglobulin A deficiency	

*More than 200 causes have been described.

Table 10.4 Causes of primary and secondary immunodeficiency

More than two infections separated by time at the same anatomical site raise suspicion of a structural abnormality. For example, vesico-ureteric reflux is suspected in children with recurrent urinary tract infections (page 229).

Diagnostic approach

A child with suspected primary immunodeficiency, or who is known to have a syndrome associated with immunodeficiency, is referred to an immunologist for detailed investigations. Baseline blood antibody measurements are done to identify low levels, and more complex investigations are usually carried out to test specific aspects of immune function.

Management

Management depends on the underlying cause of the immunodeficiency and is guided by an immunologist. Prophylactic antibiotics are frequently given to prevent infection; if infection occurs, antibiotics are given for a longer duration and often administered intravenously. Intravenous immunoglobulins are given as replacement therapy in children with congenital agammaglobulinaemia and hypogammaglobulineamia.

In severe primary immunodeficiency, bone marrow transplantation may be needed. Gene therapy is an evolving therapy with the potential to cure primary immunodeficiencies. Prognosis is variable and depends on the severity of the primary immunodeficiency.

DiGeorge's syndrome

DiGeorge's syndrome, also known as congenital thymic aplasia, is a congenital syndrome that affects 1 in 4000 children. It is the result of deletion of the long arm of chromosome 22 (22q11 deletion), which leads to a defect in embryological development of the 3rd and 4th pharyngeal pouches. This abnormal development results in absence of the thymus and abnormal parathyroid glands. The thymus is the site of maturation of T cells, a type of white blood cell with key roles in enabling the immune system to respond effectively to specific antigens. Therefore absence

of the thymus results in T-cell deficiency and impaired immune system function. Hypocalcaemia and hypoparathyroidism result from the malfunctioning parathyroid glands. DiGeorge's syndrome is also associated with palatal abnormalities (in 50%; abnormal movement or cleft palate), congenital heart abnormalities (40%) and learning difficulties (90%).

Diagnosis is made when the child has the clinical features associated with DiGeorge's syndrome and deletion of the long arm of chromosome 22 is confirmed by genetic testing. Management consists of managing the various associated conditions and providing educational support.

'CATCH-22' is the mnemonic for DiGeorge's syndrome and its associated features:

- Cardiac abnormality
- Abnormal facies (dysmorphism)
- Thymic aplasia (immunodeficiency)
- Cleft palate
- Hypocalcemia and/or hypoparathyroidism
- Chromosomal 22 abnormality

Secondary immunodeficiency

Secondary immunodeficiency is diagnosed when a disease or condition impairs the functioning of the immune system, resulting in immunocompromise. The true incidence of secondary immunodeficiency is unknown, but it is associated with certain diseases or conditions (see **Table 10.4**).

Presentation is the same as that of primary immunodeficiency. However, diagnosis can be reached more quickly than with primary immunodeficiency if the child is known to have a condition associated with secondary immunodeficiency. If the underlying disease or condition is addressed, for example when chemotherapy ends, normal immune system function is usually restored. Prognosis depends on the cause of the secondary immunodeficiency.

Childhood infections

Most of the typical childhood infections are viral, cause a characteristic rash (viral exanthem) and spread easily to others. Many childhood infections have become rare in developed countries following the introduction of vaccinations. However, outbreaks still occur if a population's vaccination rate becomes low. Routine vaccination schedules are discussed on page 421.

Immunocompromised children, including those on chemotherapy or regular steroid therapy, are particularly vulnerable to severe infections and serious complications.

The following section discusses systemic viral infections. Bacterial and viral infections that principally target single body systems, e.g. respiratory infections, are discussed in the relevant 'system' chapters.

> **Meningitis is an example of childhood infection that has both viral and bacterial causes.** Its initial presentation is usually similar to simple viral illnesses, but if it is suspected it must be promptly investigated because it can be life-threatening. It is discussed in detail on page 251.

> **Exanthem** is a widespread skin rash; **enanthem** is a rash on the mucous membranes

Measles

Measles is the disease caused by infection with the measles virus. It is transmitted by respiratory droplets. Symptoms of measles occur about 10 days after infection (**Figure 10.2**). Characteristically, the child is very miserable because they feel so unwell. Diagnosis is based on clinical signs and symptoms but can be confirmed by the presence of anti-measles antibodies in the saliva. Infection is preventable with vaccination.

> **In many developed countries, the number of children diagnosed with measles has risen over the past 15 years, because of a drop in uptake of the MMR vaccine,** which provides immunity against measles, mumps and rubella. Uptake decreased worldwide in response to publication of a 1998 report claiming a link between the MMR vaccine and autism in a study of 12 children. This research has since been discredited, with subsequent studies showing no evidence for the association. An outbreak of measles in Wales in 2013 resulted in more than 800 children diagnosed and one death, demonstrating the danger of a reduction in 'herd immunity'.

Management

Treatment of measles is supportive; however, clinicians should be vigilant for serious complications (**Table 10.5**). In high-income countries, death is rare (1 per 1000 infected). A similar number develop acute encephalitis, often resulting in permanent brain damage. Complications are increased in low- and middle-income countries, which have measles mortality rates of up to 10%. Most deaths

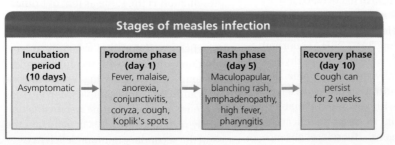

Figure 10.2 The four stages of measles infection after the average 10-day incubation period.

Complications of measles	
Category	**Complications**
Pulmonary	Bronchopneumonia
	Otitis media
Neurological	Encephalitis
	Acute disseminated encephalomyelitis (demyelinating disease of the brain during the recovery phase), with death in < 20% of cases
	Subacute sclerosing panencephalitis
Eye	Keratitis
	Corneal ulceration
Gastrointestinal	Gingivostomatitis
	Diarrhoea and gastroenteritis
	Mesenteric lymphadenitis and appendicitis
	Hepatitis
Cardiac	Myocarditis and pericarditis
Immunosuppression	Severe secondary infections

Table 10.5 Complications of measles infection

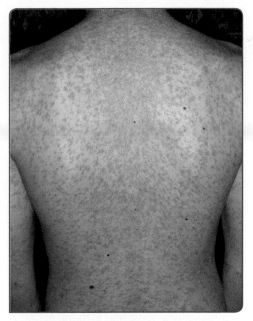

Figure 10.3 Rubella. A maculopapular blanching rash starting on the face and spreading to the neck, the trunk and then the extremities. The lesions may become confluent petechiae or haemorrhagic. After 3 days, the rash turns brown and fades. This is followed by fine desquamation (peeling), settling by 7 days.

from measles are the result of respiratory complications or encephalitis.

Koplik's spots, an enanthem, are pathognomonic for measles infection, detected in 50–70% of patients if examined 2–3 days before the measles exanthem appears. They resemble grains of salt on a red background on the buccal mucosa, opposite the molar teeth.

Subacute sclerosing panencephalitis occurs in 1 in 100,000 cases of measles. It is a progressive neurodegenerative disease and is fatal. It occurs 7–10 years after measles infection. Symptoms include personality change, myoclonus, dementia and finally a continuous (persistent) vegetative state and death within a few years.

Rubella

The rubella virus is spread by respiratory droplets. It is now less common because of rubella vaccination.

The infection is usually mild and may be subclinical. Clinical features, including pyrexia, arthralgia and coryza, occur about 14 days after infection. A maculopapular rash also develops, starting on the face before spreading to the trunk and extremities, covering the whole body within 24 h (**Figure 10.3**). The rash resolves within 3 days.

Diagnosis is based on clinical findings but can be confirmed by the presence of anti-rubella antibodies in the blood. Treatment is supportive. Rare complications include bleeding disorders due to thrombocytopaenia, and encephalitis.

Congenital rubella syndrome can occur if a woman contracts rubella during pregnancy, especially the first trimester. Rubella infection in early pregnancy can cause miscarriage or stillbirth. A baby born with congenital rubella will have severe birth defects, including congenital heart disease, hearing impairment, cataracts and developmental delay. A 'blueberry muffin rash' is a presenting sign.

Measles, mumps and rubella were made notifiable diseases in the UK after introduction of the MMR vaccine in1998. This enables monitoring for outbreaks and to evaluate the success of the immunisation programme.

Mumps

The mumps virus is highly infective, and is transmitted by respiratory droplets or direct contact. Symptoms occur 2–3 weeks after infection. Clinical features include general malaise and low-grade fever. There is characteristically a rapid and extreme parotitis, i.e. swelling of the parotid glands, as a consequence of infection of the epithelial cells lining the parotid duct. Symptoms resolve after 7–10 days. Diagnosis is clinical or confirmed by presence of mumps-specific immunoglobulin M (IgM) and/or mumps RNA in the saliva of infected individuals.

Management

Treatment is based around treating symptoms, consisting mainly of analgesia and rest. Complications include orchitis (inflammation of the testes), in 3–10% of adolescent and adult males, which causes painful testicular swelling, bilateral in up to 40%, and can lead to reduced fertility (very rarely sterility). Other rarer complications, each <1% are, pancreatitis, deafness and encephalitis.

Chickenpox

Chickenpox, varicella, is common: in temperate climates it is contracted by 9 out of 10 children by the time they reach their teenage years. It is caused by the varicella-zoster virus, which is transmitted by respiratory droplets or on direct contact with the contents of the vesicles that develop on the skin as a result of the infection. Chickenpox in childhood is usually a benign illness, but it is more severe in adolescents, adults and immunosuppressed individuals.

Chickenpox develops in four stages (**Figure 10.4**). Symptoms begin 10–21 days after infection. There may be general malaise followed shortly by the rash stage. The rash starts as small red macules, which then develop into fluid-filled vesicles (**Figure 10.5**). These continue to appear for about 3–4 days. The vesicles are intensely itchy. They begin to crust over and fall off after 2 weeks. The child is contagious from 2 days before the rash appears until the lesions have crusted over.

Management

For most patients, treatment is symptomatic and includes antihistamines to help relieve the itching. If the child is immunocompromised, antiviral medication is given to help prevent severe infection. Complications of chickenpox can be very serious (**Table 10.6**).

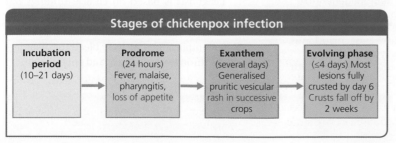

Figure 10.4 The four stages of chickenpox infection.

Stages of chickenpox infection			
Incubation period (10–21 days)	Prodrome (24 hours) Fever, malaise, pharyngitis, loss of appetite	Exanthem (several days) Generalised pruritic vesicular rash in successive crops	Evolving phase (≤4 days) Most lesions fully crusted by day 6 Crusts fall off by 2 weeks

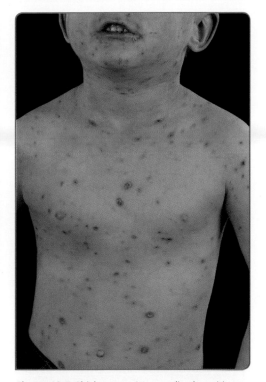

Figure 10.5 Chickenpox. A generalised pruritic vesicular rash during the exanthem stage.

Complications of chickenpox	
Category	Complications
Skin and soft tissue infections (invasive group A *Streptococcus*)	Cellulitis
	Myositis
	Necrotising fasciitis
	Toxic shock syndrome
Respiratory	Pneumonitis
	Pleural effusion
Neurological	Encephalitis or meningitis at time of rash
	Acute cerebellar ataxia 1–2 weeks after rash
Gastrointestinal	Diarrhoea
	Hepatitis
Ear, nose and throat	Pharyngitis
	Otitis media
Haemorrhagic	Purpura fulminans
Congenital anomalies	In first trimester: scarred limbs, microcephaly and ocular damage
	Near to term: severe neonatal infection

Table 10.6 Complications of chickenpox infection. The serious complications occur more commonly in infants, adults and immunocompromised people.

> **Immunosuppressed children are at risk of serious chickenpox infection with severe complications (Table 10.6).** If they have been in contact with someone who has chickenpox, they must be given zoster immune globulin promptly to prevent infection with varicella-zoster virus.

After the chickenpox infection is over, the varicella-zoster virus remains dormant in the dorsal root ganglion. If the child (or adult) becomes immunosuppressed later in childhood or in adult life, the virus can be reactivated and causes shingles (herpes zoster), a vesicular rash in a dermatomal distribution.

Glandular fever

Glandular fever, also called infectious mononucleosis, is the disease caused by infection with the Epstein–Barr virus. One in five children contract it, typically in adolescence; it is transmitted through contact with infected saliva.

Clinical features include malaise, headache and mild fever, which are followed by tonsillitis and/or pharyngitis, cervical lymph node enlargement, higher grade fever and fatigue. Some patients will be asymptomatic. Other features include palatal petechiae and periorbital oedema. Mild hepatitis occurs in about 90% of patients, and splenomegaly in 50%. Diagnosis is clinical but can be confirmed by the presence of anti-Epstein–Barr virus antibodies in serum, or a blood film showing atypical lymphocytes.

Management

Treatment is supportive. Symptoms resolve in about 2 weeks, but the fatigue can last for months. Splenic rupture is a rare but serious complication, so contact sports are avoided for a month after the infection.

Infectious mononucleosis is a viral infection, so antibiotics are not indicated. If amoxicillin is given, it causes a generalised morbilliform rash.

Herpetic gingivostomatitis

Herpetic gingivostomatitis is a painful condition in which blisters occur in and around the mouth. It is caused by infection with herpes simplex virus type 1 and is transmitted by saliva. Clinical features include a period of general malaise with inflammation of the mouth and gums, secondary to small vesicles that eventually rupture, leaving painful ulcers (**Figure 10.6**). Affected children can be very unsettled; they may not want to eat or drink, so are at risk of dehydration. Infection can be subclinical.

Diagnosis is based on clinical appearances but can be confirmed by PCR analysis of vesicular fluid, showing the presence of herpes type 1 viral DNA. Treatment is symptomatic and includes analgesia and fluids to maintain hydration. Herpes simplex virus is associated with many other infections affecting various organ systems (**Table 10.7**).

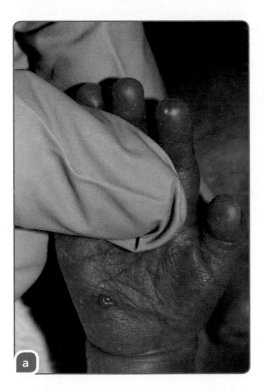

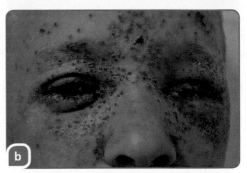

Figure 10.6 Herpetic infections. (a) Neonatal herpes simplex. (b) Eczema herpeticum on the face

Herpes simplex virus infection in children		
Illness	Disease presentation	Other features and notes
Neonatal herpes simplex virus infection Type 2 infection: from mother's genital tract during delivery Type 1 infection: from postnatal contact	Vesicular rash Seizures if central nervous system involvement (often focal onset) Hepatosplenomegaly Bleeding secondary to liver involvement and secondary coagulation problems	High morbidity and mortality: intravenous antiviral therapy is essential
Keratoconjunctivitis	Corneal dendritic ulcers	Treated with topical antiviral medication
Eczema herpeticum	Infection of skin: extensive vesicular rash Visceral dissemination, which is life-threatening but death is rare	Child has background of eczema, making skin vulnerable to infection. Prompt recognition and treatment as a dermatological emergency is vital to prevent death
Cold sores (herpes labialis): recurrent herpes simplex infection	Lesions around the mouth	Associated with upper respiratory tract infections, sun exposure, stress
Herpetic whitlow	Painful vesicular rash on digit	Usually from sucking digit when child has primary gingivostomatitis
Meningoencephalitis	Headache, fever, behavioural disturbance, reduced consciousness Focal seizures Often no skin lesions	Predominantly frontal and temporal lobe involvement shown on electroencephalography and CT

Table 10.7 Conditions caused by herpes simplex virus in children

Answers to starter questions

1. Subacute sclerosing panencephalitis (SSPE) is a degenerative disease of the central nervous system that presents 7–10 years after an initial measles infection, even though the person appears to have fully recovered from the illness, and is due to an abnormal immune response. SSPE has been divided into four stages with symptoms including myoclonus, with massive myoclonic jerks and a pathognomonic EEG. Patients end up in a continuous vegetative state, which may last for several years, before death. The relentless and fatal course of this complication reinforces the importance of measles vaccination.

2. Chickenpox is usually a fairly benign illness, but if a child is immunosuppressed, such as on regular oral steroids, they can contract a severe and life-threatening infection. If the child has not developed antibodies for chickenpox they are given zoster immune globulin (ZIG); if they develop chickenpox they are given aciclovir to reduce the severity of the infection.

Chapter 11
Genetic disorders and dysmorphism

Starter questions

Answers to the following questions are on page 322.

1. Why are some girls affected by X-linked recessive conditions?
2. Why are certain recessive conditions more prevalent in some populations than others?

Introduction

Every individual has a unique set of genes located on 23 pairs of chromosomes contained within every cell in their body. This is the person's genotype and consists of about 25,000 genes. The genotype, together with environmental factors, determines a person's phenotype, i.e. observable physical and functional features (e.g. hair colour or susceptibility to disease).

Within each pair of chromosomes one is inherited from the mother and one from the father. Pairs 1–22 are called autosomes and are alike in males and females. The 23rd pair are the sex chromosomes; females have two

X chromosomes and males have an X chromosome and a Y chromosome.

Genetic disorders arise in one of three ways:

- a change in chromosome number or structure (aneuploidy)
- a mutation in a single gene, i.e. an alteration in the DNA sequence
- interaction between a multifactorial pattern of genetic predisposition and environmental factors

Mutations are inherited from a parent, passed on via germ cells (sperm cells or oocytes), or arise spontaneously in the developing embryo.

Babies and children with genetic disorders usually present with dysmorphic features, congenital anomalies or delayed development. Some children present with several different anomalies or features that are either a random collection of conditions or part of a single syndrome. A referral to the genetics team will help diagnose an underlying unifying syndrome. Testing for the faulty gene may be possible (**Table 11.1**), but for some conditions the responsible gene has yet to be identified.

When a genetic disorder is identified in a child, the family is likely to be offered genetic counselling. This includes information on the natural history of the disease, its usual mode of inheritance and an indication of the risk of recurrence in future children. In some conditions, there is the option of preimplantation or antenatal testing. If a genetic disorder is known to occur in a family, prospective parents may consult a geneticist before conception.

There is no cure for genetic disorders.

> **Identical genotypes do not always produce the same phenotype** because of the variable expression and penetrance (the number of individuals with a given genetic mutation displaying the associated phenotype) of some genes.

Genetic investigations		
Investigation	Indications	Description
Karyotype (chromosome analysis; see Figure 11.1)	Suspected aneuploidy, e.g. Down's syndrome (trisomy 21) Multiple dysmorphic features or congenital anomalies (as an initial screen)	Lymphocytes cultured from peripheral bood; mitosis is arrested during metaphase and chromosomes are stained and studied under a microscope
Fluorescence in situ hybridisation (FISH)	Suspected defect for which a probe is available	Fluorescently labelled probe attaches to specific DNA sequence if present
Microarray comparative genomic hybridisation	Multiple congenital anomalies (to identify chromosomal duplications or deletions too small to see in traditional karyotype analysis)	Patient and control DNA samples are labelled with different dyes and compete to hybridise with 1000s of DNA probes arrayed on a slide which is scanned for computer analysis of fluorescent signals
Direct DNA analysis or sequencing	Suspected condition associated with a known DNA sequence alteration	Sequence is ascertained and compared with normal sequence
Quantitative fluorescence polymerase chain reaction	Suspected trisomies (rapid test)	Small selected sections of chromosome are copied and labelled, allowing quantification of the DNA present
Cell-free fetal DNA (non-invasive prenatal diagnosis)	Fetal sex determination, Rhesus D determination, diagnosis of some single-gene disorders, screening for aneuploidies	Analysis of small fragments of extracellular fetal DNA from the placenta, which circulate in maternal plasma

Table 11.1 Genetic investigations in clinical use

Case 15 Parents worried about a baby's poor feeding

Presentation

Tyler is 6 hours' old. He was born by normal vaginal delivery and required no resuscitation. Tyler is not interested in feeding. His parents have noticed that his tongue appears to be big and are worried that this is making it difficult for him to feed. The midwife has called the paediatric senior house officer, because she is concerned about the poor feeding and due to some characteristic facial features she suspects Tyler has Down's syndrome.

The senior house officer and consultant review the baby together.

Initial interpretation

Any newborn baby who is not feeding well requires further evaluation; there are many possible causes, including infection. Concerns regarding a baby's appearance should prompt a thorough examination by an experienced clinician.

Further history

Gemma, Tyler's mother, is a 26-year-old teacher who is normally fit and well, and she has no family history of note. The pregnancy was her first and was uneventful, with normal scans and serology. Gemma declined Down's syndrome screening, because she thought that Down's syndrome affected only babies born to older mothers.

Examination

Tyler is asleep in his cot. He is pink and well perfused. His anterior fontanelle

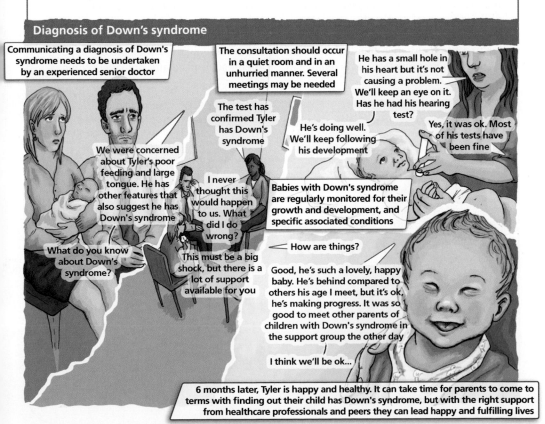

Diagnosis of Down's syndrome

Communicating a diagnosis of Down's syndrome needs to be undertaken by an experienced senior doctor

The consultation should occur in a quiet room and in an unhurried manner. Several meetings may be needed

He has a small hole in his heart but it's not causing a problem. We'll keep an eye on it. Has he had his hearing test?

The test has confirmed Tyler has Down's syndrome

He's doing well. We'll keep following his development

Yes, it was ok. Most of his tests have been fine

We were concerned about Tyler's poor feeding and large tongue. He has other features that also suggest he has Down's syndrome

I never thought this would happen to us. What did I do wrong?

Babies with Down's syndrome are regularly monitored for their growth and development, and specific associated conditions

What do you know about Down's syndrome?

This must be a big shock, but there is a lot of support available for you

How are things?

Good, he's such a lovely, happy baby. He's behind compared to others his age I meet, but it's ok, he's making progress. It was so good to meet other parents of children with Down's syndrome in the support group the other day

I think we'll be ok...

6 months later, Tyler is happy and healthy. It can take time for parents to come to terms with finding out their child has Down's syndrome, but with the right support from healthcare professionals and peers they can lead happy and fulfilling lives

Case 15 *continued*

is soft but quite large, and his posterior fontanelle is also easily palpable. Tyler's movements appear normal, but his tone is reduced. He has prominent epicanthic folds and a flat nasal bridge, and his tongue is protruding. Tyler has single palmar creases bilaterally. Cardiovascular, respiratory and abdominal examinations are all normal.

Interpretation of findings

The combination of facial features found during Tyler's examination and hypotonia strongly suggest Down's syndrome. However, genetic confirmation should be obtained.

Investigations

A definitive diagnosis of Down's syndrome requires chromosome analysis, i.e. karyotyping (**Figure 11.1**), but this can take up to 10 days. Therefore a blood sample is sent for urgent quantitative fluorescence PCR which is an accurate test and is reliable in identifying non-mosaic trisomy 21, and should give a result within 2–3 days.

Diagnosis

The PCR result confirms within 48 h that Tyler has Down's syndrome (trisomy 21). A karyotype will identify whether it is a full trisomy or an unbalanced Robertsonian translocation of chromosome 21. The implications of this diagnosis are discussed with his parents in an unhurried manner, allowing plenty of time for questions. They are directed to sources of information, provided with support from specialist nurses and are encouraged to ask questions.

Tyler is given supplementary nasogastric feeds for a few days and slowly starts to feed well from the bottle. His thyroid function is tested, and an echocardiogram and ophthalmology review are arranged (see pages 311–313 for a discussion of medical conditions associated with Down's syndrome). Tyler is discharged home, after arrangements are made for follow-up appointments at the paediatric outpatient clinic.

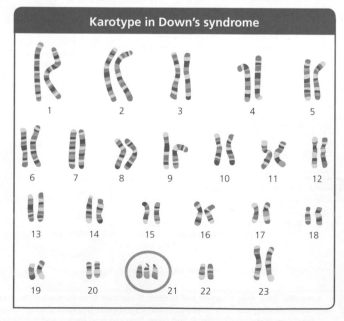

Karotype in Down's syndrome

Figure 11.1 A karyotype (chromosome map) showing the three copies of chromosome 21, rather than the normal two, in a person with Down's syndrome.

Dysmorphism

A dysmorphism is an abnormality in a structure, particularly the face, which is present from birth. It often becomes more apparent as the child gets older. Dysmorphic features include:

- malformations, for example cardiac septal defects, where the affected body part has developed incorrectly
- deformations, which occur when normally formed structures become deformed by physical forces; an example is talipes (abnormal positioning of the foot) secondary to oligohydramnios (reduced amniotic fluid volume)
- disruptions, when physical factors prevent normal development, for example when an amniotic band affects limb formation or in severe cases causes amputation of a limb

Dysmorphic features are caused by genetic disorders, exposure to teratogens (agents that can cause birth defects) environmental factors or a combination of these factors. In many patients, the cause remains unidentified.

Clinical features

A dysmorphic feature may be an isolated finding, for example simple polydactyly (extra digits), or part of a syndrome (**Figure 11.2**), association or sequence.

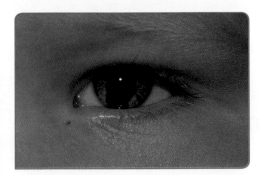

Figure 11.2 A coloboma (hole), one of the congenital malformations seen in a child with CHARGE syndrome (see **Table 11.2**).

- A syndrome is a condition in which a number of malformations occur together, secondary to a known cause
- An association is a similar combination of malformations occurring together more frequently than would be expected by chance, but for which no underlying cause has been identified
- A sequence is a group of malformations that have arisen as a consequence of an initial malformation

Examples of each are given in **Table 11.2**.

Diagnostic approach

Clinical geneticists assess children who are suspected to have a genetic disorder. A detailed history is taken, including:

- family history, especially miscarriage or stillbirths (as fetuses with certain genetic disorders are more likely to spontaneously abort) and consanguinity (biological relationships between parents)
- pregnancy events, such as illnesses or exposure to teratogens
- birthweight and growth
- developmental milestones so far

The physical examination includes checking for dysmorphic features. Some abnormalities, such as congenital vertical talus (rocker-bottom feet) and a typical hand posture in trisomy 18 (Edwards' syndrome) (**Figure 11.3**), are distinctive. Many other abnormalities are non-specific; they occur in various syndromes.

Genetic testing confirms many diagnoses, but associations, sequences and syndromes in which the responsible gene has yet to be identified may have to be diagnosed on the basis of clinical findings alone.

Examples of a syndrome, an association and a sequence

Condition	Features	Underlying cause
CHARGE syndrome	Coloboma (a hole in a structure of the eye, usually the iris) Heart defect Atresia of choanae (congenital blockage of a nasal passage) Retardation (of growth or development) Genital anomalies Ear anomalies (and deafness)	Mutation of gene on chromosome 8 (60% of cases)
VACTERL association	Vertebral anomalies Anal atresia Cardiac defects Tracheo-oesophageal fistula or oesophageal atresia Renal or radial anomalies Limb defects	Unknown
Pierre–Robin sequence	Micrognathia (small mandible) in early fetal life leads to the tongue preventing fusion of the palatal shelves, causing cleft palate and upper airway obstruction	Multifactorial; may be isolated or part of a syndrome such as fetal alcohol syndrome

Table 11.2 Examples of a syndrome, an association and a sequence: see the text for an explanation of the distinction between these

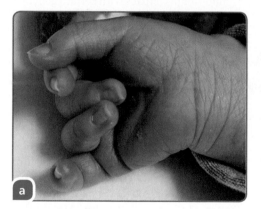
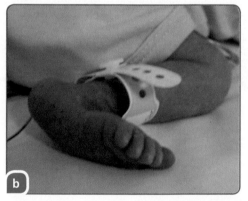

Figure 11.3 Distinctive dysmorphic features. (a) Typical hand posture in trisomy 18. (b) Rocker-bottom feet in both trisomy 18 and trisomy 13.

Chromosomal abnormalities

Many chromosome abnormalities are incompatible with life, contributing to > 50% of spontaneous abortions. The overall incidence in live-born babies is about 1 in 200. Anomalies can affect the autosomes or sex chromosomes, but sex chromosome abnormalities tend to have a less severe phenotype and are more likely to be live-born.

Chromosomal abnormalities are broadly considered numerical or structural. The most common numerical abnormalities are:

- trisomy, i.e. an extra chromosome
- monosomy, i.e. a missing chromosome

The most common structural abnormalities are:

- deletions, duplications and inversions of part of a chromosome
- translocations, when a whole chromosome or segment of a chromosome inappropriately joins with another chromosome

A chromosomal abnormality can be de novo, i.e. new to the individual; it can then be passed on to their offspring. Alternatively, it can be inherited from a parent, for example in the case of translocation. For this reason, when a child is found to have a chromosomal abnormality, chromosome studies are often offered to the parents.

The most common chromosomal abnormalities are trisomies and sex chromosome abnormalities. These occur because of errors during cell division and gametogenesis (**Figure 11.4**). The most frequently occurring trisomy is Down's syndrome (trisomy 21); other, rarer examples are trisomy 18 (Edwards' syndrome) and trisomy 13 (Patau's syndrome) (**Table 11.3**).

The commonest sex chromosome abnormality in girls is Turner's syndrome (see page 313). In boys it is Klinefelter's syndrome (see page 310), with a prevalence of 1 in 600 males. Features of Klinefelter's syndrome are not apparent until puberty, and it is often not diagnosed until adulthood, during investigations for infertility. The features of Turner's syndrome and Klinefelter's syndrome are shown in **Figure 11.5**.

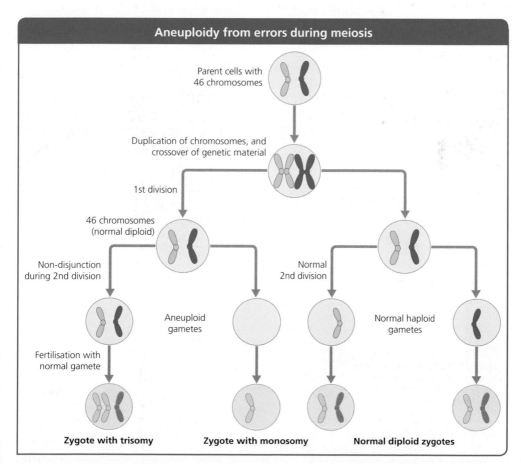

Figure 11.4 Aneuploidy resulting from non-disjunction during meiosis, which can occur during the 1st or 2nd division.

Trisomy 18 and trisomy 13			
Syndrome	Physical characteristics	Associated features	Prognosis
Trisomy 18 (Edwards' syndrome) 1 per 10,000 live births	Intrauterine growth restriction Microcephaly Facial dysmorphism: micrognathia, cleft lip and/or palate, hypertelorism Rocker-bottom feet Clenched fist with index and 5th fingers overriding 3rd and 4th Thumb aplasia	Cardiac anomalies Renal anomalies Gastrointestinal anomalies Severe learning disability	95% of affected babies die within a year
Trisomy 13 (Patau's syndrome) 0.3 per 10,000 live births	Intrauterine growth restriction Microcephaly Holprosencephaly (failure of division of the forebrain into two hemispheres) Facial dysmorphism with midline defects including cleft lip and/or palate Congenital vertical talus (Rocker-bottom feet) Postaxial polydactyly	Cardiac anomalies Renal anomalies Omphalocele Cutis aplasia (areas of missing skin) Severe developmental problems and learning disability	50% of affected babies die within 1 week and 90% within a year

Table 11.3 Clinical features of trisomy 18 (Edwards' syndrome) and trisomy 13 (Patau's syndrome)

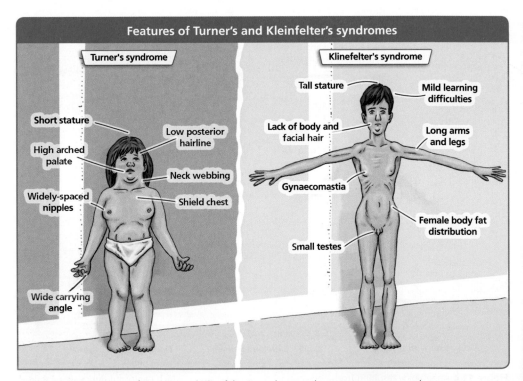

Figure 11.5 Phenotypes of Turner's and Klinefelter's syndromes, the most common sex chromosome abnormalities

The risk of aneuploidy, i.e. an abnormal number of chromosomes, increases dramatically with increasing maternal age.However, since just over half of sex chromosome abnormalities are paternal in origin, maternal age does not have such a significant effect on their incidence.

Down's syndrome

Down's syndrome is characterised by typical facial dysmorphism, hypotonia and delayed development. It is the result of an extra copy of chromosome 21. Affected individuals have three copies rather than two, so the condition is also known as trisomy 21.

The overall incidence worldwide varies from 1:600 to 1:1100 live births. Incidence increases with maternal age, rising from 1 in 2000 live births at 20 years to 1 in 100 live births at 40 years. The incidence of Down's syndrome in live births is lower than that in pregnancy, due to a high rate of spontaneous abortion in affected fetuses. However the main reason for the variability in live birth incidence between countries is the differing rates of selective termination following antenatal diagnosis.

Clinical features

Down's syndrome is associated with various characteristic facial and body features (**Figure 11.6**), although not all features are present in all affected individuals. Typical facial features are prominent epicanthic folds, a flat nasal bridge and a large tongue. Other characteristic features are a flat occiput, a single palmar crease and a sandal gap (increased space between the big toe and the other toes).

Babies with Down's syndrome are hypotonic and usually slow to feed. Growth and developmental milestones are delayed; most people with Down's syndrome have mild to moderate learning difficulties (IQ, 35–70) (see page 427). There is a higher incidence of behavioural disorders (e.g. attention deficit hyperactivity disorder), autism and other medical problems (**Table 11.4**).

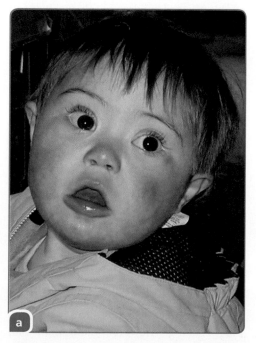
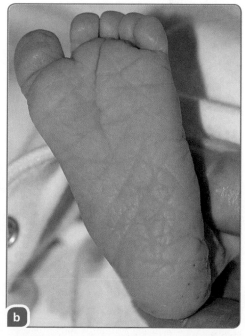

Figure 11.6 Dysmorphic features of Down's syndrome in a toddler (a) and a baby (b) The typical sandal gap between the big toe and the other toes.

Down's syndrome: associated medical conditions

System	Condition
Cardiovascular	Congenital heart disease (50% of cases) most commonly:
	Ventriculoseptal defect
	Atrioventriculoseptal defect
Gastrointestinal	Duodenal atresia
	Hirschsprung's disease
Immune	Autoimmune disease (e.g. hypothyroidism, diabetes mellitus, coeliac disease)
Haematological	Acute lymphoblastic leukaemia
Visual	Long-sightedness
	Congenital cataracts
Auditory	Otitis media with effusion (glue ear)
Musculoskeletal	Atlantoaxial and atlanto-occipital instability*

*Not screened for, but children advised not to perform forward rolls or other 'head over heels' manoeuvres, and care needs to be taken in supporting the neck when moving an unconscious child.

Table 11.4 Medical conditions associated with Down's syndrome

Diagnostic approach

Down's syndrome is identified by antenatal screening or diagnosed soon after birth, when the presence of typical phenotypic features have been noted.

Antenatal screening

In most developed countries, screening for Down's syndrome is offered to pregnant women in the first trimester. Currently, a combined test involving measurements of pregnancy-associated plasma protein-A and β-human chorionic gonadotrophin in the maternal blood, along with an US measurement of the fetal nuchal translucency (a collection of fluid at the back of the fetal neck), are used to calculate the likelihood of the pregnancy being affected by Down's syndrome. If the result is >1 in 150, diagnostic testing is offered. For this, a sample of fetal cells is obtained by chorionic villus sampling or amniocentesis for karyotyping and a definitive result.

However, advances in technology mean that non-invasive screening (with a high sensitivity and specificity for Down's syndrome in addition to Edward's and Patau's syndromes) by identification of free fetal DNA in maternal blood, is likely to replace the combined test in the near future.

> **Atrioventricular septal defect, a congenital heart abnormality that can be diagnosed antenatally, strongly suggests Down's syndrome (40–50% of fetuses with an AVSD have Down's syndrome).**

Postnatal diagnosis

Clinical suspicion of Down's syndrome at birth is confirmed by blood karyotype or quantitative fluorescence PCR. The karyotype shows three copies of chromosome 21 (see **Figure 11.1**).

Management

The aims of management are to manage any associated conditions (see **Table 11.4**) and to enable affected children to achieve their full potential at school and develop the skills they need to live as independently as possible in adult life. Following diagnosis an echocardiogram should be performed to identify any congenital heart disease, and throughout childhood, regular hearing and vision tests, along with screening for hypothyroidism and coeliac disease, are required to optimise development and growth. Surgery may be indicated for any cardiac or gastrointestinal abnormalities.

Prognosis

This depends on the severity of any associated medical conditions, such as congenital heart disease or acute lymphoblastic leukaemia. Most children with Down's syndrome are able to lead happy and fulfilling lives, and with appropriate support can attend mainstream schools and grow up to live fairly independently. However, more than half of people with Down's syndrome develop Alzheimer's disease in their fifties, and life expectancy is reduced.

Although the likelihood of a pregnancy being affected by Down's syndrome is higher in women with increasing age (especially over 35 years), Down's syndrome is also common in younger mothers. This is because more babies in total are born to younger mothers.

Turner's syndrome

Turner's syndrome affects girls and is characterised by short stature and primary ovarian failure as a consequence of gonadal dysgenesis; the ovaries are replaced by streaks of fibrous stroma. It is the most common sex chromosome abnormality, affecting 1 in 2000 live female births.

The condition arises because an X chromosome is missing, giving a 45XO karyotype. Mosaicism is present in up to half of all cases; this means that there are two cell lines, one with the chromosomal abnormality and one without it, so that half the cells are XO and the other half are XX.

Clinical features

Presentation usually follows parental concerns regarding short stature or delayed puberty. Turner's syndrome may also be diagnosed soon after birth, when suggested by oedema of the feet, a low hairline or coarctation of the aorta. The other phenotypic features, as shown in **Figure 11.6a**, are variable.

Associated conditions include cardiac abnormalities, most commonly aortic valve disease or coarctation of the aorta, and renal abnormalities, such as a horseshoe kidney. Problems with otitis media and hearing loss are common. Although intelligence is usually normal, there is increased risk of mild learning difficulties, particularly mathematical abilities and visual-spatial skills. There is a higher risk of autoimmune diseases, especially hypothyroidism, coeliac disease and inflammatory bowel disease.

Diagnostic approach

In Turner's syndrome, a blood karyotype shows the absence of one of the X chromosomes in a female patient. Therefore karyotyping is one of the investigations performed when a girl presents with short stature or delayed puberty, and it may also be considered in girls with aortic valve anomalies or coarctation.

Abdominal US shows the 'streak gonads' and small uterus. Renal abnormalities may also be found. Echocardiography is used to detect associated congenital heart disease.

If a girl presents with delayed puberty, the results of biochemical blood tests indicate hypergonadotropic hypogonadism. This is caused by the failure of the ovaries to respond to pituitary hormones.

Management

Turner's syndrome is managed by an endocrinologist and requires regular monitoring of growth and screening for complications. Growth hormone treatment during childhood helps girls with Turner's syndrome achieve an adult height that is closer to that of their peers. Most also require cyclical oestrogen therapy to achieve puberty and healthy uterine growth. Oestrogen is also extremely important for maintenance of normal bone density.

Prognosis

This depends on any associated cardiac anomaly; for example, there is an increased risk of death from aortic dissection. There is also a high risk of hypertension and cardiovascular disease in adulthood. The majority of girls with Turner's syndrome are infertile, but pregnancy is possible using IVF and donor eggs.

Single-gene disorders

Genes are sections of DNA encoding particular proteins. Mutations in the DNA sequence of a single gene result in the alteration or absence of the protein it encodes, thereby resulting in a single-gene disorder. Single-gene disorders cause syndromes with a wide range of features. Most show a Mendelian pattern of inheritance, i.e. they are either autosomal dominant or autosomal recessive (**Table 11.5**).

In genetic disorders, other factors in addition to genotype may determine the phenotype.

- Because of variable penetrance, an individual with the abnormal genotype may not be greatly affected by the disease
- Because of variable expression, the severity of the disease phenotype varies between individuals with the same genotype

Generally, carriers are unaffected, but they may have a mild version of the disease in some conditions.

> **In the vast majority of metabolic conditions**, such as inborn errors of metabolism, the inheritance pattern is autosomal recessive.

Noonan's syndrome

Noonan's syndrome is often called 'the male Turner's syndrome', because of similar phenotypic features. However, Noonan's syndrome affects an equal number of females as males, and unlike Turner's syndrome it is not caused by a sex chromosome abnormality but a single-gene defect.

Noonan's syndrome is autosomal dominant, but it arises from a spontaneous mutation in up to half of cases. About 50% of cases result from a single-gene defect on chromosome 12; defects in genes on other chromosomes have also been detected but many other defects remain unidentified. Noonan's syndrome affects about 1 in 1500 live births.

Clinical features

Typical facial features become more apparent in early childhood. They include:

- hypertelorism
- down-slanting eyes
- low-set ears
- short webbed neck

Children with Noonan's syndrome have short stature, cubitus valgus (wide carrying angle at the elbow) and both pectus carinatum and excavatum (a chest deformity in which the sternum appears to protrude or is sunken). A large proportion have cardiac anomalies, most commonly pulmonary stenosis, and 20–30% develop cardiomyopathy. About 10% have mild developmental delay. Puberty may be delayed. Some males may be infertile, but females have normal fertility. Patients with Noonan's syndrome have a tendency to bruise or bleed easily because of thrombocytopenia (platelet deficiency), platelet dysfunction and coagulation factor abnormalities (most commonly factor XI deficiency).

Diagnostic approach

> **Noonan's syndrome** is considered in any child, male or female, with **pulmonary stenosis** or **short stature**.

Noonan's syndrome is confirmed genetically by the presence of any of the mutations known to be associated with the disorder. However, defects in some unidentified genes also cause Noonan's syndrome, so the absence of a known mutation does not exclude the diagnosis, which is still often based on clinical features. Once the diagnosis is made, assessment for associated conditions includes echocardiography and vision and hearing assessment.

Management

Management includes surveillance for and treatment of any complications. Growth hormone therapy is a treatment option for severe growth failure.

Prognosis

This depends on the associated problems, especially any cardiac anomaly, which can be

Comparison of autosomal dominant and autosomal recessive conditions		
Feature	Autosomal dominant conditions	Autosomal recessive conditions
Status of parents in order to transmit disease	One affected parent	Two carrier parents
Chance of offspring inheriting the disease	1 in 2	1 in 4
Chance of becoming a carrier	No carrier status	1 in 2
Examples	Achondroplasia	Cystic fibrosis
	Marfan's syndrome	Sickle cell disease
	Noonan's syndrome	Thalassemia
	Neurofibromatosis type 1	Congenital adrenal hyperplasia
	Tuberous sclerosis	Most inborn errors of metabolism

Table 11.5 Differences between autosomal dominant and autosomal recessive inheritance

life-threatening. However, most individuals with Noonan's syndrome lead normal lives.

Marfan's syndrome

Marfan's syndrome is a disorder affecting the strength and elasticity of various connective tissues that results in abnormalities in the skeleton, eyes and cardiovascular system. It is an autosomal dominant condition affecting the *FBN1* gene on chromosome 15, which encodes fibrillin, a glycoprotein in the extracellular matrix required for healthy connective tissue formation. This leads to a decrease in the amount of functional fibrillin produced.

The condition affects about 1 in 5000 people, 25% of whom have a spontaneous mutation. It may present in childhood or be undiagnosed until adulthood. Many patients are diagnosed through screening after a member of their family has been found to have Marfan's syndrome, as a diagnosis of Marfan's has the potential for serious cardiovascular complications.

Clinical features

Marfan's syndrome is easily recognised clinically by a patient's tall stature and wide arm span; however, the phenotype is variable. Typical features include:

- aortic root abnormalities (particularly dilatation)
- lens dislocation
- skeletal abnormalities

Diagnostic approach

More than 1000 fibrillin gene mutations have been identified, almost all of which are unique to an affected family. A diagnosis is made by a combination of family history, the presence of one of the *FBN1* mutations and clinical criteria, based on the revised Ghent classification.

If no family history is identified the presence of aortic dilatation and either lens dislocation or *FBN1* genetic mutation is diagnostic. The diagnosis can also be made in the presence of aortic dilatation and other clinical features based on a scoring system.

If a family history is present, diagnosis can be made in the presence of lens dislocation or aortic dilatation alone, or by a variety of other clinical features based on a scoring system.

Management

Complications reflect the various connective tissues affected. The most serious complication is aortic root dilatation with the possibility of aortic dissection. Regular monitoring of the width of the aortic root with echocardiography is required. Beta-blockers are useful in adults to decrease mean arterial pressure and therefore the progression of aortic dilatation and risk of aortic rupture; however, their efficacy in children is unclear. Prophylactic surgery may be required. At least half of individuals with Marfan's syndrome have ectopia lentis (lens dislocation), so regular ophthalmological screening is required. Other complications include spontaneous pneumothorax and recurrent hernias.

Prognosis

Marfan's syndrome may affect a patient's lifestyle, with restrictions on strenuous activity and contact sports. Aortic rupture underlies increased mortality, but the prognosis is much improved with careful management.

Imprinted gene disorders

Each individual inherits two active copies of most genes, one from their father and one from their mother. However, for a small percentage of genes, only one active copy is inherited. This is because either the paternal copy or the maternal copy is inactivated (silenced) by genetic imprinting, a normal process in which methyl groups are added to DNA to inactivate certain genes during formation of the sperm cell or oocyte, respectively. Errors in imprinting result in imprinted gene disorders, which do not follow Mendelian patterns of inheritance.

A cluster of imprinted genes is present on chromosome 15q11. Disorders affecting these genes cause two disorders with different phenotypes, depending on whether the affected genetic material is paternally or maternally derived.

- In Prader–Willi syndrome, paternal genes are missing or, less commonly, there are two sets of maternal copies
- In Angelman's syndrome, a maternal gene is missing or defective or, less commonly, there are two paternal copies of the gene

Prader–Willi syndrome

Prader–Willi syndrome is characterised by hypotonia, obesity and hypogonadism. It occurs when there is a loss of the paternal genes in a small area of the long arm of chromosome 15, a region labelled q11–q13. The paternal gene is inactive because of microdeletion of a specific area on the paternal chromosome 15 (75% of cases); alternatively, there is no paternal

chromosome 15 because of maternal uniparental disomy, i.e. both copies of the chromosome come from the mother (25% of cases). Prader–Willi syndrome affects 1 in 15,000 children.

Clinical features

Prader–Willi syndrome normally presents in infancy with hypotonia, poor feeding and slow growth. However, between the ages of 1 and 6 years children with Prader–Willi syndrome develop an excessive appetite driven by a permanent feeling of hunger; they become progressively obese in consequence. They also have:

- short stature
- hypogonadism
- characteristic facial features, such as almond-shaped eyes and a thin upper lip
- moderate learning difficulties
- difficult behaviour
- sleep disorders (the lack of sleep can worsen behaviour)

Diagnostic approach

A checklist of clinical features typical of Prader–Willi syndrome is used to identify children for whom genetic testing is appropriate. The number of clinical features required increases with increasing age.

Fluorescence in situ hybridisation (FISH) and PCR are used to identify a deletion on chromosome 15 and uniparental disomy 15, respectively.

Management

Growth hormone treatment is indicated for children with Prader–Willi syndrome due to its beneficial effects on body composition and bone density in addition to improving linear growth. Management also includes avoidance of excessive weight gain through exercise and limiting access to food. Support with schooling and behavioural difficulties is also required.

Prognosis

Life expectancy may be reduced because of the complications associated with obesity or gastric rupture.

> Positive behavioural support is an evidence-based approach used by those working with both children and adults with learning disabilities and challenging behaviour. First, information is collected to understand the purpose of the behaviour. This is used to create a positive behaviour support plan so that they can learn better ways of having their needs met. The plan may include teaching the individual new skills, more positive ways to communicate and coping strategies for situations they find stressful. Family and other people in the individual's life also learn how best to provide support, for example by avoiding things that distress them.

Angelman's syndrome

Angelman's syndrome affects the nervous system, causing severe physical and intellectual disability. About 80% of cases occur because of the loss or mutation of maternal chromosomal material at the q11 region of chromosome 15; 20% of cases are caused by paternal uniparental disomy of chromosome 15. Angelman's syndrome has a prevalence of 1:10,000 to 1:40,000 children.

Clinical features

Angelman's syndrome presents from 6 months, with severe developmental delay and jittery movements. If walking is later achieved, the child usually has problems with balance and coordination, with an ataxic gait. Children with Angelman's syndrome typically have a happy and excitable personality but minimal speech. Most have microcephaly and develop seizures by the age of 3 years.

Diagnostic approach

Angelman's syndrome may be suspected if a child's development is delayed and any of the characteristic clinical features are present. A deletion or inactivity on chromosome 15 is identified using FISH or array comparative genomic hybridisation (CGH).

Management

Management includes specialist schooling and medication to control seizures and muscle twitching. Life expectancy is normal, but the child requires lifelong care.

X-linked disorders

The X chromosome is a sex chromosome. Females inherit two: one from the father and one from the mother. Males inherit one X chromosome, either paternal or maternal.

An autosomal recessive condition arises only if both parents are carriers of the mutated gene. In contrast, in X-linked recessive conditions the son of a carrier mother has a 50% chance of having the disease, regardless of the father's carrier status; this is because boys have only one X chromosome. Daughters become silent carriers, i.e. they have no symptoms, unless both parents carry the mutation. Most X-linked diseases are recessive.

Females inherit one X chromosome from their mother and one from their father. Early in embryonic development either the paternally or maternally derived X chromosome is inactivated, usually in roughly equal proportions of cells. This is known as 'X-inactivation'.

Males only inherit one X chromosome (either from their mother or father) therefore if that X chromosome carries the gene responsible for an X-linked recessive condition, they will be affected. In contrast, females who are heterozygous for the condition may be affected to a variable degree if the normal X chromosome is inactivated in ≥ 75% of cells (skewed X-inactivation).

■ If the X chromosome carrying the mutated gene is inactivated in most cells, a heterozygous female may be unaffected by the disorder or have only minor symptoms
■ If the X chromosome carrying the normal gene is inactivated in most cells, she may have more severe symptoms, similar to those in a male who has inherited the mutated gene

X-inactivation is also known as lyonisation, in honour of the geneticist Mary Lyon, who proposed the original hypothesis.

The more variable patterns of inheritance for X-linked recessive conditions, such as haemophilia and muscular dystrophy, in females than in males can be explained by X-inactivation (lyonisation).

X-linked dominant conditions are rare. They are usually lethal in males (resulting in miscarriage), so are encountered only in females.

Examples of X-linked conditions are haemophilia (see page 379) and muscular dystrophy (see page 261).

Fragile X syndrome

Fragile X syndrome is the most common cause of inherited learning disability, affecting about 1 in 4000 boys and 1 in 8000 girls. It is caused by a single-gene mutation on the long arm of the X chromosome, and is a recessive disorder. The abnormality is an unstable CGG triplet repeat expansion in the *FMR1* gene. Carriers of the faulty gene may have a full mutation or an area of instability considered a premutation.

Fragile X syndrome is so called because early cytogenetic analysis showed 'fragile sites', i.e. areas that, when stained, appeared as thin strands on the long arm of the X chromosome in affected individuals. Therefore it was originally considered a chromosomal abnormality. Newer molecular techniques show no structural abnormality, but the name has remained.

Fragile X syndrome is the most common inherited cause of moderate learning disability. Although Down's syndrome is a more common genetic disorder, most cases of Down's syndrome occur sporadically.

Clinical features

All boys with a full mutation have learning disabilities, especially in language, and cognitive impairment. Typical physical features, which are often not apparent until adolescence, include:

■ a long, thin, asymmetrical face with prominent forehead, jaw and ears
■ joint hyperlaxity
■ large testicles
■ behavioural traits suggesting attention deficit hyperactivity disorder and autism (see page 429–431)

Up to 50% of girls with the full mutation have mild learning difficulties.

Various genetic disorders are associated with autism spectrum disorder.

Diagnostic approach

Array CGH analysis of blood is the first-line test to detect chromosomal imbalances in children with moderate to severe learning disability, developmental delay or behavioural problems. If the result is normal, further testing for fragile X syndrome includes PCR analysis to detect expansion of CGG repeats on the X chromosome.

Management

Management is supportive, and includes educational and speech and language support. Life expectancy is normal but most males will require lifelong support with activities of daily living.

Microdeletion syndromes

Some deletions of genetic material are too small to be seen under a conventional microscope, so they are termed microdeletions. Although little genetic material is lost, they can cause syndromes if they affect a few contiguous genes in a critical region. The most common microdeletion syndrome is 22q11 deletion, also known as DiGeorge's syndrome (see page 295). Williams' syndrome is caused by a microdeletion affecting chromosome 7.

Williams' syndrome

Williams' syndrome is associated with several characteristics that become apparent in the pre-school years, including typical facial features and delayed development. It is usually the result of a spontaneous microdeletion of genetic material on chromosome 7q11.23 , but a small number are inherited from a parent in an autosomal dominant pattern. The incidence is about 1 in 18,000 children.

Clinical features

Children with Williams' syndrome are generally short. An 'elfin' face, with a short nose, a long philtrum and a wide mouth with big lips, is characteristic (**Figure 11.7**). The iris typically has a stellate (lace-like) pattern. Cardiac anomalies may be present, most commonly supravalvular aortic stenosis. There may be mild learning difficulties and difficulties with fine motor and visuospatial tasks, but children with Williams' syndrome characteristically have good language skills and are very outgoing and sociable, despite a hypersensitivity to noise. Other associations include renal anomalies, hypertension and hypercalcaemia.

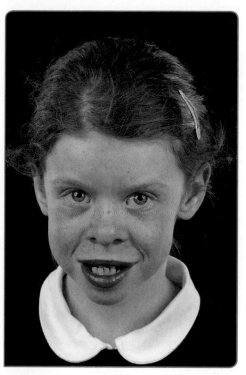

Figure 11.7 The typical 'elfin' facial features of Williams' syndrome, an example of a microdeletion syndrome.

Diagnostic approach

Detection of the chromosome 7q11.23 microdeletion by a genetic blood test, either the specific FISH test or the array CGH test, confirms the diagnosis. Screening for complications include blood tests for hypercalcaemia in the first few years of life, and if hypercalcaemia is present, measurement of urinary calcium and renal US scans to detect nephrocalcinosis. Echocardiography confirms or excludes associated cardiac anomalies.

Management

Progression of aortic stenosis and blood pressure are monitored and treated if necessary.

Hypercalcaemia is managed with a low calcium diet. With appropriate management of complications and extra educational support, most will be able to lead an active life.

Mitochondrial disease

The mitochondrial diseases are genetic disorders in which cells are unable to function because they have insufficient energy in the form of adenosine triphosphate (ATP).

Mitochondria are intracellular organelles that produce ATP via the mitochondrial respiratory chain pathway. Most genetic material is contained in cell nuclei, but 37 genes are encoded in the mitochondria (13 of these for polypeptide components of the respiratory chain). Different types of mitochondrial disease arise from mutations in the DNA, either nuclear or mitochondrial, encoding enzymes and substrates of the respiratory chain pathway.

Mitochondrial disorders arising due to mitochodrial gene mutations are always maternally inherited as sperm contains very little mitochondria. However, most respiratory chain proteins are encoded by nuclear DNA and mitochondrial disorders arising due to a mutation in these genes follow usual mendelian patterns.

Clinical features

Symptoms vary greatly between conditions and between individuals, depending on the ratio of functional mitochondria to those that are non-functional within each cell. The organs most commonly affected are those with the highest energy demands, i.e. the brain, muscles, liver, heart and kidneys.

Symptoms are usually progressive and involve multiple systems (most commonly neurological and muscular). Children present with faltering growth, motor regression, profound weakness, encephalopathy, seizures, swallowing difficulties and apnoea-like breathing problems.

Diagnostic approach

If the clinical picture is suggestive of a particular disease pattern, specific genetic testing may be possible. However, in most cases in children the symptoms are non-specific and the diagnosis is reached through a series of investigations which may include the following:

Biochemistry

An increase in blood lactate concentration, i.e. lactic acidosis, is usually present in around 30% of cases; however, it is a non-specific sign and could be indicative of many other conditions. Measurement of creatine kinase is also useful, and is usually normal or only slightly elevated (whereas it is usually high in other myopathies). Lactate in the cerebrospinal fluid is increased in some conditions. Urine amino acids and organic acids may be increased.

Histology

Muscle or skin biopsy usually show 'ragged red fibres' (abnormal accumulation of mitochondria in muscle fibres using a special stain) in cases secondary to mitochondrial DNA mutations but may be normal in other cases. Tests can be performed to assess the electron transport chain activity.

Imaging

Brain MRI shows characteristic patterns in some types of mitochondrial disease, affecting the central nervous system.

> **Next-generation sequencing uses modern techniques that can quickly sequence the whole human genome and identify even the smallest mutations in DNA**. It is currently mainly used for research purposes but has enormous potential for future clinical use.

Genetic testing

Next-generation sequencing can determine the location and type of mutation in the mitochondrial DNA. However, in most countries it is currently available only through research projects.

Management

Treatment is supportive, for example medication is used to control seizures. Any stress on the body, for example infection, can worsen symptoms. Regular aerobic exercise is beneficial in mitochondrial myopathies. Respiratory chain cofactors such as coenzyme Q10 and thiamine, and special diets may occasionally make the respiratory chain more efficient, but benefits are limited.

It is now possible to use replacement techniques ('three-person in vitro fertilisation') to prevent mitochondrial diseases being passed on via maternal mitochondrial DNA. Not all countries have legalised this technique yet; the UK is one that has. In one such technique, nuclear DNA from the prospective mother is placed in a donor oocyte from which the nucleus has been removed. The oocyte is then fertilised by sperm from the prospective father.

Prognosis

Many children with mitochondrial diseases do not reach adulthood, often dying in the early years.

Multifactorial inheritance

Many inherited conditions are caused by an identified chromosome or gene abnormality and have a predictable pattern of inheritance, such as Mendelian or X-linked inheritance. However, many other conditions recur in families, and their inheritance pattern is not predictable. This is because of multifactorial inheritance: the condition arises because of a combination of several genes (i.e. these conditions are polygenic), often interacting with environmental factors. Disorders with multifactorial inheritance are more common than single-gene or chromosomal abnormalities, and include:

- autoimmune conditions (e.g. type 1 diabetes)
- cleft lip and palate or isolated cleft palate
- neural tube defects
- pyloric stenosis
- asthma and atopy
- epilepsy

It is difficult to predict the exact risk of an individual in a family developing a condition with multifactorial inheritance, because of the complex interplay between genetic factors (including the expression and penetrance of the defective genes), environmental factors, sex and lifestyle. However, the risk is usually quite low (e.g. the risk of recurrence of a cleft in sibling is around 2–5% versus 0.17% in the general population). The risk is higher if:

- several members of the family are affected
- a first-degree relative is affected
- the proband (first affected individual) has severe disease
- the proband is the opposite sex to the sex more commonly affected

Answers to starter questions

1. Although women have two copies of the X chromosome, and therefore two copies of the gene, only one X chromosome is 'active' (lyonization). Women can therefore still be affected by X-linked recessive conditions when they have a 'normal' copy of the gene if the recessive copy is the one that is active (see Box on page 318)

2. A recessive mutation may be more prevalent if it confers a benefit to the population, for example sickle cell trait is more common in African populations because it gives resistance to malaria. Another explanation is due to genetic drift: in a small population a rare mutation can become more common simply by chance differences in the rates of reproduction of different individuals or consanguineous reproduction within a community. For example, the Ashkenazi Jew population has significantly higher incidences of Tay–Sachs disease and Gaucher's disease.

Chapter 12
Endocrine disorders

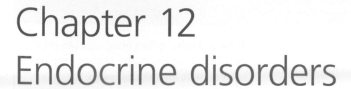

Starter questions

Answers to the following questions are on page 348.

1. Why does early puberty lead to a shorter final height?
2. Why are babies with ambiguous genitalia at risk of having low blood sugar?

Introduction

The endocrine system consists of several glands that secrete a variety of hormones (chemical messengers). Hormones circulate in the body to maintain homeostasis and regulate physiological activities via their effects on metabolism, growth and development, sexual function and reproduction, sleep and mood. The endocrine glands are the hypothalamus, pituitary gland, thyroid gland, pineal gland, parathyroid gland, adrenal gland, pancreas and gonads (ovaries or testicles). Each type of hormone is targeted towards certain organs and tissues, and some glands signal to each other in sequence, such as those in the hypothalamic–pituitary–thyroid axis (see page 26). Endocrine disorders can arise as a consequence of excessive or insufficient levels of a hormone.

Case 16 Excessive thirst and urination in a 14-year-old

Presentation

Emma is 14 years old. She has been referred to the paediatric assessment unit by her general practitioner (GP), having complained of lethargy for 2 weeks and because of her mother's concern that she has lost weight. The GP had carried out a urine dipstick test, which gave a +++ result for glucose.

Initial interpretation

Diabetes mellitus needs to be considered in any child presenting with glycosuria, especially with associated lethargy and weight loss. Therefore further history is needed.

Further history

On further questioning, Emma admits to feeling thirstier than usual over the past few weeks; as a consequence, she is drinking more and passing lots of urine, even occasionally during the night. Her appetite has been normal, but her clothes are now loose. She denies any abdominal pain or vomiting.

Examination

Emma appears alert and comfortable. A plot of her height places it on the 50th centile, and her weight is on the 9th centile. She has a normal respiratory rate, and her breath smells normal. Emma's mucous membranes are moist (she has been drinking water during the consultation). Her abdomen is soft and non-tender. There are no abnormal features on general examination.

Interpretation of findings

The history of lethargy, glycosuria, thirst, polyuria and weight loss (despite a normal appetite) strongly suggests new onset

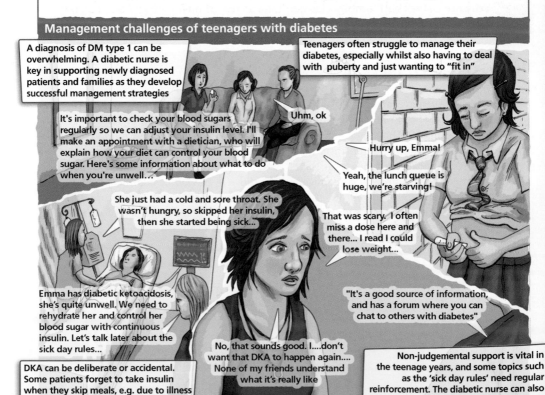

Management challenges of teenagers with diabetes

A diagnosis of DM type 1 can be overwhelming. A diabetic nurse is key in supporting newly diagnosed patients and families as they develop successful management strategies

Teenagers often struggle to manage their diabetes, especially whilst also having to deal with puberty and just wanting to "fit in"

It's important to check your blood sugars regularly so we can adjust your insulin level. I'll make an appointment with a dietician, who will explain how your diet can control your blood sugar. Here's some information about what to do when you're unwell...

Uhm, ok

Hurry up, Emma!

Yeah, the lunch queue is huge, we're starving!

She just had a cold and sore throat. She wasn't hungry, so skipped her insulin, then she started being sick...

That was scary. I often miss a dose here and there... I read I could lose weight...

Emma has diabetic ketoacidosis, she's quite unwell. We need to rehydrate her and control her blood sugar with continuous insulin. Let's talk later about the sick day rules...

"It's a good source of information, and has a forum where you can chat to others with diabetes"

DKA can be deliberate or accidental. Some patients forget to take insulin when they skip meals, e.g. due to illness

No, that sounds good. I....don't want that DKA to happen again.... None of my friends understand what it's really like

Non-judgemental support is vital in the teenage years, and some topics such as the 'sick day rules' need regular reinforcement. The diabetic nurse can also direct patients to other sources of support

Case 16 *continued*

type 1 diabetes mellitus. Although there are no suggestive clinical signs, diabetic ketoacidosis must still be considered because about 25% of new cases of type 1 diabetes mellitus present with diabetic ketoacidosis.

Investigations

Laboratory measurement of blood glucose, blood gas measurements and assessment of ketones in either blood or urine are mandatory in the assessment of a new diagnosis of diabetes mellitus. Emma's blood glucose concentration is 18 mmol/L, but her blood gas results are normal and there are no ketones in her urine.

Diagnosis

A diagnosis of type 1 diabetes mellitus

is confirmed. Emma and her family are upset by the news.

The normal blood gases and absence of ketones confirm Emma does not currently have diabetic ketoacidosis, so she does not require treatment with intravenous fluids or intravenous insulin. She is started on subcutaneous insulin therapy in a basal bolus regimen (four insulin injections daily). Emma is admitted for education on self-management.

The next day, the diabetic specialist nurse comes to the ward to provide advice and information booklets. Emma and her family are taught how to administer insulin via a pen device and how to monitor her blood glucose levels. She is discharged home, after regular visits from the diabetic nurse have been planned to provide additional support and advice.

Case 17 Short stature in a 12-year-old

Presentation

Sophie is 12 years old. Her GP has referred her to the paediatric outpatient department because she and her parents are worried that she is much shorter than her friends and is 'not developing'. Only one previous measurement is available, taken during a previous hospital admission for asthma aged 8 showing her height to have been on the 25th centile. However, Sophie's current height is plotted between the 0.4th and 2nd centile. Her weight is on the same centile.

Initial interpretation

Sophie's height has fallen across two centile lines, which is an indication for further assessment. However, if she has yet to enter puberty she will not have had the normal pubertal growth spurt and will

therefore appear shorter than friends who have already entered puberty.

Further history

Sophie is normally fit and well. She reports a good level of energy and is doing well at school. She has a healthy appetite, eats a varied diet and has no constipation or loose stools. Sophie's mother recalls being slow to enter puberty herself, reaching menarche at about the age of 16 years.

Examination

Sophie looks well. Her cardiovascular, respiratory and abdominal examinations are normal. She has no dysmorphic features and her body (limb versus trunk length) looks in proportion. Examination of her chest and genital area (chaperoned by her mother and a nurse) reveal that

Case 17 *continued*

she is prepubertal (see page 29). Her parents' heights are plotted using her mother's measured height in clinic and her father's reported height: the mid-parental centile is between the 25th and 50th centile.

Interpretation of findings

Sophie shows no signs or symptoms of a pathological cause for her short stature (see **Table 12.4**). She is still prepubertal, which is acceptable for a girl of her age and with a family history of puberty at an older age. Although her height is three centiles below her mid-parental centile, this is acceptable in this case. On balance, the most likely diagnosis is constitutional delay of growth and puberty.

Investigations

In view of the likely diagnosis, extensive investigations are not indicated at this time. A period of observation will be most informative. However, a radiograph of the left hand is performed to look for delayed bone age, which is useful to support the diagnosis.

Should Sophie's growth remain delayed, other investigations to consider include thyroid function tests and screening for coeliac disease. A karyotype is performed in all girls with short stature and delayed puberty, to rule out Turner's syndrome (see page 313).

Diagnosis

Sophie and her parents are reassured by a diagnosis of constitutional delay and

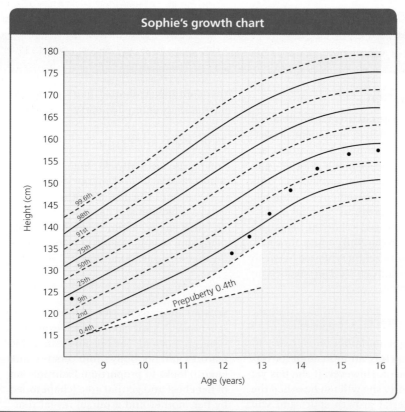

Figure 12.1 Sophie's growth chart, showing constitutional delay of growth and puberty.

Case 17 *continued*

return to the clinic 6 months later. By this time, she has some breast development and a few pubic hairs have appeared. Her growth is monitored over the next couple of years and shows a growth spurt that plateaus after she reaches menarche at the age of 15 years (**Figure 12.1**). These findings confirm the diagnosis as constitutional delay of growth and puberty.

Diabetes mellitus

In diabetes mellitus, the body is unable to metabolise glucose appropriately. Glucose in the bloodstream is normally regulated by the hormones insulin and glucagon (**Figure 12.2**).

■ Type 1 diabetes mellitus is caused by a deficiency of insulin
■ Type 2 diabetes mellitus is characterised by insulin resistance, i.e. the reduced ability of body tissues to respond to insulin

Epidemiology

In contrast to in adults, most diabetes diagnosed in children is type 1 (97% of cases). The annual incidence in the UK is 24 cases per 100,000 children.

The incidence of both type 1 and type 2 diabetes mellitus has been increasing in Europe in recent years. The reason for the increase in type 1 is unknown, whereas in type 2 it is linked to the increase in obesity.

Aetiology

Both types of diabetes are polygenic (influenced by several different genes) in origin. Type 1 diabetes mellitus is an autoimmune condition in which the beta cells of the pancreatic islets are destroyed; the exact trigger for this is unknown. The major risk factors for type 2 diabetes mellitus are obesity and a sedentary lifestyle; South Asian and African children are at higher risk than white children (the reasons for this are unknown).

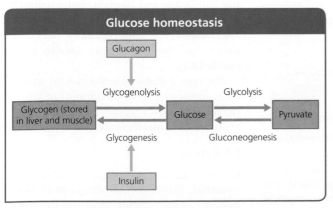

Figure 12.2 Regulation of blood glucose levels by insulin and glucagon.

Diabetes may also occur as a consequence of other conditions that affect the pancreas, such as cystic fibrosis (see page 163).

Clinical features

In diabetes mellitus, the higher level of glucose in the blood increases its osmolarity (a measure of solute concentration), thereby leading to many of the primary symptoms.

1. The threshold for renal glucose reabsorption is exceeded, leading to glycosuria
2. Glycosuria leads to an osmotic diuresis, which causes polyuria, i.e. voiding of large volumes of urine
3. Polyuria leads to polydipsia, i.e. excessive thirst leading to the consumption of large amounts of fluid; in younger children, both polyuria and polydipsia may result in nocturnal bedwetting in those who were previously continent

In addition, the inability of cells to use glucose leads to general lethargy. Eventually weight loss occurs, despite a good appetite, as a result of lipolysis (lipids are broken down to provide substrates for gluconeogenesis) and the depletion of the body's nutrients via urinary losses.

Investigations

The detection of glucose on dipstick urinalysis or a high glucose level in capillary blood (obtained by finger prick test) suggests diabetes mellitus. However, the diagnosis requires either of the following laboratory test results:

- blood glucose concentration ≥ 11.1 mmol/L on a random glucose test, i.e. on blood from a non-fasting individual
- fasting plasma glucose ≥ 7 mmol/L

The proportion of children who have diabetic ketoacidosis at presentation varies worldwide; in the UK it is 25%. It is detected by the finding of ketones in the urine or blood, and acidosis on a blood gas sample. It is a medical emergency (see page 409).

Diabetic ketoacidosis is a potentially life-threatening condition that is most common in type 1 diabetes. It arises when a severe lack of insulin means that the body is unable to use blood glucose and therefore breaks down fatty acids (components of lipids) to produce energy. This process produces ketones, which accumulate to cause acidosis.

Management

Type 1 diabetes is managed by control of the diet, particularly intake of carbohydrate and fats, and administration of exogenous insulin, guided by regular monitoring of blood glucose concentration. The priority in type 2 diabetes is lifestyle change.

Education

Advice on diet and exercise and an explanation of their effects on blood glucose are crucial for successful management of diabetes. Education on the symptoms and management of hypoglycaemia, a consequence of the use of exogenous insulin, is also vital.

Medication

Management of type 1 diabetes mellitus requires multiple daily doses of subcutaneous insulin, self-injected using a pen device. Different regimens are used, depending on the child's age and lifestyle. Some regimens are a combination of longer and shorter acting insulin via multiple daily injections, and some children use an insulin pump (**Table 12.1**).

For type 2 diabetes mellitus, oral antidiabetic medication (e.g. metformin) or subcutaneous insulin is occasionally required if lifestyle change is insufficient or not achieved.

Monitoring

Careful monitoring of blood glucose is essential. This is done by finger prick blood testing before meals and maintenance of a diary record. Blood concentration of

Insulin: types and regimens	
Type (all given subcutaneously)	**Features**
Rapid-acting insulin	Onset of action: 10–20 min
	Peak action: 1–2 h
	Duration of action: 2–4 h
Short-acting insulin	Onset of action: 30–60 min
	Peak action: 2–4 h
	Duration of action: up to 8 h (only 30 min when given intravenously)
Intermediate-acting insulin	Onset of action: 1–2 h
	Peak action: 4–12 h
	Duration of action: 16–35 h
Long-acting insulin	If given regularly at the same time each day, concentrations reach a steady state and remain constant, with no peaks and troughs

Insulin regimens		
Regime type	**Insulin type**	**Advantages/disadvantages**
Basal bolus regimen (injections four times daily)	Short-acting insulin at mealtimes and long-acting insulin at bedtime (most common regimen)	Improved control and greater flexibility, because of ability to adjust timing and dose of short-acting insulin to coincide with meals
Twice-daily injections	Biphasic insulin (mixture of short- and intermediate-acting insulin)	More restrictive of lifestyle – less flexibility for adjusting the timing and content of meals
		Preferred by some patients because fewer daily injections
Continuous subcutaneous infusion via an insulin pump	Delivers a continuous background dose of short- or rapid-acting insulin, and additional boluses with food	Can help improve control and reduce number of hypoglycaemic episodes; understanding of carbohydrate counting is essential

Table 12.1 Different types of insulin and insulin regimens

haemoglobin A1c (glycosylated haemoglobin A) provides a measure of glycaemic control over a longer period of time. The target is a haemoglobin A1c concentration < 7.5% to reduce the risk of diabetic complications.

Complications of diabetes include serious health problems and can be fatal, so screening is essential. At each annual review, the patient's blood pressure is measured, their urine is screened to detect microalbuminuria (leakage of small amounts of albumin into the urine) thereby identifying the early stages of diabetic nephropathy, their blood is screened to detect thyroid disease and an eye examination is carried out to look for signs of diabetic retinopathy.

Prognosis

Average life expectancy in people with diabetes mellitus is reduced by about 10 years because of diabetic complications in adulthood, such as heart and microvascular disease.

> **Paradoxically, a child's insulin requirement is usually increased during illness, even if they are not eating.** This is because of the effect of stress hormones on gluconeogenesis. Therefore 'sick day rules' for children with diabetes mellitus advise that insulin injections should be continued during illness, and blood glucose carefully monitored, to avoid diabetic ketoacidosis or hypoglycaemia.

Thyroid disorders

The thyroid is a gland located in the neck. It produces thyroxine, a hormone that stimulates the metabolism of virtually all cells of the body. The thyroid gland itself is under the hormonal control of the hypothalamus (**Figure 12.3**), so thyroid disorders result from conditions affecting the hypothalamus or the thyroid. Disorders of the thyroid affect several systems; in children, the effect on growth and development is of particular importance, because of potentially serious lifelong consequences.

Hypothyroidism (underactive thyroid) in children is either congenital or acquired.

- In congenital hypothyroidism, a reduced amount of thyroxine, or none at all, is produced from birth
- In acquired hypothyroidism, the amount of thyroxine produced is reduced, usually as a result of autoimmune conditions (as in adults)

Hyperthyroidism (overactive thyroid) is usually acquired, mainly from autoimmune conditions. However, it can occur transiently in a neonate if their mother has hyperthyroidism.

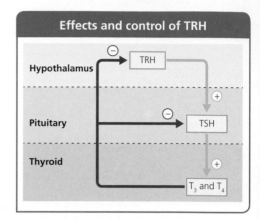

Figure 12.3 Secretion of thyrotrophin-releasing hormone (TRH) from the hypothalamus, and its effects on the anterior pituitary gland. T3, tri-iodo-thyronine; T4, thyroxine; TSH, thyroid-stimulating hormone.

- poor feeding
- constipation
- hypotonia
- a large fontanelle
- prolonged jaundice

Congenital hypothyroidism

Congenital hypothyroidism affects about 1 in 3500 live births. The commonest cause is agenesis or dysgenesis of the thyroid gland (75% of cases), which is usually sporadic. Other causes include disorders of thyroxine synthesis or function, which are often hereditary, and central disorders of the hypothalamus or pituitary gland.

Clinical features

Most children with congenital hypothyroidism are diagnosed at an asymptomatic stage, via the newborn screening programme (see page 425). Babies with the condition are often described as 'good' or 'quiet', because they sleep for longer periods and have decreased activity in comparison to normal newborns. Other features include:

Diagnostic approach

Babies with congenital hypothyroidism are identified through the newborn screening programme, when the blood spot card shows increased thyroid-stimulating hormone (TSH). Serum TSH and thyroxine are then measured; the diagnosis is confirmed by increased blood TSH and decreased thyroxine levels.

Management

The treatment for congenital hypothyroidism is lifelong thyroxine replacement. If it is detected early, during the asymptomatic stage, and appropriate treatment is provided, the prognosis is good, with most children achieving normal growth and development. However, untreated babies (rare since the advent of screening but see box) develop severe developmental disabilities, which are irreversible, hence the importance of newborn screening.

Be aware that the newborn blood spot screening programme does not detect central congenital hypothyroidism. This is because blood TSH levels are not increased in this rarer form of congenital hypothyroidism. A high index of suspicion is required when assessing babies with symptoms of hypothyroidism but normal screening results.

Acquired hypothyroidism

Acquired hypothyroidism can develop at any age. The most common cause is Hashimoto's thyroiditis, an autoimmune condition in which autoantibodies are produced against thyroid peroxidase, thyroglobulin and TSH receptors. Acquired hypothyroidism is rarely secondary to hypothalamic–pituitary problems, such as a benign pituitary tumour, or treatment for hyperthyroidism. The prevalence of childhood acquired hypothyroidism is highest in adolescent girls, affecting about 1 in 1000 teenagers overall, but with a male to female ratio of 1:2.8.

Clinical features

Many symptoms of hypothyroidism in children are similar to those in adults (**Table 12.2**), but there are some notable differences. The most common presentation is with slow growth and short stature, delayed puberty or declining school performance.

Diagnostic approach

The diagnosis of hypothyroidism is confirmed by thyroid function test results: a high serum concentration of TSH (unless there is a central cause, in which case TSH is low) and a low serum concentration of thyroxine. The presence of thyroid autoantibodies confirms an autoimmune cause.

Management

All children with hypothyroidism require oral thyroxine replacement therapy with levothyroxine, titrated to maintain a euthyroid state. On treatment, they have normal growth and development, leading normal lives.

Hypo- and hyperthyroidism: signs and symptoms	
Hypothyroidism	Hyperthyroidism
Slow growth or short stature (delayed bone age)	Normal or accelerated growth or tall stature (advanced bone age)
Delayed puberty (occasionally precocious puberty)	No effect on puberty (but may develop secondary amenorrhoea)
Goitre	Goitre
Lethargy and/or sluggishness	Hyperactivity and/or decreased attention span
Constipation	Loose stools or diarrhoea
Cold, dry skin	Warm, moist (sweaty) skin
Facial puffiness	Exophthalmos (protrusion of the eyeballs)
Bradycardia	Tachycardia and/or palpitations

Table 12.2 Signs and symptoms of hypothyroidism and hyperthyroidism

Hypothyroidism is associated with other autoimmune conditions, such as diabetes mellitus and coeliac disease. It is also associated with conditions caused by chromosomal abnormalities, such as Down's or Turner's syndrome. Therefore children with certain autoimmune conditions or chromosomal abnormalities require regular screening for hypothyroidism.

Hyperthyroidism

In hyperthyroidism, excess thyroxine is produced. The most common cause in children is Graves' disease, with an incidence of 1 in 100,000 children; adolescent girls are mainly affected.

Graves' disease is an autoimmune condition in which TSH receptor antibodies stimulate the TSH receptor, thereby causing excessive production of thyroxine. It is very unusual in younger children. However, transient neonatal thyrotoxicosis is occasionally encountered in babies born to mothers with Graves' disease, because of high levels of maternal TSH receptor antibodies, which cross the placenta (see page 148).

Clinical features

Hyperthyroidism in children presents with similar signs and symptoms to those in adults, with the addition of accelerated growth and advanced bone age (see **Table 12.2**).

Diagnostic approach

In hyperthyroidism, thyroid function tests show high thyroxine and low TSH levels. The presence of TSH receptor antibodies confirms Graves' disease.

Management

The aim of treatment is to reach a euthyroid state; however, achieving this may require complete blockage of thyroid gland activity and replacement with synthetic thyroxine.

Medication

First-line treatment is with carbimazole, which inhibits production of thyroid hormones. Most children become euthyroid within 8–12 weeks of starting treatment. A beta-blocker can help control symptoms until carbimazole takes effect.

Radioactive iodine therapy

This is considered if medical management is unsuccessful. The radioactive iodine is selectively absorbed by the thyroid gland, which then causes radioactive damage to the thyroid cells so that they are no longer able to produce thyroid hormones. However, secondary hypothyroidism frequently develops, requiring thyroxine replacement in most cases.

Surgery

Occasionally, when other management options have failed, all or part of the thyroid gland is removed surgically, particularly in children under 5 years when radioactive iodine treatment is contraindicated. This is also likely to cause hypothyroidism.

Prognosis

Carbimazole is usually continued for several years and then stopped once the patient is in remission, although many patients will relapse. All patients require lifelong monitoring of their thyroid function test results; a significant proportion develop hypothyroidism in later years, mainly as a consequence of treatments they receive but also due to autoimmune destruction of the thyroid gland.

Growth disorders

Growth disorders relate to the causes of short and tall stature. Growth is determined by nutrition, genetics and hormones. A diagnosis of short or tall stature requires assessment of growth velocity, which is calculated by using serial measurements of height.

Short stature

Short stature is defined as a height that is more than two standard deviations below the mean compared with others of the same age and sex (i.e. below the 3rd percentile on a growth chart), or a height that is more than three centiles below the mid-parental height centile (see page 22). Only in a minority of clinic referrals for short stature will there be a pathological cause.

Aetiology

In most children, the underlying cause is familial short stature or constitutional delay in growth and puberty. However, short stature may be the presenting feature of an endocrine disease, any chronic disease or genetic condition that affects growth (**Table 12.3**).

Clinical features

Children with familial short stature are otherwise healthy. Their growth chart shows normal growth, albeit on a lower centile, within two centiles of their mid-parental height centile.

Those with constitutional delay of growth and puberty are also healthy. Their growth chart shows a reduced growth velocity between the ages of around 6 months and 3 years, which

Short stature: causes	
Age group	Causes
Babies and young children	Intrauterine growth restriction
	Nutritional deficiency or poor food intake
	Chronic illness (e.g. significant congenital heart disease)
	Neglect, or emotional or physical abuse
Adolescents	Constitutional delay of growth and puberty
All ages	Familial short stature
	Chronic illness (e.g. renal disease, cystic fibrosis, inflammatory bowel disease)
	Coeliac disease
	Hypothyroidism
	Growth hormone deficiency or hypopituitarism
	Chromosomal abnormalities (e.g. Turner's or Down's syndrome) or other genetic disorders
	Skeletal dysplasias (e.g. achondroplasia)
	Iatrogenic (e.g. chronic use of steroids)

Table 12.3 Causes of short stature

may normalise during childhood. However, during early adolescence growth velocity is again reduced, with a delayed pubertal growth spurt.

In pathological short stature, the clinical findings depend on the underlying cause. The history and examination include birthweight and birth history, body mass index, any dysmorphic features (including disproportion of limb length), pubertal staging and symptoms of signs of chronic disease (**Table 12.4**).

Diagnostic approach

Familial short stature is diagnosed clinically, based on the history and examination, serial growth measurements and plotting of the mid-parental height centile. Investigations are not indicated.

The diagnosis of constitutional delay is also mainly clinical. However, a bone age is useful to support the diagnosis.

Children with short stature of unknown cause require a thorough clinical history, examination and further investigation.

Short stature: features suggesting a pathological cause		
Body region	Clinical feature	Underlying pathology
Midline	Cleft palate	Occasionaly associated with hypothalamic/pituitary problems
	Hypogonadism (may be associated with growth hormone deficiency)	
Limbs and trunk	Disproportionate in size	Skeletal dysplasia
Head and face	Papilloedema, visual field defects	Brain tumour
	Dysmorphic features	Genetic conditions e.g. Turner's syndrome
Gastrointestinal	Diarrhoea	Inflammatory bowel disease
		Coeliac disease
All over body	Increased or decreased fat or muscle mass	Low BMI: poor nutrition secondary to eating disorder, chronic illness
		High BMI: possible endocrine disease
	Signs of chronic disease (e.g. clubbing, heart murmur, tachycardia)	Any chronic illness, e.g. severe congenital heart disease

Table 12.4 Features suggesting a pathological cause of short stature

Generally, **a weight over the 99.6th centile is more likely to be pathological** if the child is short than if their height is also on a higher centile.

Investigations

Investigations are not indicated in a healthy child if the history is suggestive of familial short stature. However, if the history is suggestive of a pathological cause, patients should have a full range of investigations.

Measure each parent's height when they attend clinic with their child, because reported heights can be misleading. Fathers often believe they are taller than they truly are!

Radiology

The results of a radiograph of the left hand to assess bone age (degree of a child's bone maturity) is useful to support the differential diagnoses reached based on the clinical history and examination. It may be delayed, advanced or correspond to the child's chronological age, depending on the underlying condition (**Table 12.5** and page 46).

Blood tests

Abnormal results for full blood count, renal function or inflammatory markers suggest chronic disease, such as chronic kidney disease. Screening should be performed for coeliac disease and thyroid function tests will identify hypo/hyperthyroidism. In girls, karyotyping excludes Turner's syndrome.

Other specialist investigations include a growth hormone stimulation test to rule out growth hormone deficiency.

Dynamic growth hormone stimulation tests are required in children with suspected growth hormone deficiency. This is because growth hormone is released in pulses. Levels of growth hormone circulating in the blood fluctuate throughout the day and are also affected by exercise, sleep, stress and diet. Therefore a random measurement of growth hormone concentration is not very useful; a low level may be normal if the blood was drawn at the end of a pulse.

Management

Reassurance alone is required in children with familial short stature or constitutional delay. Other causes of short stature require treatment of the underlying condition.

Medication

Synthetic growth hormone, given daily via subcutaneous injection, promotes growth in children with growth hormone deficiency. It may also increase height in children with Turner's syndrome, Prader-Willi syndrome or chronic renal disease.

Prognosis

Children with constitutional delay achieve a normal adult height. Many children with chronic disease or an endocrine deficiency have 'catch-up growth', i.e. a period of accelerated growth enabling them to achieve the height determined by their genetic potential,

Relationship of bone age to chronological age in different conditions		
Delayed	Advanced	Equivalent to chronological age
Constitutional delay	Precocious puberty	Familial short stature
Hypothyroidism	Hyperthyroidism	Intrauterine growth restriction
Growth hormone deficiency	Obesity (in young children)	Familial tall stature
Chronic disease		

Table 12.5 Bone age compared with chronological age in different conditions

once their underlying condition is treated; however, some will always remain short.

Tall stature

Tall stature is defined as a height two standard deviations above the mean when compared with others of the same age and sex, equivalent to being above the 97th percentile on a growth chart, or a height more than three centiles above the mid-parental height centile. It presents less commonly than short stature, because of both a lower incidence and society's perception that tall stature is not a problem.

Aetiology

The commonest causes of tall stature are familial tall stature and, especially in younger children, obesity. Rarer causes include:

■ genetic conditions, for example Klinefelter's or Marfan's syndrome
■ endocrine causes, for example growth hormone excess or hyperthyroidism
■ precocious puberty

Clinical features

Children with familial tall stature are healthy. Their height is within two centiles of the mid-parental height centile, and they have normal growth velocity. Young children who are obese are usually tall for their age, although it is not fully understood why this is.

An underlying endocrine disorder such as precocious puberty, hyperthyroidism, growth hormone excess or a pituitary problem may present with increased growth velocity and associated signs and symptoms of the underlying condition, (see pages 331 and 337). Features of a genetic condition, such as Klinefelter's or Marfan's syndrome, may be apparent (see pages 310 and 315).

Diagnostic approach

A child's body mass index is always calculated in those with tall stature. No investigations are required if the child is clinically well and has normal growth velocity, a height within the target parental height centiles and pubertal development within the normal range. These features lead to a clinical diagnosis of familial tall stature. Calculating the body mass index is useful to identify tall stature secondary to obesity.

Investigations

Investigations are guided by the clinical history and examination. A bone age is useful in most cases, but the choice of blood tests depends on the suspected underlying cause.

Radiology

A radiograph of the left hand is useful for determination of bone age (see **Table 12.5**). An MRI of the brain is necessary if a pituitary adenoma is suspected.

Blood tests

Karyotyping rules out Klinefelter's syndrome in boys. For both sexes, specific genetic testing can be carried out if clinically indicated, for example in children with suspected Marfan's syndrome. Thyroid function tests and other endocrine tests are carried out if clinically indicated.

Management

In the absence of an underlying pathology, management is with reassurance only. Rarely, if tall stature is causing psychological distress (usually in girls), early induction of puberty may be considered to limit final adult height by causing premature fusion of the bone epiphyses.

Prognosis

Growth normalises with treatment of any underlying endocrine condition, such as hyperthyroidism.

Disorders of puberty

Puberty is the period of sexual maturation during which a child's body undergoes physical changes to become an adult body with functional reproductive organs (see page 25). The normal age range for entering puberty is 8–13 years in girls and 9–14 years in boys. Outside these ages, puberty is considered to be precocious or delayed. Delayed puberty is more common in boys, whereas precocious puberty is more common in girls.

Delayed puberty

Delayed puberty is the lack of any breast development by the age of 13 years in girls, and in boys a testicular volume of < 4 mL by 14 years of age. The prevalence is about 3% of children.

Aetiology

In both sexes, the most common cause of delayed puberty is constitutional delay. Pathological causes are categorised as central or peripheral (**Table 12.6**).

■ Central causes are problems affecting the pituitary or hypothalamus

■ Peripheral causes are problems affecting the gonads

A pathological cause for delayed puberty is more common in girls than boys.

Clinical features

Adolescents with constitutional delay may have short stature, but they are otherwise healthy and often have a family history of late or delayed puberty. In delayed puberty with a pathological cause, the clinical history should elicit any symptoms of an underlying chronic disease or a previous illness that may have resulted in hypogonadism, such as testicular torsion.

> **Examination in children with delayed puberty** should include formal pubertal staging and assessment of growth, body composition, dysmorphic features and chronic disease stigmata.

Diagnostic approach

If constitutional delay is confirmed, no further investigations are required. However, a

Delayed or precocious puberty: causes		
Category	Delayed puberty	Precocious puberty
Central causes	Intact hypothalamic–pituitary axis ■ Constitutional delay in growth and puberty ■ Chronic disease ■ Malnutrition or anorexia nervosa	Gonadotrophin-dependent (with otherwise normal central nervous system) ■ Familial early puberty ■ Hypothyroidism ■ Obesity (in girls) ■ Idiopathic
	Secondary hypogonadism: impaired secretion of gonadotrophins (luteinising hormone and follicle-stimulating hormone) ■ Pituitary problems (e.g. tumours, after radiotherapy) ■ Congenital gonadotrophin-releasing hormone deficiency	Gonadotrophin-dependent, secondary to central nervous system disease ■ Brain tumour ■ After brain injury or radiotherapy ■ Congenital (e.g. hydrocephalus)
Peripheral causes	Gonadal dysgenesis ■ Turner's syndrome ■ Klinefelter's syndrome Bilateral testicular damage (e.g. torsion or mumps infection)	Gonadotrophin-independent ■ Ovarian, testicular or adrenal tumours ■ Congenital adrenal hyperplasia

Table 12.6 Causes of abnormal timing of puberty

Delayed puberty: investigations		
Category	Investigation	Suspected underlying pathology
Blood tests	LH	Primary hypogonadism: if sex hormones are low, with normal or high LH and FSH – a problem with the gonads
	FSH	
	Testosterone (boys)	Secondary hypogonadism (hypogonadotrophic): if sex hormones, and LH and FSH, are low – problem with the pituitary or hypothalamus
	Oestradiol (girls)	
	Thyroid function	Hypothyroidism
	Inflammatory markers	Chronic inflammatory illness, e.g. juvenile idiopathic arthritis or inflammatory bowel disease
	Karyotype	Turner's syndrome
		Klinefelter's syndrome
Radiology	Pelvic US	Absence or abnormalities of uterus and ovaries
	Brain MRI	Abnormalities of pituitary gland
FSH, follicle-stimulating hormone; LH, luteinising hormone.		

Table 12.7 Investigations to identify pathological causes of delayed puberty

bone age radiograph can be useful to support the diagnosis.

If a pathological cause is suspected, initial tests may include blood tests and radiology (**Table 12.7**).

Management

All adolescents with constitutional delay eventually enter puberty spontaneously, without treatment. However, if the delay is causing psychological distress, puberty can be induced by a short course of testosterone or oestrogen. Children with delayed puberty secondary to chronic disease also enter puberty spontaneously once the underlying condition is treated. Those with primary hypogonadism or gonadotrophin (hormones that stimulate the reproductive organs) deficiency require induction of puberty, with the use of exogenous hormones followed by maintenance hormone replacement.

Precocious puberty

Precocious puberty is defined as signs of puberty before the age of 8 years in girls and 9 years in boys. However, puberty may occur earlier than this in certain ethnic groups,

without being pathological. For example, African-Caribbean girls start puberty at a younger age than white girls, on average.

Aetiology

Precocious puberty may originate centrally (involving the hypothalamic-pituitary axis) or peripherally (from the sex organs or adrenal glands), however only those central causes are considered true precocious puberty. True central precocious puberty is gonadotrophin-dependent; it is caused by the normal release of gonadotrophin-releasing hormone in response to early activation of the hypothalamic–pituitary axis. It will follow the same pattern, or sequence of events, as normal puberty. Peripheral precocious puberty, also known as precocious pseudopuberty, is gonadotrophin independent and is the consequence of an excess of sex hormones originating from the testes, ovaries or adrenal glands. The causes of central and peripheral precocious puberty are shown in **Table 12.6**. Central precocious puberty is usually idiopathic in girls, whereas a pathological cause is much more common in boys. Peripheral precocious puberty is usually pathological in both sexes.

Precocious puberty has an overall prevalence of 1 in 5000, but it is 10 times more common in girls.

> **Premature pubarche, i.e. isolated pubic hair development, is usually benign.** It is associated with adrenarche, the prepubertal increase in androgen production by the adrenal glands. The rest of the history and examination will be normal and levels of gonadotrophins will be prepubertal. However, in rare cases it is caused by excess systemic androgens secondary to conditions such as congenital adrenal hyperplasia or a virilising tumour.

Clinical features

Central precocious puberty (gonadotrophin-dependent) starts and progresses in a similar fashion to normal puberty (see page 25), except that it occurs too early. Associated symptoms may provide clues to indicate a central trigger; for example, headaches may raise the possibility of a brain tumour.

In peripheral precocious puberty (gonadotrophin-independent), sex steroids originating from the adrenal gland or gonads without stimulation from the hypothalamic–pituitary axis for example in those with congenital adrenal hyperplasia, can produce different signs in both sexes. Girls can develop clitoromegaly (abnormal enlargement of the clitoris) and hirsutism, whereas boys can develop increasing penile length (from the effect of testosterone) without testicular enlargement (which requires secretion of the gonadotrophin follicle-stimulating hormone).

> **In precocious puberty, the growth spurt is often very noticeable.** The child may have become much taller than their peers.

Diagnostic approach

Further investigation is not always required, particularly in girls with idiopathic central precocious puberty. In other children, investigations should be considered.

Investigations

Blood tests are used to establish whether the child has pubertal levels of sex hormones and establish whether the origin is central or peripheral. Radiological tests, such as a radiograph to assess bone age, are helpful to establish whether the child truly has precocious puberty or a benign variant, and further imaging may identify any pathological causes.

> **Premature thelarche, i.e. isolated breast development, is usually idiopathic and benign.** There is no associated growth spurt and the bone age is usually equivalent to the chronological age.

Blood tests

In boys, measurement of early morning testosterone levels is a reliable indicator of whether they have entered puberty and how far it is advanced. In girls, measurement of oestradiol is less useful because levels naturally fluctuate, but once it reaches a certain level it does indicate that a girl is in puberty. Very high levels of both testosterone or oestradiol, with suppressed gonadotrophin levels, suggests peripheral precocious puberty.

Serum LH concentration is at pubertal levels in central precocious puberty and this is the most useful initial test. Random FSH levels can be difficult to interpret. The gonadotrophin releasing hormone (GnRH) stimulation test is useful if the picture is unclear; in central precocious puberty there will be a rise in LH and FSH following GnRH administration, but there will be no change in peripheral precocious puberty.

In both sexes 17-hydroxyprogesterone is measured if congenital adrenal hyperplasia is being considered.

Radiology

A radiograph shows advanced bone age if a child has precocious puberty. MRI of the brain is indicated in all boys, and girls under the age of 6, as a pathological cause for precocious puberty is more likely in these groups. It is also indicated in any older girls with symptoms suggesting central nervous system pathology. Pelvic US is used to assess whether uterus size is pubertal and to exclude ovarian pathology.

Management

In children with idiopathic precocious puberty, the decision to initiate treatment depends on individual circumstance. Some children may choose to progress through puberty; however, in others precocious puberty is halted by using gonadotrophin agonists. In pathological cases of precocious puberty,

management of the underlying cause is required. Gonadotrophin agonists do not work in peripheral precocious puberty.

> **Although precocious puberty means that affected children are initially tall for their age, its main complication is a diminished final adult height.** This is because the early pubertal growth spurt means that closure of the bone epiphyses at the end of puberty occurs prematurely, leading to less total time to grow overall.

Adrenal disorders

The adrenal gland has two parts, which produce different substances.

- The adrenal cortex produces steroid hormones
- The adrenal medulla produces catecholamines

The manifestations of adrenal disorders depend on the hormone pathway affected. Adrenal insufficiency or excess hormone production are either the result of a primary adrenal disorder or secondary to a central pituitary problem affecting secretion of adrenocorticotrophic hormone (ACTH) (see page 343).

Congenital adrenal hyperplasia

Congenital adrenal hyperplasia is an autosomal recessive condition caused by deficiency of an enzyme in the corticosteroid synthesis pathway, which occurs in the adrenal gland. The condition affects about 1 in 16,000 live births. The classic form of congenital adrenal hyperplasia (95% of cases) is the result of 21-hydroxylase deficiency, leading to a decreased cortisol production and in around 75% of cases aldosterone deficiency. Cortisol deficiency in turn leads to further ACTH secretion which results in

excessive testosterone production as the pathway continues in the other direction.

Clinical features

In females, classic congenital adrenal hyperplasia presents at birth, because the excess testosterone causes virilisation, resulting in ambiguous genitalia. The genitalia in baby boys usually appear normal at birth. In both sexes, if there is associated aldosterone deficiency, the baby develops 'salt wasting', which can present with:

- hypoglycaemia
- hyponatraemia
- hyperkalaemia
- acidosis
- dehydration
- collapse

This is easy to anticipate in females presenting with ambiguous genitalia, but not in males who appear otherwise normal at birth. For this reason salt wasting, which is akin to an addisonian crisis (see page 341), is the commonest presentation of congenital adrenal hyperplasia in male infants. Males who have the non salt-losing form may present with signs of virilisation or precocious puberty between the ages of 2 and 4 years.

> **In children with ambiguous genitalia, do not guess the child's sex.** It cannot be assigned until all investigations are complete and clinical opinions have been sought. The genetic sex, usually determined by the sex chromosomes, may not be the best one to assign to the child.

Diagnostic approach

In children with ambiguous genitalia, an initial set of investigations are performed as quickly as possible to allow sex of rearing to be assigned at the earliest opportunity, and avoid a salt-losing crisis (**Table 12.8**). Classic congenital adrenal hyperplasia is confirmed by an increased level of 17-hydroxyprogesterone. Blood glucose and electrolytes are also monitored.

Management

Urgent hydrocortisone replacement is required; the dose is adjusted to a level sufficient to suppress excessive androgen production without causing development of Cushing's syndrome (see page 341). Fludrocortisone and salt supplements are also required if salt wasting is confirmed. Severe virilisation may require surgical correction.

Prognosis

Appropriate steroid replacement ensures normal growth and development. In later childhood, the effects of excess androgens may become more apparent, for example with the development of acne or hirsutism in females. This may be the only manifestation of mild or non-classic congenital adrenal hyperplasia. Fertility may be suboptimal in females with congenital adrenal hyperplasia.

Addison's disease

Addison's disease is primary adrenal insufficiency not caused by congenital adrenal hyperplasia. It is rare in childhood; there are about 35 children diagnosed per year. It is usually the consequence of autoimmune destruction of the adrenal gland, which is then unable to produce sufficient corticosteroid in response to stress, for example from infection, surgery or trauma. Addison's disease may be associated with other autoimmune diseases.

> **Adrenal insufficiency can also occur secondary to inadequate stimulation of the adrenal gland** due to a hypothalamic or pituitary problem.

Clinical features

Addison's disease presents with non-specific symptoms, which include:

- lethargy
- weight loss
- loss of appetite
- nausea and vomiting
- pigmentation of the skin and mucous membranes

Because of the non-specificity of the symptoms, diagnosis is often delayed. Extreme weight loss, along with other symptoms, such as reduced appetite, can lead to teenagers with Addison's disease being incorrectly thought to have anorexia nervosa.

Ambiguous genitalia at birth: baseline investigations	
Investigation	Purpose
Karyotype	Establish whether genetically male or female
Blood glucose and electrolytes	Hypoglycaemia and salt wasting can develop in congenital adrenal hyperplasia
Pelvic US	Establish presence or absence of sexual organs (e.g. the uterus) and gonads (testes or ovaries)
Blood 17-hydroxyprogesterone	Increased in congenital adrenal hyperplasia
Blood 11-deoxycortisol	Increased in some types of congenital adrenal hyperplasia
Blood testosterone	Increased in congenital adrenal hyperplasia

Table 12.8 Baseline investigations in ambiguous genitalia at birth

> The hyperpigmentation in Addison's disease is the result of pituitary overproduction of ACTH. ACTH stimulates melanocytes, which produce melanin, the pigment responsible for skin colour.

An addisonian crisis presents with collapse as a result of severe dehydration, hypotension, shock and hypoglycaemia. It is precipitated by stress, such as from infection, trauma or surgery. It can be the initial presentation of Addison's disease and can be life-threatening.

Diagnostic approach

The results of blood biochemical investigations show hyponatraemia, hyperkalaemia and hypoglycaemia.

Morning blood cortisol concentration is low confirming adrenal insufficiency. A high ACTH concentration implies adrenal disease rather than a central cause. A Synacthen (Synthetic ACTH) stimulation test differentiates between primary adrenal insufficiency and a central cause. Measurement of cortisol levels pre- and post-administration of synacthen shows a poor cortisol response, because the defect is in the adrenal gland, not secondary to insufficient ACTH from the pituitary.

An US or CT scan of the adrenal glands identifies any other cause of adrenal insufficiency, such as haemorrhage, calcification or infiltrative disease. All such causes are very rare in childhood.

Management

Lifelong hydrocortisone and fludrocortisone replacement is required, with increased steroid dose in times of illness or traumatic stress. An addisonian crisis is a medical emergency; management consists of intravenous dextrose, saline and hydrocortisone.

> Children on maintenance hydrocortisone therapy must always carry a steroid card detailing their dose and what they and others should do if they become unwell. Never stop steroids suddenly, and always double the dose during acute illnesses.

Cushing's syndrome

Cushing's syndrome is caused by excess circulating glucocorticoids (which may be endogenous or exogenous). It is rare in children and is usually iatrogenic secondary to prolonged corticosteroid therapy (e.g. for the management of certain autoimmune or inflammatory conditions), so the incidence is variable. Endogenous Cushing's syndrome can be ACTH dependent or independent. The most common cause of endogenous Cushing's syndrome in children over the age of 7 is an ACTH-producing pituitary tumour (known as Cushing's disease). The most common ACTH independent cause is an adrenal tumour, and this is the most frequent cause of Cushing's syndrome in children under 4 years.

Clinical features

The onset of symptoms is usually insidious but Cushing's syndrome (**Figure 12.4**) is characterised by:

- poor linear growth
- facial and truncal obesity
- striae
- hirsutism
- delayed sexual development
- easy bruising

Diagnostic approach

The most reliable screening test for Cushing's syndrome is measurement of free cortisol in urine samples collected over 24 h. The concentration of free cortisol is increased if Cushing's syndrome is present.

The normal circadian rhythm for blood cortisol is a low level at midnight and a high level first thing in the morning. This diurnal pattern is lost in Cushing's syndrome: serum cortisol levels are high both at midnight and in the morning. Measurement of early morning ACTH will usually distinguish between ACTH dependent and independent causes (it will be high in ACTH dependent causes and suppressed in ACTH independent causes). An MRI scan to look for pituitary tumours or an ultrasound scan looking for adrenal tumours should then be arranged.

If the cause is clearly iatrogenic no further investigation is required.

Clinical features of Cushing's syndrome

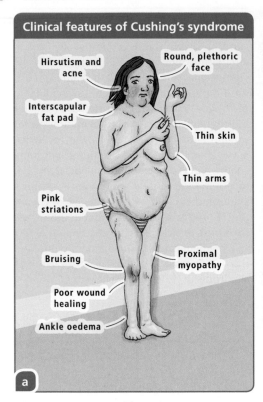

Hirsutism and acne

Round, plethoric face

Interscapular fat pad

Thin skin

Thin arms

Pink striations

Bruising

Proximal myopathy

Poor wound healing

Ankle oedema

a

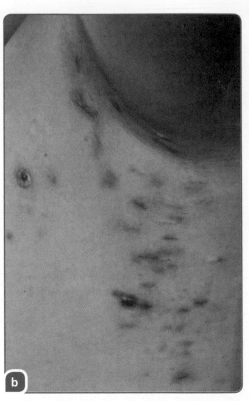

b

Figure 12.4 (a) Clinical features of Cushing's syndrome. (b) Underarm striae in a child with Cushing's disease.

> Random measurement of cortisol level is not a useful test due to the physiological fluctuations associated with the circadian rhythm.

Management

Exogenous Cushing's syndrome is managed by gradual withdrawal of the corticosteroid, with the aim of discontinuation, if possible. If necessary, steroid-sparing agents are considered, for example cyclophosphamide in nephrotic syndrome or methotrexate in juvenile idiopathic arthritis.

Steroid medication should not be stopped suddenly, because this may precipitate an adrenal crisis due to suppression of the hypothalamic pituitary-adrenal axis. Gradual reduction will allow the HPA axis to recover its function.

If an adenoma is identified, this can be removed by trans-sphenoidal surgical excision. Adrenal tumours are also removed surgically.

> When considering Cushing's syndrome or Addison's disease, remember the mnemonic CCCAAA:
>
> Copious Cortisol causes Cushing's and Absence of Aldosterone (and cortisol) causes Addison's.

Pituitary disorders

The pituitary gland is situated at the base of the brain. It is connected to, and regulated by, the hypothalamus, via the pituitary stalk. The pituitary produces hormones that act throughout the body (**Table 12.9**). Damage to the anterior pituitary results in hypopituitarism; an insult to the posterior pituitary results in diabetes insipidus. Hyperpituitarism is very rare.

Hypopituitarism

Hypopituitarism, i.e. partial or complete insufficiency of multiple pituitary hormones, may derive from pituitary or hypothalamic disease or damage. Causes include genetic conditions, congenital anomalies, perinatal asphyxia, intracranial tumours and infiltration, or it may be secondary to radiation treatment.

Multiple pituitary hormone deficiency is rare in childhood, with an estimated 30 children per year diagnosed. Isolated growth hormone deficiency is much more frequent, affecting 1 in 3500 children.

Clinical features

The clinical features of hypopituitarism depend on the age of onset and the functions of the hormone affected (**Table 12.10**). Neonates may present with dysmorphic features, especially midline facial defects (because the pituitary is midline).

Diagnostic approach

If hypopituitarism is suspected, evaluation of the hypothalamic-pituitary axis is required. This consists of blood hormone assays measuring:

- hormones directly produced by the pituitary, for example TSH
- hormones indirectly produced by the pituitary, for example cortisol (measured in the morning)

Pituitary stimulation tests, such as the Synacthen test and the thyrotrophin-releasing hormone test, are also useful, to measure the ACTH response and the thyrotrophin response, respectively.

Imaging studies may include a contrast head MRI to rule out a brain tumour.

Management

Replacement of the deficient hormone is usually required. Tumours may be resected;

Pituitary gland hormones		
Site of production	Hormone	Primary effect
Anterior pituitary gland	Growth hormone	Promotes growth of bone and tissues
	Adrenocorticotrophic hormone	Stimulates adrenal gland to produce cortisol
	Prolactin	Stimulates lactation
	Gonadotrophins:	
	Luteinising hormone	Triggers ovulation (females) and stimulates testes to produce testosterone (males)
	Follicle-stimulating hormone	Stimulates ovaries to produce eggs (females) and stimulates testes to produce sperm cells (males)
	Thyroid-stimulating hormone	Stimulates thyroid to produce thyroxine
Posterior pituitary gland	Oxytocin	Stimulates contractions during childbirth
	Antidiuretic hormone	Stimulates thyroid to produce thyroxine

Table 12.9 Hormones produced by the anterior and posterior pituitary gland

Hypopituitarism in children: signs and symptoms		
Age	Symptom	Cause
Infants	Hypoglycaemia	ACTH deficiency
	Hyponatraemia	ACTH deficiency
	Microgenitalia	Gonadotrophin deficiency
	Dysmorphic features and/or midline defects	Associated congenital anomalies
Children	Growth failure with delayed bone age	Growth hormone deficiency or central hypothyroidism
	Lethargy	ACTH deficiency or central hypothyroidism
	Hypoglycaemia	ACTH deficiency
	Delayed or absent puberty	Gonadotrophin deficiency
	Polyuria and polydipsia	ADH deficiency
ACTH, adrenocorticotrophic hormone.		

Table 12.10 Signs and symptoms of hypopituitarism in children

however, surgery to the pituitary gland can itself lead to hypopituitarism.

Prognosis

Hypopituitarism is usually lifelong, but with appropriate hormone replacement children can lead a normal life. However, the underlying cause may have an effect on life expectancy, e.g. a brain tumour may lead to increased morbidity and mortality. There may also be sequelae from complications prior to diagnosis, e.g. profound hypoglycaemia leading to brain damage.

Diabetes insipidus

Diabetes insipidus occurs as a result of either of the following:

- deficiency of antidiuretic hormone from the posterior pituitary (central diabetes insipidus)
- renal tubular unresponsiveness to antidiuretic hormone (nephrogenic diabetes insipidus)

Both result in the kidneys failing to reabsorb water, which leads to polyuria, rapid hypernatraemia and dehydration.

Central diabetes insipidus is usually acquired, secondary to head injury, tumours or neurosurgery. Rarely, it may be genetic in origin.

Nephrogenic diabetes insipidus usually develops in neonates, and usually is genetic in origin. In children, central diabetes insipidus is more common than nephrogenic diabetes insipidus, but both are rare.

> **Diabetes insipidus is so called because the urine of those affected has low sodium content and is therefore tasteless (Latin: insipidus, 'without taste').** In contrast, the urine of those with diabetes mellitus is sweet, because it contains glucose (Latin: mellitus, 'sweet').

Clinical features

Children with diabetes insipidus have polyuria (> 4 mL/kg/h), polydipsia and faltering growth. Babies cannot help themselves to water so may present with irritability, a vigorous suck and weight loss. In older children, the polydipsia may be uncontrollable; children may even try to drink from toilets. If the child is unable to get the water their body requires, they may have seizures as a result of severe hypernatraemia and dehydration.

Investigations

Initial investigations such as 24-hour urine collection showing polyuria and paired morning serum sodium and urine osmolality (showing an inappropriately dilute urine, and high serum sodium concentration) is suggestive of diabetes insipidus, but a water deprivation test is required to confirm the diagnosis.

Water deprivation test

In addition to confirming the diagnosis the water deprivation test will differentiate between a nephrogenic and central cause. To perform the test the patient is deprived of water for up to 8 hours (or 5% weight loss), with regular monitoring of urine and serum osmolality and weight. In diabetes insipidus these show increased serum osmolality with inappropriately dilute urine. There is also marked weight loss caused by excessive urine output. The patient is then given desmopressin (synthetic ADH) and the urine osmolality repeated; the urine becomes concentrated if there is a central cause, but not if there is a nephrogenic cause.

> **In primary polydipsia because of compulsive water drinking, which is psychogenic,** initial testing with a water deprivation test may suggest central diabetes insipidus, due to the 'down-regulation' of ADH release over a long period. However, after a period with controlled access to water, the test results will normalise.

Radiology

Imaging may include a contrast MRI for diabetes insipidus with a suspected central cause, or US or CT for those with a suspected nephrogenic cause.

Management

Central diabetes insipidus is treated with oral synthetic antidiuretic hormone replacement therapy, i.e. desmopressin, given daily.

Nephrogenic diabetes insipidus is more difficult to treat. The combination of diuretics and a low-solute diet is used.

Prognosis

In central diabetes insipidus, the outcome depends on the cause. With treatment, primary (genetic) central diabetes insipidus has an excellent prognosis.

In nephrogenic diabetes insipidus, as long as water is always available long-term survival is also excellent.

Hypoglycaemia

Hypoglycaemia occurs when, because of a defect in the pathway for glucose metabolism and homeostasis (see **Figure 12.2**), the level of blood glucose becomes insufficient to maintain cell function. A blood glucose concentration of < 2.5 mmol/L in a non-diabetic child warrants further investigation.

Epidemiology and aetiology

Hypoglycaemia is most common in the neonatal period (see page 153). Its incidence decreases with increasing age. In children with diabetes mellitus, hypoglycaemia is a consequence of excess exogenous insulin.

Age is helpful in guiding the most likely cause. The most common cause of hypoglycaemia in a child aged 18 months to 5 years is ketotic hypoglycaemia (accelerated starvation), a condition of unknown cause in which

children are unable to tolerate periods of fasting, even overnight. The prevalence is estimated at 12 per 100,000 in children younger than 5 years. Ingestion of substances, such as ethanol and salicylates, can lead to hypoglycaemia in children.

Other rare causes include inborn errors of metabolism, adrenal or pituitary disorders and hyperinsulinism, all of which are more frequent in infants and young children. In adolescents, insulin-producing pancreatic tumours, although rare, are the most common cause of true hypoglycaemia.

Clinical features

The presenting features of hypoglycaemia vary, depending on a child's age and the underlying cause.

- Early symptoms are manifestations of the autonomic response, for example sweating, tremulousness, hunger and tachycardia
- Later symptoms are the effects of neuroglycopenia, for example confusion, changes in behaviour and lethargy
- Prolonged or severe hypoglycaemia can cause seizures, coma and death

The clinical history includes the timing of symptoms in relation to the last meal, previous episodes of hypoglycaemia, general growth and development, and any family history of sudden unexpected death in infancy (see page 438).

Diagnostic approach

Handheld bedside blood glucose monitors are used to detect hypoglycaemia. It is essential to collect blood and urine samples for a hypoglycaemia screen (**Table 12.11**) before the correction of hypoglycaemia, because interpretation of the results of some constituents of the screen is possible only in the presence of hypoglycaemia.

> Ketones are used by the brain as an alternative fuel when glucose is scarce. Ketosis is a normal response to hypoglycaemia. The absence of ketones in non-ketotic hypoglycaemia suggests excessive insulin or a fatty acid oxidation defect as the cause of the hypoglycaemia.

Management

Prompt recognition of hypoglycaemia is essential to avoid serious but avoidable neurological complications. Treatment includes giving a sugary drink or snack, oral glucose gel or intravenous dextrose solution, depending on the child's clinical condition.

Ketotic hypoglycaemia is a diagnosis of exclusion. The treatment is regular meals and a snack of complex carbohydrate at bedtime. It usually resolves spontaneously by 5–9 years of age.

Hypoglycaemia screen: constituents		
Sample	Investigations	Interpretation
Blood	Cortisol	Inappropriately low in adrenal insufficiency
	Insulin	Inappropriately present/raised in hyperinsulinism
	C-peptide	Present in endogenous, but not exogenous, sources of insulin
	Growth hormone	Decreased in growth hormone deficiency
	Ammonia Lactate Ketone bodies Amino acids Organic acids	Levels variable depending on the type of inborn errors of metabolism. Ammonia often raised to varying degrees
Urine	Urinary ketones	Inappropriately absent in hyperinsulinism or disorders of fatty acid metabolism
	Urinary metabolic screen (amino acids and organic acids)	Different metabolites raised dependent on type of inborn errors of metabolism

Table 12.11 Constituents of the hypoglycaemia screen

> In children with hypoglycaemia, a bolus of glucose (IV or oral) should not be given in isolation, because it would lead to a surge of endogenous insulin and thereby cause rebound hypoglycaemia. It is followed with a maintenance infusion of dextrose or a complex carbohydrate snack.

Prognosis

Prompt management should result in full recovery, but prolonged symptomatic hypoglycaemia can lead to irreversible neurological damage, which may cause developmental delay, learning difficulties or seizures. Prognosis otherwise depends on the underlying cause.

Inborn errors of metabolism

Inborn errors of metabolism, also called inherited metabolic diseases, are a group of conditions caused by the absence or defect of enzymes or transport proteins controlling a metabolic pathway, resulting in a block in the pathway. As a consequence, the body is unable to create essential substrates, or toxic metabolites accumulate. Categories of inborn errors of metabolism are shown in **Table 12.12.**

Most inborn errors of metabolism are single-gene disorders and are autosomal recessive. Individually, the disorders are rare, but the cumulative incidence is about 1 in 1500 live births. Incidence is increased in some ethnic groups and in individuals with cosanguinous parents. Phenylketonuria is the most common inborn error of metabolism, affecting 1 in 10,000 live births.

Screening for several inborn errors of metabolism is included in the routine newborn screening programme. It enables treatment to be started in the asymptomatic phase of these conditions (see page 425).

The incidence of recessive genetic disorders such as inborn errors of metabolism is higher in communities in which marriage between cousins or other close blood relatives is more common. This is because consanguineous couples are more likely to carry the gene for the same recessive disorder. Recessive disorders affect about 33 in 1000 babies born to cousin couples, compared with 2 in 1000 born to unrelated couples.

Clinical features

Presentation of inborn errors of metabolism not detected by the newborn screening test is non-specific and varied:

- collapse or encephalopathy in the neonatal period or during an episode of intercurrent illness in childhood
- neurodevelopmental problems
- organomegaly
- family history of sudden unexplained death
- hypoglycaemia

Inborn errors of metabolism		
Type of disorder	Subcategories	Examples
Disorders that result in toxic accumulation	Disorders of protein metabolism	Phenylketonuria and other amino acid disorders
		Organic acid disorders
		Urea cycle defects
	Disorders of carbohydrate intolerance	Galactosaemia
	Lysosomal storage disorders	Gaucher's disease
Disorders of energy production or utilisation	Fatty acid oxidation defects	Medium-chain acyl-coenzyme A dehydrogenase deficiency
	Disorders of carbohydrate utilisation or production	Glycogen storage disorders
		Disorders of gluconeogenesis
		Disorders of glycogenolysis
	Mitochondrial disorders	Leigh's syndrome
		Mitochondrial encephalomyopathy with lactic acidosis and stroke-like episodes (MELAS)
	Peroxisomal disorders	X-linked adrenoleukodystrophy

Table 12.12 Categories of inborn errors of metabolism

Diagnostic approach

Hypoglycaemia and metabolic acidosis (high levels of lactate) are the usual findings in acute presentations of inborn errors of metabolism. A high index of suspicion is necessary, so that appropriate further tests are ordered to make a diagnosis.

Diagnosis of an inborn error of metabolism does not require extensive knowledge of biochemical pathways or individual diseases. Blood and urine samples are sent for metabolic screening, and the blood is also tested for ammonia. If the test results are suggestive of an inborn error of metabolism, more definitive tests are carried out, with guidance from a metabolic specialist.

> **Biochemical abnormalities in inborn errors of metabolism may be transient and occur only when the child is acutely unwell.** Therefore the diagnosis must be considered in a child who seems too unwell for the precipitating illness, such as gastroenteritis, and the appropriate samples collected.

A metabolic screen is also considered in children presenting with developmental delay (see page 427).

Management

Inborn errors of metabolism are usually managed by dietary manipulation to avoid the substrate that cannot be metabolised. For example, individuals with phenylketonuria follow a strict phenylalanine-restricted diet (primarily low protein). Glucose supplementation may be required during periods of illness. Specific enzyme replacement therapy is possible in a few conditions.

Prognosis

The earlier an inborn error of metabolism is diagnosed, the better the outcome; a normal life is possible in most children if the condition is detected on newborn screening and treated appropriately. However, in many inborn errors of metabolism the child is asymptomatic until irreversible brain damage has occurred; the condition then presents with delayed milestones. Affected children may develop severe developmental delay and seizures.

Answers to starter questions

1. Although sex hormones initiate the pubertal growth spurt by stimulating growth hormone secretion, they also trigger the closure of the epiphyseal growth plates at the end of puberty. This means that those children who enter (and therefore complete) puberty early have less time for growth and achieve a shorter adult height. This is also one reason why men are taller than women on average.

2. Congenital adrenal hyperplasia, reduces cortisol production and is a common cause of ambiguous genitalia. Cortisol raises blood glucose; without adequate cortisol neonates become hypoglycaemic during periods of fasting.

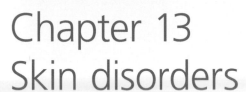

Chapter 13
Skin disorders

Starter questions

Answers to the following questions are on page 365.

1. What do Mikhail Gorbachev, Portugal and birthmarks have in common?
2. When are worm infections treated with anti-fungals?

Introduction

Skin disorders affect children of all ages. Some are benign and transient, particularly in neonates, and no treatment is required. Others cause symptoms that are difficult to relieve and are more likely to be chronic, for example eczema, which varies greatly in its severity. Eczema and the other common chronic skin disease in children, psoriasis, can be causes of significant morbidity and have a considerable impact on a child's quality of life. Patient education is an essential part of their management because both require meticulous daily care of the skin.

Describing and documenting skin disorders requires a specialised vocabulary: **Table 13.1** lists common terms used in dermatology. Many illnesses present with symptoms such as rash, chickenpox, measles and meningococcal septicaemia, but are not skin disorders. These are usually recognisable by the appearance of the rash and any other associated symptoms. These are discussed in the relevant chapters, however the terms in **Table 13.1** are still used to describe rashes in these systemic illnesses.

Dermatological terms

Term	Definition
Erythema	Redness of the skin
Macule	Flat and non-palpable area of change in skin colour
Papule	Raised, and therefore palpable, discrete lesion < 5 mm in size
Maculopapular	Combination of macules and papules
Nodule	Raised, discrete lesion > 5 mm in size, usually solid
Pustule	Papule containing pus
Vesicle	Papule containing fluid (usually serous fluid)
Plaque	Flat lesion that is slightly raised, and therefore palpable
Bulla	A fluid-filled blister
Comedones:	Hair follicles that become blocked and dilatated with keratin debris and sebum
Open (blackhead)	Black appearance due to oxidised melanin (oxidation occurs as contents are exposed to air)
Closed (whitehead)	Contents remain below skin surface

Table 13.1 Descriptive terms in dermatology

Case 18 Red lump on a baby's face

Presentation

William, a 1-month-old baby, is taken to the general practitioner by his mother. She is concerned about a red lump on his right lower eyelid.

Initial interpretation

Pink or red skin lesions in neonates are likely to be vascular birthmarks. Vascular birthmarks include port wine stains, 'stork bites' and capillary haemangiomas. The age at which the skin lesion is noticed gives a clue to the diagnosis.

Further history

William's mother noticed the mark 2 weeks ago. She does not remember it being present at birth. She is concerned because it has been rapidly increasing in size. William is otherwise well.

Examination

William has an obvious red swelling, measuring about 3 by 1 cm, on his right lower eyelid (**Figure 13.1a**). It is raised, has an irregular surface, is bright red and has the appearance of a strawberry. There are no other lesions, and the rest of the examination is normal.

Interpretation of findings

A red, raised area of skin with an irregular surface, which was not present at birth, is more typical of a capillary haemangioma. Port wine stains and stork bites are flat and present at birth.

Investigations

No investigations are required. Capillary haemangiomas are diagnosed based on visual inspection alone.

Case 18 *continued*

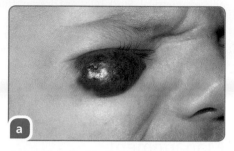
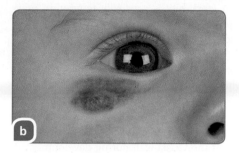

Figure 13.1 Capillary haemangioma. (a) A large, red and raised capillary haemangioma encroaching on the visual field. (b) Excellent response of lesion to treatment.

Diagnosis

A capillary haemangioma is diagnosed, based on the appearance and the age at which the lesion appeared.

Following its natural history, the haemangioma would be expected to continue to grow until William is 18 months old, so there is a risk of it encroaching on the eye, leading to visual impairment (amblyopia). Under the guidance of a dermatologist and ophthalmologist, William is given a course of the beta-blocker propranolol, which leads to shrinkage of the haemangioma so that visual impairment is avoided (**Figure 13.1b**).

Congenital skin lesions

Birthmarks are skin lesions that are identifiable at birth or shortly after. They are usually isolated findings. However, a minority are associated with other abnormalities and indicate the presence of a syndrome, for example facial port wine stain in Sturge–Weber syndrome.

Birthmarks are divided into vascular and pigmented lesions. They are diagnosed by visual inspection.

Vascular birthmarks

Vascular birthmarks are caused by abnormal changes to any type of vessel, including lymphatic vessels, but blood vessels are usually affected. It is not known why these changes occur.

Types

Vascular birthmarks are further subdivided into vascular 'tumours' and vascular malformations.

Vascular tumours are caused by abnormal proliferation of blood vessels and lymphatics and include:

- infantile haemangioma (strawberry haemangioma or capillary haemangioma)

Vascular malformations are caused by changes to the structure of blood vessels and lymphatics and include:

- stork bite (naevus simplex or 'salmon patch')
- port wine stain (naevus flammeus)

Epidemiology and aetiology

An infantile haemangioma is a benign tumour caused by proliferation of endothelial cells. It is the commonest birthmark, affecting 10% of Caucasian babies, and 1% of black and Asian babies. Girls and premature babies (25% of babies <1 kg at birth) are most frequently affected.

A stork bite is a usually temporary mark caused by dilatation of certain blood vessels. About one third of babies have one.

A port wine stain is abnormal morphogenesis of capillaries and postcapillary venules with increased vessel density, not proliferation of vessels. Evidence supports a neural role (sympathetic nervous system) which influences the composition and functional properties of the vessel wall during development. It affects about 3 in 1000 children. Females are twice as likely as males to have a port wine stain although the reason for this is unknown.

Clinical features

Infantile haemangiomas are rarely present at birth; they appear as a small red or blue lump at about 2–4 weeks of age. They can be superficial (most cases) or deep.

- Superficial haemangiomas are bright red, irregular, raised lesions (see **Figure 13.1a**)
- Deep haemangiomas are swellings with a bluish discoloration

A minority of haemangiomas are the combination of both superficial and deep lesions.

Infantile haemangiomas occur anywhere on the body, including internally. Common sites are the head and neck. In a minority, particularly if the lesion is large, the surface of the haemangioma becomes ulcerated and may bleed.

A stork bite is an irregular, pink, macular lesion commonly seen on the forehead, eyelids or back of the neck (**Figure 13.2**). The size varies among individuals. Multiple lesions may be present, in which case they are usually symmetrical. Stork bites are present from birth.

A port wine stain is most often unilateral, affecting the head and neck in about two thirds of cases. At birth, it is a flat and irregular red lesion. With increasing age, it becomes a deeper purple colour, bumpy and thickened (**Figure 13.3**).

Management

For most infantile haemangiomas, no treatment is required. They grow rapidly until about 6 months of age; this is followed by a period of stasis before involution (shrinkage in size until it disappears). Most (70%) disappear completely by 5 years of age, 90% by 7 years.

A large haemangioma may require further imaging to assess its extent. Imaging of other organs, particularly the liver, is required in children with multiple haemangiomas, because hepatic haemangiomas are common in these children.

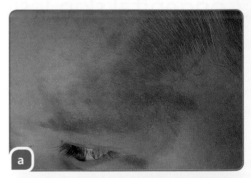

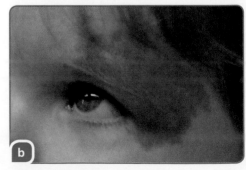

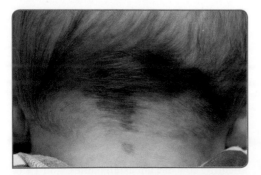

Figure 13.2 'Stork bite' on the back of the neck.

Figure 13.3 A port wine stain. The affected area is pale in infancy (a) but the colour usually deepens with age (b).

Treatment is warranted if a haemangioma is in an area which can lead to secondary complications, for example the airway, where there is a risk of airway obstruction, or the periorbital area, in which case visual development could be affected. First-line treatment is usually with oral propranolol (a beta-blocker), but the mechanism of action for this condition is unknown. Other options include laser therapy, steroid injections and, rarely, surgery.

> **Before propranolol treatment is started, a baseline electrocardiogram is usually obtained to ensure no contraindication to the drug use.** The first dose is administered in hospital, with half hourly monitoring to detect potential adverse effects of propranolol which peak at 2 hours following an oral dose. These are significant and include hypotension, bradycardia and hypoglycaemia.

Stork bites on the forehead generally fade by 18 months of age. However, those on the back of the neck usually persist. No treatment is required as they are of no consequence.

Port wine stains around the eye and forehead can be associated with Sturge-Weber syndrome (8% of patients) and glaucoma (rare). Therefore follow-up with neurologists and ophthalmologists is required.

> **Sturge–Weber syndrome is a neurocutaneous syndrome characterised by a facial port wine stain, in the distribution of the first or second trigeminal nerve, and seizures. There may be an associated ipsilateral leptomeningeal capillary–venous malformation.** Other complications include glaucoma, developmental delay and hemiparesis.

Port wine stains grow with the child and persist into adulthood. They can be disfiguring, and may cause significant psychological distress to the child. Cosmetic camouflage may be helpful. Laser treatment under the guidance of a dermatologist can achieve a good result by causing the birthmark to fade.

Pigmented birthmarks

Pigmented lesions occur as a result of excessive skin pigmentation with melanin. Melanin is produced by melanocytes, neural crest derived cells, most of which are located in the epidermal layer of the skin.

Types

Pigmented birthmarks include:

- Mongolian blue spot (congenital dermal melanocytosis)
- café au lait spots
- congenital melanocytic naevi (moles)

Epidemiology and aetiology

Mongolian blue spots are caused by the persistence of melanocytes in the dermis during intrauterine development. They are most often encountered in babies of Indian, Asian and African ethnic origin.

Café au lait spots are caused by a localised increase in melanin concentration. They affect 13% of white and 27% of black children.

Congenital melanocytic naevi are lesions in which there is a proliferation of melanocytes. They occur in 1 in every 100 neonates worldwide.

Clinical features

Mongolian blue spots are flat, blue-grey lesions of varying size. They are commonly located on the buttocks or lower back (**Figure 13.4**), and are present at birth.

Café au lait spots are light to dark brown–coloured macular lesions (see Figure 8.6). They vary in size and occur anywhere on the body. They may present at birth but more commonly develop in early childhood.

Congenital melanocytic naevi are macular or papular, and brown to black. Their border and texture are irregular, and they are generally < 1.5 cm diameter in size (**Figure 13.5**). They occur in about 3% of newborns. Naevi > 20 cm diameter in size are called giant naevi and are usually hairy. Congenital melanocytic naevi are present at birth or develop in the first year of life.

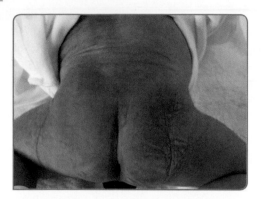

Figure 13.4 Mongolian blue spot on the lower back and buttocks.

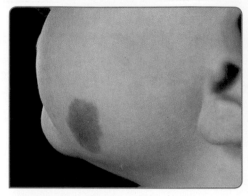

Figure 13.5 Congenital melanocytic naevus.

Management

Mongolian blue spots fade by adolescence. Because of this, and the fact that they are in an inconspicuous area and are not associated with other conditions, no investigation or treatment is necessary.

Isolated café au lait spots are benign. However, the presence of multiple ones may be associated with a neurocutaneous syndrome, including neurofibromatosis (see page 265).

Small congenital melanocytic naevi need no intervention. However, giant naevi are monitored by a dermatologist for signs of malignant change which occurs in up to 6% of cases.

> **Mongolian blue spots can be mistaken for bruises, raising the possibility of child abuse.** Therefore clear documentation of the site and extent of any Mongolian blue spot identified during the newborn examination is essential to avoid any misinterpretation of the lesion and subsequent unnecessary investigations at a later date.

Common neonatal skin rashes

Skin rashes are common in the neonatal period, affecting most newborns. Their underlying causes are uncertain, but they have been attributed to hormonal changes and immaturity of the skin. Rashes can be present at birth or appear within the first month of life. Diagnosis is usually based on clinical examination. Most neonatal rashes are benign and self-limiting.

Milia

Milia, also known as 'milk spots', are small keratin-filled papules. They appear as small white spots, commonly on the nose and

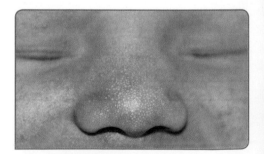

Figure 13.6 Milia on the bridge of the nose.

cheeks (**Figure 13.6**), and disappear within a few weeks. About 50% of newborns have milia.

Erythema toxicum neonatorum

Erythema toxicum neonatorum is a common rash; it occurs in 50% of full-term babies within a few days of birth. It has the appearance of red macules with a small central yellow papule or pustule. The extent of the lesion varies from a few spots to a widespread rash. Any part of the body can be affected, but the palms and soles are usually spared.

The cause is unknown. Erythema toxicum neonatorum resolves spontaneously.

Nappy rash (napkin dermatitis)

Nappy rash is a form of contact dermatitis secondary to irritation from the urine and faeces present in the nappy (**Figure 13.7**). The skin is red and inflamed in patches or over the whole area. The affected areas are either dry or moist, and sometimes look shiny, with pimples or blisters. Characteristically the flexures are spared as they are not in contact with the nappy. It is a common finding in babies. Frequent nappy changes and good hygiene help prevent nappy rash. Barrier creams are also effective; they protect the skin from contact with the irritants, often containing water repellent substances such as paraffins.

The affected area can become secondarily infected, usually with *Candida* but occasionally with a bacterial infection. Differentiation between simple nappy rash and *Candida* infection is usually clinical. In simple nappy rash the skin folds, areas that are not in contact with the irritants, are usually spared. In nappy rash with *Candida* infection, the skin folds are often affected, and satellite lesions (characteristic of fungal infections) may be present (**Figure 13.8**). White plaques on the tongue are characteristic of coexistent oral Candida infection (thrush), so the mouth is also examined in children with nappy rash.

Secondary infections are treated with topical antifungal or antibacterial creams, as appropriate.

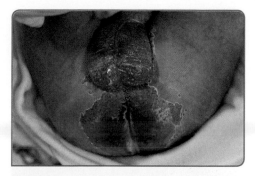

Figure 13.7 Nappy rash caused by contact irritation.

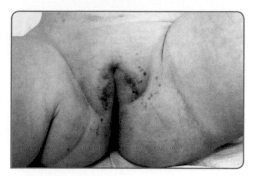

Figure 13.8 Candidal nappy rash, showing the typical satellite lesions.

> Fungal nappy rash may occur as an adverse effect of antibiotic treatment. It is managed with oral antifungal suspension in addition to topical antifungal cream applied to the perineum; the oral agent treats fungal infection of the bowel.

Baby acne (neonatal cephalic pustulosis)

Acne in neonates is characterised by multiple small inflammatory papules and pustules, usually on the nose, forehead and cheeks (**Figure 13.9**). It develops at about 3 weeks of age and is thought to be caused by colonisation with *Malassezia*, a type of fungus. In contrast to the 'true' acne seen in adolescents, there are no comedones (blackheads).

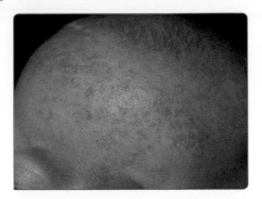

Figure 13.9 Baby acne across the forehead.

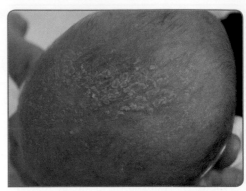

Figure 13.10 Cradle cap: greasy yellow plaques on the top of the head.

The condition gradually resolves, so no intervention is required. However, topical ketoconazole (an antifungal agent) may expedite resolution in children with severe acne.

Cradle cap (infantile seborrhoeic dermatitis)

Cradle cap consists of greasy yellow plaques that form on the scalp as a consequence of overactivity of the sebaceous glands (**Figure 13.10**). It affects infants from about 6 weeks of age and normally resolves spontaneously by 6–12 months of age. Washing with gentle shampoo helps treat the condition.

Childhood rashes

A rash, i.e. exanthema, is a change in the colour or texture of the skin. It is a common clinical presentation in paediatrics and can indicate benign self-limiting conditions, usually secondary to a viral infection, or severe life-threatening illnesses. Diagnosis is guided by the appearance and distribution of the rash, and any associated features or systemic upset (see **Table 13.1** for terms used to describe a rash).

Erythema multiforme

Erythema multiforme is a skin eruption characterised by distinctive lesions resulting from an immune-mediated hypersensitivity reaction. It varies in severity and affects all ages. There are many causes, the commonest being the herpes simplex virus (**Table 13.2**).

Erythema multiforme in children: causes		
Infection	Drugs	Idiopathic
Herpes simplex	Penicillin	Unknown trigger thought to often be due to subclinical herpes simplex infection
Mycoplasma pneumoniae	Tetracyclines	
	Sulfonamides	
Adenovirus	Phenytoin	
Tuberculosis	Barbiturates	

Table 13.2 Causes of erythema multiforme in children. Of the identified causes, herpes simplex is by far the most common cause in children

Children typically present with symmetrically distributed pink macular lesions that become raised and enlarge to about 2 cm. The centre of each lesion becomes paler, but the outer ring remains pink; this produces the typical 'target lesion' appearance (**Figure 13.11a**). Lesions begin on the extensor

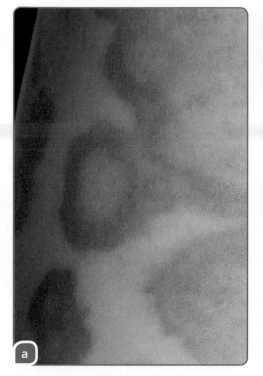

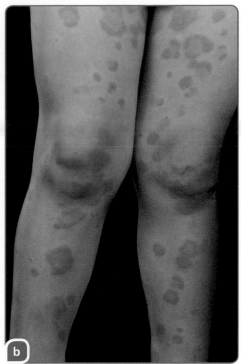

Figure 13.11 Erythema multiforme. (a) Close-up of the typical 'target lesions'. (b) Rash covering a wide area.

surfaces of hands and feet and spread centrally (**Figure 13.11b**). The oral mucosa may also be involved.

The condition is self-limiting, generally resolving after 2–3 weeks and without scarring. Treatment of the underlying cause, for example *Mycoplasma*, can be helpful.

Stevens–Johnson syndrome

Stevens–Johnson syndrome is a severe immune complex-mediated hypersensitivity reaction of the skin. It is very rare, affecting only two per million of the population worldwide with a mean age of 25 years, but it is also seen in children. In up to 75% of cases the trigger is the use of certain drugs, particularly anticonvulsants and some antibiotics. However, the syndrome can be secondary to infection, for example with *Mycoplasma* or cytomegalovirus, or rarely vaccinations.

Patients usually experience a prodrome of malaise, fever and sore throat before the onset of a rapidly spreading and painful rash.

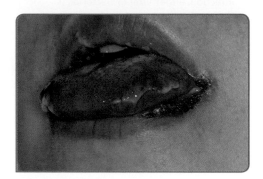

Figure 13.12 Stevens–Johnson syndrome.

The rash consists of macules that evolve into blisters before the skin begins to slough. Mucosal involvement is widespread and severe; it includes conjunctivitis and oral ulcers (**Figure 13.12**). The breakdown of skin can lead to severe dehydration and infection.

The condition has a mortality of 10–25% at all ages, determined by the extent of skin sloughing, but there is no specific treatment. Management includes withdrawal of the triggering drug and supportive care in an intensive care or burns unit setting.

Toxic epidermal necrolysis is a more severe variant of Stevens–Johnson syndrome.

Urticaria and angioedema

Urticaria is a rash that occurs secondary to the release of histamine from mast cells; it is typically triggered by an allergy, infection or use of a certain drug. The rash consists of wheals, which are raised white lesions on a red background. The wheals form in the upper dermis, vary in size and are intensely itchy. There may be associated angioedema, which is swelling secondary to fluid extravasation deeper in the skin tissue, i.e. the dermis and subcutaneous tissues.

Urticaria is acute if it is present for < 6 weeks, or chronic if present for > 6 weeks. Acute urticarial lesions are usually present for only minutes or hours and resolve spontaneously. Chronic urticaria is rarely caused by one specific allergen and can be a manifestation of an autoimmune disease.

> **Infection, either viral or bacterial, is the most common cause of urticaria in children.** In cases in which an antibiotic is prescribed to treat an infection that causes urticaria, the development of urticaria may be incorrectly attributed to use of the antibiotic rather than the infection. It is therefore incorrectly documented that the child is allergic to that antibiotic. Careful interpretation of the history should distinguish between infection and antibiotic use as the cause.

In children, angioedema is usually associated with urticaria or anaphylaxis (see page 402). It most commonly affects the lips and eyes but can involve the skin or any mucous membranes.

> **Isolated angioedema is rarely encountered in children but can be the presentation of hereditary angioedema.** This is an autosomal dominant condition in which there is either a reduced level of the protein C1 esterase inhibitor, or the C1 esterase inhibitor that is present is dysfunctional. The main function of C1 esterase inhibitor is to prevent spontaneous activation of the complement system.
>
> Hereditary angioedema affects the larynx or bowel mucosa, causing respiratory compromise or abdominal pain, respectively.

Diagnosis of acute urticaria and angioedema is based on a careful history and examination. No routine investigations are necessary. However, if a specific allergen is suspected an allergen-specific immunoglobulin E test is useful to confirm this.

The most effective aspect of management is avoidance of known triggers. Episodes are generally self-limiting, but antihistamines can help reduce itching. Management of anaphylaxis is discussed on page 404.

Viral rashes

Non-specific viral illnesses are common in children, and many of these illnesses are associated with a rash. Typically, it appears as a non-pruritic, widespread, erythematous maculopapular blanching rash. If the child has symptoms of a viral illness and no other features of serious illness (see page 398), reassurance can be given that the rash will resolve spontaneously. Rashes associated with specific childhood infections are discussed in Chapter 10.

Infections and infestations

The skin acts as a barrier to infection. However, the skin and subcutaneous tissue can themselves be infected, and this is common in children. The infection can be bacterial, viral, fungal or parasitic. The term infestation is used when arthropods, such as lice and mites, live on the surface of the skin.

Some infections and infestations, such as impetigo and head lice, spread rapidly between children because of close contact at nursery or school. Diagnosis of most skin infections and infestations is by clinical examination.

Bacterial infections

Bacterial skin infections are usually caused by bacteria, such as *Staphylococcus aureus* and *Streptococcus pyogenes*, which live harmlessly on the skin surface in up to a third of the population. Any breach of the skin, for example a cut or graze, can lead to infection of the epidermis, dermis or subcutaneous tissues. Deeper infection can cause systemic symptoms.

Types

Common bacterial skin infections in children are:

- impetigo
- cellulitis

A rare but important skin infection due to its prevalence in children and neonates and its life-threatening potential is staphylococcal scaled skin syndrome

Epidemiology and aetiology

Impetigo is a superficial infection of the skin that commonly occurs in children especially aged 3-5 years. It is caused by the bacteria *Staph. aureus* and *Strep. pyogenes*.

Cellulitis is an infection of the dermis and subcutaneous tissue. In children, it is usually secondary to a minor injury, including insect bite, or other breach in the skin that allows bacteria to enter. The usual causative organisms are *Staph. aureus* and *Strep. pyogenes*.

Staphylococcal scaled skin syndrome is a blistering disease caused by exotoxins released by Staph. aureus. The toxins cause breakdown and exfoliation of the epidermis. The condition affects young children, generally those younger than 5 years.

Clinical features

The commonest form of impetigo is non-bullous impetigo. It typically starts as a papule or vesicle that grows rapidly before breaking down to develop the characteristic honey-coloured crust (**Figure 13.13**).

In cellulitis, the skin will typically be red, hot, swollen and painful.

In staphylococcal scaled skin syndrome, the child is typically irritable and feverish. There is generalised erythema before development of large, thin-walled bullae, which are very fragile. Nikolsky's sign is positive. After rupture of the blister, the skin has the characteristic appearance of a scald.

> **Nikolsky's sign** is when rubbing or gentle pressure on the skin causes redness, peeling and blistering.

Management

Impetigo is highly contagious until the lesion has dried. It is treated with a topical antibacterial cream such as fusidic acid. Good hand hygiene helps prevent cross-infection.

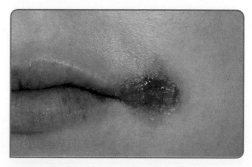

Figure 13.13 Non-bullous impetigo.

Cellulitis is treated with either oral or IV antibiotics, commonly flucloxacillin, depending on its severity.

Management of staphylococcal scaled skin syndrome consists of IV antibiotics and analgesia, with particular attention to ensuring adequate hydration. Children with large affected areas are particularly at risk of sepsis, superinfection, and dehydration or electrolyte imbalance and may require management in an intensive care setting. Mortality is up to 5% in children.

Viral infections

Local infection of the skin by viruses is common in children. These viral infections are not associated with systemic symptoms. Also, although a viral infection may last 1–2 years in a child, this is a shorter duration than in adults, because a child's immune system is more active in producing antibodies.

Types

Common viral infections in children are:

- warts
- molluscum contagiosum

Epidemiology and aetiology

Warts are skin growths caused by the human papillomavirus. They are common, affecting up to 10% of children. They are spread by direct contact.

Molluscum contagiosum is caused by the pox virus. It is transmitted by direct skin contact or contact with an infected surface. It primarily affects children aged 1–11 years old.

Clinical features

Warts are hard, rough growths of skin, commonly occurring on the fingers or soles. In the latter case, they are known as verrucae.

The classic appearance of molluscum contagiosum is small (5 mm), pearly, dome-shaped papules with a central umbilication (**Figure 13.14**). The number of lesions varies between individuals; those with eczema tend to have more lesions; these are often spread by scratching which leads to auto-inoculation of unaffected skin. The lesions normally occur on the face and neck.

Management

Warts are treated with topical salicylic acid. Cryotherapy can help if the wart is causing discomfort or significant cosmetic problems; however, most specialists advise conservative management, because 90% of warts disappear within 2 years without treatment.

For molluscum contagiosum, conservative management is advised. Lesions usually spontaneously resolve within 18 months.

Fungal infections

Tinea is the general name for infections caused by dermatophytes, a group of fungi that live on the skin. Individual conditions are named according to the site affected:

- tinea capitis affects the scalp
- tinea corporis affects skin on any part of the body, but particularly the non-hairy areas
- tinea pedis affects skin on the feet

Tinea capitis (scalp ringworm) is commonest in prepubertal children. Typical features are a scaly scalp, sometimes with broken hair within the scaly area. Less commonly there is a smooth bald patch. Occasionally, the mass turns into a boggy abscess-like swelling called a kerion.

Tinea corporis (ringworm) is characterised by large, round and scaly lesions. These later develop central clearing, giving rise to a 'ring'

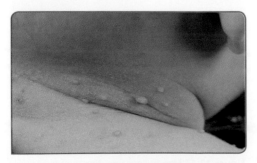

Figure 13.14 Molluscum contagiosum.

appearance. Lesions are seen on the trunk and limbs.

Tinea pedis (althlete's foot) leads to itchy, scaly and cracked skin between the toes.

In up to 70% of cases the infected area shows a yellow-green fluorescence under examination with a filtered ultraviolet (Wood's) light. Rapid diagnosis is made by microscopic examination of skin scrapings for fungal hyphae. Definitive identification of the fungus is by culture.

> The term 'ringworm' is a misnomer. It was originally thought to be caused by a worm due to the annular appearance of the lesion, but is now known to be due to fungi.

Management

Tinea capitis requires oral antifungals and topical antifungal shampoo. Tinea corporis and tinca pedis are treated with topical antifungal treatment, or oral antifungals for severe infection, for several weeks.

Parasitic infestations

In developed countries the commonest infestations affecting children are head lice and scabies. They both spread easily by close contact; a whole class of children often need to be treated as a group. Scabies is a global public health problem, affecting persons of all ages, races and socioeconomic groups. It is endemic in many tropical and subtropical regions (resource-poor populations). Natural disasters, war and poverty lead to overcrowding and increased rates of transmission.

Epidemiology and aetiology

Head lice are small (≤ 3 mm) parasitic insects that live on the scalp of humans, feeding on their blood. Infestation with head lice is extremely common in childhood; up to 50% of children are affected at one or more points

in their life. The incidence peaks at 7 years. Lice cannot jump, so they are passed to others by head-to-head contact.

Scabies is caused by small parasitic mites that infest the skin. The females burrow into the epidermis and lay eggs. Scabies is a common problem worldwide: 1.5% of the world's population have had the infestation and an estimated 300 million cases occur annually. Prevalence rates are higher in children. It is spread by touch.

Clinical features and diagnostic approach

Head lice cause itching and irritation of the scalp, which may be the first sign of infestation. Lice may be spotted moving in the hair. After hatching, the empty eggs ('nits') laid by the lice appear white and therefore by becoming more visible than the brown filled eggs they can be spotted attached to the hair, normally near the scalp. A Wood's light examination of the infested area shows yellow–green fluorescence of lice and nits.

The mite infestation in scabies causes an intensely itchy rash. The mites' burrows appear as wavy lines in the skin. These are commonly seen on the wrist and interdigital web spaces. The itching tends to be worse at night. Diagnosis is made clinically and can be confirmed by visualising the mite by microscopy.

Management

Head lice infestation is treated by a combination of regular combing of wet hair with a very fine-toothed comb and treatment with an insecticidal shampoo. It is recommended that the chemical treatments are repeated after 7 days to target any surviving lice.

Scabies is treated with the use of chemical washes, for example permethrin. The initial treatment is repeated 7 days later.

For both types of infestation, all members of the household are treated at the same time and all clothing and bedding thoroughly washed.

Chronic skin conditions

Some skin conditions affecting children are persistent and chronic, such as eczema and psoriasis. In children with severe skin conditions, they cause significant morbidity and reduce quality of life. Diagnosis is based on clinical examination, by looking for typical features and assessing cutaneous distribution (**Table 13.3**).

Atopic eczema

Atopic eczema is a chronic, itchy, inflammatory disease of the skin. It is common, affecting up to 20% of children. Most children with eczema present before 1 year of age. The condition is caused by a combination of genetic and environmental factors. Most children have other atopic conditions or at least one parent with atopy.

Clinical features

Clinical features vary between individuals. Typically, the skin is dry and red and itchy. Acute exacerbations ('flare-ups') of eczema cause lesions that are usually red, weepy and crusty. In chronic eczema, the skin has a dry and thickened appearance (lichenified) as a consequence of frequent scratching (**Figure 13.15**). Sites affected depend on the age of the child (see **Table 13.3**).

Severe eczema can significantly reduce a child's quality of life because of the constant itchiness, scratching and disturbed sleep.

Management

Management of eczema has multiple elements but is based mainly on the use of topical therapies. Phototherapy (i.e. ultraviolet light therapy), oral corticosteroids and systemic immunosuppressants are rarely indicated; their use is reserved for severe conditions. They are prescribed by consultant dermatologists only.

Medication

The most essential part of management is

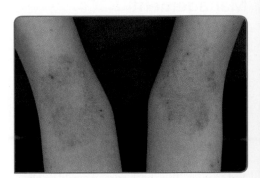

Figure 13.15 Eczema on the flexor surfaces of the elbows (the typical pattern) in a teenager.

Comparison of eczema and psoriasis		
Feature	Atopic eczema	Psoriasis
Age at onset	85% in first year and 95% before 5 years	Teenage years
Typical appearance	Pruritic dry areas with red, weepy and crusty areas in flare-ups and lichenification in long-standing disease	Pink or red, slightly raised, well-circumscribed plaques with a classic silvery scale on top
Typical distribution	Infants (<1 year): begins on face, before progressing (can become widespread) Toddlers (1–5 years): patches on extensor surfaces of wrists, elbows, ankles and knees Older children (>5 years): flexures of knees and elbows	Symmetrical Extensor surfaces of knees and elbows Lower back Scalp (but rare on face)
Natural history	95% of children 'grow out' of eczema	Persists into adulthood (life-long)

Table 13.3 Differences between eczema and psoriasis

emollient (moisturisers) therapy, because emollients hydrate and soften the skin and act as a barrier to water and external irritants. Children with eczema must use emollients rather than soap, which is too drying to the skin, for washing and bathing. Emollients are also used for moisturising, applied liberally at least three times a day as their effects are short lasting. Their use should continue even after the eczema has cleared.

Flare-ups are treated with topical corticosteroid creams, such as hydrocortisone, which reduce skin inflammation. Topical corticosteroids vary in potency; the potency prescribed should be appropriate to the severity and site of the eczema. Generally mild corticosteroids are for the face and flexures, and more potent ones for thickened lichenified areas (due to repeated scratching) or severe eczema (not facial). Topical corticosteroids should only be given as short courses as prolonged use causes thinning of the skin and may also be absorbed into the circulation, rarely causing adrenal suppression. Therefore, topical corticosteroids should be applied thinly, using the fingertip unit guide, to affected areas only and a maximum twice daily.

> One fingertip unit (FTU) is the amount of topical corticosteroid that is squeezed out from a standard tube along an adult's fingertip (from the very end of the finger to the first crease in the finger). One FTU is enough to treat an area of skin twice the size of the flat of the adult's hand with the fingers together.

Topical calcineurin inhibitors, which are topical immunosuppressants, are rarely used under the guidance of a dermatologist in children that are unresponsive to topical corticosteroids. An example is tacrolimus in ointment form. Eczematous skin is at risk of secondary infection with bacteria or viruses, for example resulting in eczema herpeticum, which occurs when eczematous skin is infected with herpesvirus. Secondary infection is treated with topical or oral antibiotic or antiviral agents, as appropriate.

Education

Exposure to irritants or particular allergens is avoided.

Dressings

Bandages or dressings placed over the affected skin help prevent scratching. 'Wet wrapping' is the application of wet bandages to the skin, over a thick layer of emollient. This helps cool and hydrate the skin. Dressings and clothing soaked with paraffin ointment are easily ignited by a naked flame so patients should keep away from fire, flames and cigarettes.

Psoriasis

Psoriasis is an inflammatory disease of the skin caused by an autoimmune process that stimulates overproduction of skin cells, resulting in the characteristic rash. It affects about 2–3% of the population worldwide, is commoner in Caucasians, with a prevalence of 0.5–1% of children. It begins at any age (up to 15% of cases starting at under 10 years of age) with a median age of onset of 28 years. There is thought to be a genetic link. Girls are affected more often than boys.

Clinical features

The commonest type of psoriasis is plaque psoriasis which appears as a well-circumscribed area of thickened pink or red skin with a silver scaly surface (**Figure 13.16**). In children, the plaques are less thick than in adults. Nail changes, such as pitting or discoloration under the nail, are present in up to 50% of cases. Severity varies, but the condition can significantly reduce the individual's psychological well-being, because of the visible appearance (often mistaken as being contagious by others) and the chronic nature of the condition.

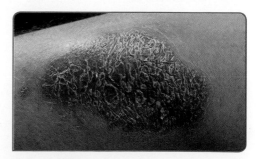

Figure 13.16 Psoriasis.

Koebner's phenomenon is the appearance of psoriatic lesions at a site of injury to the skin.

Management

The first-line treatment is topical use of corticosteroids and tar preparations. Phototherapy, i.e. ultraviolet light therapy, can be helpful. Systemic immunosuppressants and biological therapies are reserved for severe conditions.

Psoriasis is a lifelong illness with remissions and exacerbations, and is sometimes refractory to treatment. About 10% of individuals with psoriasis go on to develop psoriatic arthritis, usually in adulthood, but it can occur in childhood and in some cases the arthritis precedes the psoriasis by many years (see page 279).

The incidence of psoriasis affecting flexures and the face is higher in children than adults.

Acne

Acne is characterised by blocked and inflamed sebaceous glands. It affects 90% of teenagers at some point during adolescence. Increased androgen release at puberty causes both increased keratinocyte activity and increased release of sebum from the sebaceous glands, which blocks the glands and causes comedones to form. Inflammation driven by the skin commensal *Propionibacterium acnes*, which thrives with the increased sebum, leads to development of papules and pustules.

Clinical features

The characteristic appearance of acne is greasy skin with a mixture of open and closed comedones, papules, pustules and, more severely, nodules. Most lesions are seen on the face, but the back and chest can also be affected. Severity varies between individuals. Acne can be painful and cause psychological distress.

Management

Mild acne can be treated with over-the-counter topical benzoyl peroxide products. Useful prescribed treatments for mild to moderate acne are:

- topical retinoids, i.e. vitamin A derivatives that break down comedones and normalise keratinocyte activity
- topical antibiotics, especially when inflammatory lesions are prevalent

Systemic treatment is considered in children with moderate to severe acne and can include a prolonged course of an oral antibiotic, for example doxycycline, or hormonal antiandrogen treatment with the combined oral contraceptive pill (contains both oestrogen and progesterone) which decreases circulating androgens. Oral retinoic acid, i.e. isotretinoin, is effective but is used only under consultant direction due to its toxic nature, and only when other treatments have been ineffective.

Prognosis is usually good. Acne eventually resolves, although nearly 1% have acne scarring, with 1 in 7 of these considered to have 'disfiguring scars'.

Retinoic acid, a medication for acne, is highly teratogenic. Therefore girls must avoid pregnancy while on this treatment. Appropriate contraception should be used if they are sexually active.

Answers to starter questions

1. Mikhail Gorbachev, the first president of the USSR had a port wine birthmark on his scalp. The name port wine comes from the deep red colour of port wine birthmarks resembling the colour of the fortified red wine produced in Portugal.

2. The condition called ringworm (tinea) is not a 'worm' but a skin infection caused by dermatophytes, a group of fungi that live on the skin. Therefore, although the skin appearance in ringworm looks like it is made by a 'round worm' under the skin it is a fungal infection and is treated with topical or systemic antifungal medication.

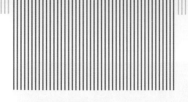

Chapter 14
Haematological disorders

Starter questions

Answers to the following questions are on page 380.

1. Why do multiple blood transfusions cause organ damage?
2. Why do children with reduced platelet counts not have platelet transfusions?

Introduction

This chapter covers all the major paediatric haematological disorders with the exception of haematological malignancy, which is discussed in Chapter 15 (see page 386).

The commonest haematological disorder is iron deficiency anaemia, affecting a significant proportion of the population. Other blood disorders, especially those with a genetic basis, may be rare overall but common in specific populations because of the evolutionary advantages they conferred. A paediatrician's experience of these diseases depends on the population they serve.

The management of different blood disorders varies greatly. Some are easily treated and therefore managed in primary care. Others, for example sickle cell disease, have many complications, which may necessitate frequent admissions to hospital. Such chronic conditions can reduce a child's overall quality of life, including their psychological well-being, so are usually managed by specialised teams.

Case 19 Pallor and tiredness in a 2-year-old

Presentation

Joseph, a 2-year-old boy of African–Caribbean origin, is taken to see the general practitioner (GP) by his mother. She explains that he is sleeping more than usual. Initially, she put this down to him being worn out from starting playschool, but she became concerned after noticing that he is looking paler than usual.

Initial interpretation

Lethargy and pallor are symptoms of anaemia. There are multiple causes of anaemia in a child (see **Figure 14.1**); further history must narrow these down to establish the underlying cause. A good way to start thinking about them is to consider those related to decreased production of red blood cells and those in which there is increased destruction of red blood cells.

Further history

Joseph is usually fit and well, although he is recovering from a cold and has recently started to have constipation. He was born at term and had an uneventful neonatal period. His mother does not remember him being jaundiced. There is no family history of blood disorders. Joseph has never left the UK.

His mother reports that he is a fussy eater and refuses to eat vegetables. He enjoys drinking cows' milk and can drink up to 2 pints a day. He opens his bowels once every 3 days, and his mother has noticed a small amount of bright red blood in his nappy.

Examination

Joseph is not very cooperative during the examination, but the GP notes that he has pale conjunctivae. A few small cervical lymph nodes are palpable, but there is no inguinal or axillary lymphadenopathy. There is no organomegaly. A small anal fissure is present.

Interpretation of findings

There are several diagnostic possibilities in Joseph's case. His African–Caribbean origin raises the suspicion of sickle cell disease. However, this condition would normally have presented earlier than 2 years of age. Also, sickle cell anaemia is inherited, and the absence of a family history of blood disorders make a hereditary cause for the anaemia less likely.

Joseph has not been to any country in which malaria is endemic; certain types of malaria cause severe anaemia in children. Although there is a history of gastrointestinal bleeding, the small amount of blood loss from an anal fissure is unlikely to cause anaemia.

Iron deficiency anaemia is a strong possibility in view of the volume of cows' milk that Joseph is drinking and the lack of iron in his diet. Cervical lymphadenopathy without hepatosplenomegaly is more in keeping with a viral upper respiratory tract infection, but malignancy affecting the blood is always considered in a child presenting with lethargy and pallor.

Investigations

Investigations, comprising a full blood count, blood film, ferritin test, transferrin test, total iron-binding capacity test and reticulocyte count, are arranged. A haemoglobin concentration of 85 g/L confirms the diagnosis of anaemia. Blood film shows a microcytic hypochromic picture, i.e. small blood cells that are paler than normal. The reticulocyte (newly-produced, immature red blood cells) count

Case 19 *continued*

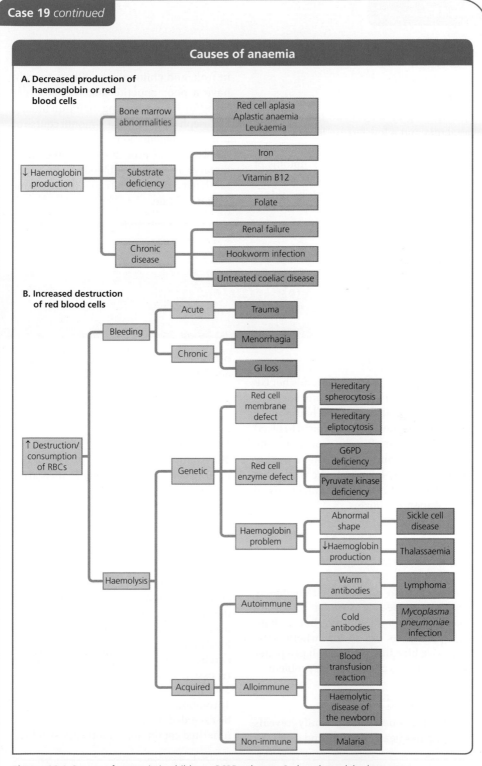

Figure 14.1 Causes of anaemia in children. G6PD, glucose 6-phosphate dehydrogenase.

Case 19 *continued*

and ferritin level are low. Total iron-binding capacity and transferrin level are high.

Diagnosis

The finding of microcytic hypochromic anaemia and a low ferritin level are consistent with a diagnosis of iron deficiency anaemia. In the absence of symptoms of malabsorption, the anaemia is secondary to poor dietary intake of iron. This is typically encountered in children who drink lots of cows' milk. Cows' milk is low in iron, and children who fill up on milk have a poor appetite and therefore eat little, further decreasing their iron intake.

Joseph is started on a 3-month course of iron supplementation and referred to the dietician, who provides his mother with dietary advice. Repeat blood tests to check his haemoglobin levels are arranged for 3 months' time.

Case 20 Bleeding after dental work in a 13-year-old

Presentation

Emily, who is 13 years old, attends her GP surgery following advice from her dentist. The previous week, she had a tooth extracted and her gum continued to bleed for over an hour after the procedure. She is normally fit and well. She has a history of nose bleeds, for which she visited an ear, nose and throat consultant, but these settled spontaneously.

Initial interpretation

The history of prolonged bleeding after trauma on a background of epistaxis (bleeding from the nose) immediately suggests a bleeding disorder. There are many possible diagnoses, but a logical approach is to consider whether the excessive bleeding is the result of a platelet problem or a clotting factor problem.

Further history

On further questioning, Emily reveals that she has heavy periods and seems to bruise easily after trivial bumps. Emily is adopted and has little information about her birth parents, so no family medical history is available.

Examination

The examination is normal except for the finding of a few bruises over Emily's arm, which she attributes to a minor injury sustained during netball practice.

Interpretation of findings

Heavy periods and easy bruising increases the probability of a bleeding disorder. Without a family history, there is no information to suggest a genetic cause for Emily's symptoms. However, haemophilia can be ruled out because it is an X-linked recessive condition; girls can carry the causative gene but not have the disease. Thrombocytopenia (low platelets) needs to be excluded. Von Willebrand's disease, an inherited condition, is another possibility.

Case 20 *continued*

Investigations

A full blood count shows a normal platelet count, at 200,000 platelets/mL. Prothrombin time test results are normal. Activated partial thromboplastin time is slightly prolonged. Bleeding time is significantly prolonged.

Diagnosis

The prolonged bleeding time with normal coagulation and platelet count suggests a diagnosis of von Willebrand's disease. This is confirmed by low levels of von Willebrand factor. The condition will have little effect on Emily's life, but she will require (desmopressin) before any surgery.

Anaemia

Anaemia is characterised by a low circulating level of haemoglobin or red blood cells. The level used to define anaemia varies according to the age of the child (**Table 14.1**).

> **Haemoglobin exists in different forms with varying oxygen-carrying capacity.** Normal forms include haemoglobin A, usually up to 98% of total haemoglobin in adults, and haemoglobin F (fetal haemoglobin). Haemoglobin F is the major component of haemoglobin in the fetus; its production stops at birth, and it makes up only a small fraction of total haemoglobin in adults.
>
> Abnormal haemoglobins resulting from mutations of the genes encoding the two α and two β globin chains that comprise the haemoglobin molecule can be pathological, for example haemoglobin S ('S' for 'sickle') in sickle cell disease.

Anaemia is a common diagnosis in children and has many causes (including hereditary eliptocytosis, **Figure 14.2**). These can be divided into decreased production of haemoglobin or red blood cells, and increased destruction of red blood cells (**Figure 14.1**).

Iron deficiency anaemia

Iron deficiency anaemia is the commonest cause of anaemia.

Epidemiology and aetiology

Iron deficiency anaemia affects up to a quarter of the world's population, and up to 5% of toddlers and teenage girls in high-income countries.

Anaemia: age-specific definitions	
Age	Haemoglobin concentration (g/L)
Birth	< 165
6 months to 5 years	< 110
5–11 years	< 115
12–14 years	< 120

Table 14.1 Age-specific definitions of anaemia

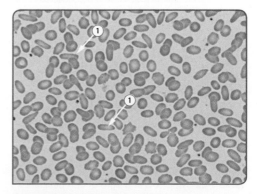

Figure 14.2 Blood film showing abnormal elliptical or oval red blood cells ① in hereditary eliptocytosis.

The commonest cause is inadequate dietary intake of iron. Iron deficiency is encountered in children who drink large amounts of unmodified (i.e. not formula) cows' milk, which contains very little iron. In teenage girls, the combination of the rapid period of growth associated with puberty and heavy periods is a contributing factor. Malabsorption of dietary iron, for example in coeliac disease, may also cause iron deficiency anaemia. In low- or middle-income countries, infestation with intestinal parasitic worms is a common cause.

Clinical features

The clinical features of iron deficiency anaemia vary depending on its severity. It is not uncommon for the child to be asymptomatic if the anaemia has developed gradually, even in the presence of significant anaemia. **Table 14.2** lists the symptoms and signs of iron deficiency anaemia.

There is some evidence that severe iron deficiency anaemia can affect cognitive development in infants and young children.

> **Pica is an eating disorder characterised by eating non-food substances, such as soil or ice, for > 1 month.** It can be encountered in children with iron deficiency anaemia.

Iron deficiency anaemia: symptoms and signs	
General	Specific
Fatigue	Pallor
Headache	Angular cheilitis (an inflammatory lesion affecting the corners of the mouth)
Irritability	
Poor feeding	
	Kolionychia (abnormally thin, concave nails)
	Tachycardia
	Flow murmur
	Pica

Table 14.2 Symptoms and signs of iron deficiency anaemia. Many children with mild anaemia are asymtomatic

Diagnostic approach

A full blood count shows a low haemoglobin concentration, and a blood film shows a microcytic hypochromic (small and pale red blood cells) picture. Reticulocyte count is low. The level of ferritin, a marker of iron stores, is low. Transferrin (a protein which binds and transports iron in the blood) level and total iron-binding capacity are high.

A thorough history, particularly related to diet, menorrhagia and symptoms of gastrointestinal bleeding, is helpful in identification of the underlying cause. If the history suggests malabsorption or gastrointestinal bleeding, then appropriate investigations, for example a coeliac screen, must be carried out.

> **Iron deficiency anaemia is often an incidental finding** on blood tests carried out for other reasons.

> **Ferritin is a very sensitive marker of iron stores.** However, caution is needed when interpreting the result of ferritin tests, because ferritin is an acute phase reactant and can be increased in inflammation.

Management

Increasing the amount of iron-rich food in the diet, such as red meat, dark green leafy vegetables and fortified cereals, and limiting excessive milk intake are the first steps in the treatment of dietary iron deficiency anaemia. Oral iron supplementation is also usually required. A gluten-free diet improves anaemia associated with coeliac disease.

> **Vitamin C increases iron absorption.** Therefore individuals with iron deficiency anaemia are advised to eat iron-rich food or take iron supplements with vitamin C, for example in orange juice. Iron absorption is reduced by milk (specifically the calcium and phosphate) and tea, so these should be avoided with iron-rich food or iron supplements.

Sickle cell disease

Sickle cell disease is a genetic disorder in which the red cells are abnormally-shaped, making them more easily destructible. This leads to vaso-occlusion and haemolytic anaemia. It is inherited in an autosomal recessive manner. There are many variants, but those who are homozygous for haemoglobin S are most severely affected; the condition is known as sickle cell anaemia.

Epidemiology and aetiology

Sickle cell disease is most prevalent in sub-Saharan Africa (up to 1 in 4 West Africans and 1 in 10 Afro-Carribeans are carriers), because of the evolutionary advantage it conferred to carriers: partial protection against malaria. It is also found in the Middle East, the Mediterranean and Asia. Overall 1 in 2000 births in England are affected, but the prevalence of the disease is highest in areas with a higher proportion of affected ethnic groups.

In sickle cell disease, a genetic mutation results in production of abnormal haemoglobin called haemoglobin S, with the amino acid valine at position 6 on the β globin chain (see page 376), rather than the glutamic acid that is normally present.

Haemoglobin S tends to form an abnormal sickle shape when deoxygenated (**Figure 14.3**). This sickling makes the haemoglobin less able to pass through small capillaries, thereby leading to vaso-occlusion. Haemoglobin S is also more prone to premature breakdown.

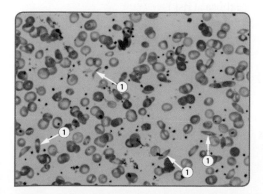

Figure 14.3 Blood film showing sickle cells in a patient with sickle cell anaemia ①.

Clinical features

Dactylitis, i.e. painful, swollen hands and feet, secondary to vaso-occlusion, is a common presentation, along with episodes of pain from vaso-occlusion elsewhere, especially the spleen. There may be symptoms of anaemia (see **Table 14.2**) or failure to thrive. Jaundice may occur secondary to haemolysis of the abnormally shaped red blood cells.

Clinical signs include splenomegaly in young children. From about 5 years of age, there is gradual autosplenctomy (fibrosis, shrinkage and loss of function) secondary to recurrent episodes of vaso-occulsion leading to infarction. This results in increased susceptibility to infection with encapsulated organisms, such as *Streptococcus pneumoniae*, which can lead to life-threatening sepsis. Gallstones can develop, especially from the second decade onwards. Their prevalence increases with age.

Sickle cell disease can lead to several serious complications. These are known as acute crises (**Table 14.3**).

Diagnostic approach

If the parents are known carriers, sickle cell disease may be diagnosed antenatally. Other children with the disease are identified in the neonatal period by the newborn screening programme. Full blood count shows a normocytic anaemia and high reticulocyte count. Blood film shows sickle cells (see **Figure 14.3**). Haemoglobin electrophoresis confirms the presence of haemoglobin S.

Management

There is no cure for sickle cell disease, so the aims of management are prevention and treatment of complications. Factors that may precipitate vaso-occlusive crises must be avoided:

- cold temperature
- dehydration
- infection
- hypoxia
- stress
- alcohol consumption

Sickle cell disease: acute crises			
Complication	Description	Signs and symptoms	Treatment
Vaso-occlusive crisis	Blood cells sickle and become stuck in capillaries, leading to ischaemia of organs Multiple triggers (see page 373)	Pain Swollen joints Tachypnoea (if lung involved) Neurological symptoms (if brain involved)	Oxygen Analgesia Hydration Warmth
Acute chest syndrome	Vaso-occlusion of pulmonary blood vessels Commonest cause of death in sickle cell disease Triggered by pulmonary infection Hypoxia worsens sickling	Chest pain Tachypnoea Dyspnoea New sputum production	As above, and: ■ with antibiotics ■ with or without exchange transfusion
Splenic sequestration crisis	Pooling of sickle cells in spleen Sudden splenic enlargement and decrease in haemoglobin	Hypovolaemia	Supportive Blood transfusions often needed
Aplastic crisis	Severe anaemia secondary to bone marrow failure Precipitated by infection with parvovirus Resolves spontaneously	Features of severe anaemia	Supportive Blood transfusion

Table 14.3 Acute crises associated with sickle cell disease

Folic acid is required because of the high turnover of red blood cells. Prophylactic penicillin is given to prevent infection with encapsulated organisms. Children with sickle cell disease should be fully immunised, due to their increased susceptibility to infection. Blood transfusions may be required for anaemia. Hydroxyurea can help reduce complications by increasing production of haemoglobin F, thereby lowering the concentration of haemoglobin S and reducing the frequency of sickling crises.

Individuals with some blood disorders require multiple blood transfusions. This puts them at risk of iron overload, with excess iron deposited in organs. Chelation agents are administered to avoid this complication.

Physicians must be alert for complications of sickle cell disease:

■ salmonella osteomyelitis
■ gallstones
■ priapism
■ stroke (screening with transcranial doppler is performed annually to identify those at risk)
■ renal failure
■ iron overload (secondary to recurrent transfusions)

Prognosis

Prognosis is variable but has dramatically improved with the introduction of screening and comprehensive care. Mean survival is about 50 years.

Thalassaemia

Thalassaemia is a genetic disorder characterised by defects in genes encoding either the α- or β-globin chain (see page 376). It is inherited in an autosomal recessive manner. There is a reduction in the number of normal globin chains produced, and this variation results in anaemia of varying severity.

Thalassaemia is common with around 5% of the world population being carriers of one variant or other. It is especially prevalent in individuals of South and Southeast Asian, and Middle Eastern origin, e.g up to 1 in 7 individuals in Cyprus are carriers for β-thalassaemia.

There are two types of thalassaemia, α and β; β-thalassaemia is the more common type. There are four subtypes of α-thalassaemia and three subtypes of β-thalassaemia (**Table 14.4**).

Clinical features

The features of thalassaemia depend on the severity of the associated anaemia (see **Table 14.4**). Unless the condition is diagnosed antenatally, children with β-thalassaemia major present with severe anaemia and failure to thrive at about 6 months of age, when the amount of haemoglobin F has diminished significantly. They develop hepatospenomegaly because of extramedullary haemopoiesis. There is overgrowth of bones secondary to bone marrow hyperplasia (in response to increased haematopoetic requirements), particularly affecting the maxilla and skull bones and leading to characteristic frontal bossing and 'thalassaemia facies'.

Mild thalassaemia may present as an incidental finding when the full blood count is checked for another reason.

Thalassaemia: classification			
Type	Description	Subtypes	Clinical features
α-Thalassaemia	Reduced α globin chain production due to gene deletions, causing excess of β globin (there are 2 loci for α globin, 4 genes per cell) Severity of anaemia depends on how many α chains are present	One deletion	Asymptomatic
		Two deletions	Thalassaemia trait (e.g. microcytosis with our without mild anaemia)
		Three deletions (haemoglobin H disease)	Severe anaemia with target cells and Heinz bodies
		Four deletions: no α haemoglobin produced	Incompatible with life Pregnancy often ends in miscarriage or birth of neonate with hydrops fetalis
β-Thalassaemia	Reduced production of β globin chains because of mutations in genes encoding β globin chains Two β alleles per cell Severity of anaemia depends on nature of mutation	β-Thalassaemia minor: one β allele has a mutation	Mild microcytic anaemia or no anaemia Often asymptomatic and no treatment required
		β-Thalassaemia intermedia: one β allele has a mutation	Moderate anaemia Blood transfusion may be needed
		β-Thalassaemia major: both alleles encoding the β globin chains are mutated	Severe microcytic anaemia

Table 14.4 Classification of thalassaemia

There are different types of normal haemoglobin (Hb):

- **Hb A (adult)** is the predominant Hb type (>95%) from 6 months of age. It contains two α- and two β-globin chains

- **Hb F (fetal)** is found in the fetus. It contains two α- and 2 γ-globin chains, and has a higher affinity for oxygen than Hb A. The transition to Hb A starts from birth, but around 1% of Hb in adults is still fetal

- **Hb A2 (minor adult)** contains two α- and two δ-globin chains. It makes up 2–3% of Hb in both fetal and adult life

Diagnostic approach

There is a microcytic hypochromic anaemia and increased reticulocyte count. Target cells are present; these are red cells with characteristic central staining making them resemble targets. Electrophoresis allows identification of different haemoglobin types, such as increased levels of haemoglobin F and haemoglobin A2, and low levels of haemoglobin A.

Management

Milder forms of thalassaemia do not require treatment. Patients with β-thalassaemia major or the Hb H type of α-thalassaemia require regular blood transfusions, with iron chelation to prevent complications from iron toxicity. Prognosis depends on the type of thalassaemia. Death in β-thalassaemia major occurs in the thirties, usually secondary to heart failure.

Hereditary spherocytosis

Hereditary spherocytosis is a genetic condition that causes defects in red blood cell membrane proteins, most commonly spectrin and ankyrin, thereby giving rise to red blood cells with an abnormal spherical shape (spherocytes). The abnormal shape is less flexible leading to the spherocytes becoming lodged in and destroyed by the spleen.

The condition is inherited in an autosomal dominant manner. It is common in European populations, and affects 200 per million of the Northern European population.

The clinical features occur secondary to haemolysis and include anaemia, jaundice and abdominal pain secondary to gallstones (which form due to build up of bilirubin). Neonates may develop severe jaundice. Splenomegaly may also be present. An aplastic crisis (resulting in temporary failure of the bone marrow to produce new red cells) can occur with parvovirus B12 infection.

After splenectomy, children are at risk of serious infection with encapsulated organisms. To avoid these infections, they are vaccinated against *Pneumococcus* and take long-term prophylactic penicillin.

Hereditary spherocytosis is suspected in the presence of anaemia with spherocytes on blood film (**Figure 14.4**), a high reticulocyte count and other evidence of haemolysis (**Table 14.5**). Diagnosis can be made clinically with a positive family history.

Folic acid supplementation is required to support increased erythropoiesis. Splenectomy is required when the condition is severe. Babies with severe haemolysis may require a blood transfusion.

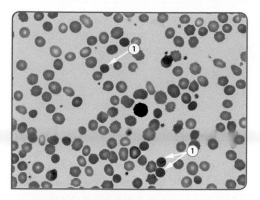

Figure 14.4 Spherocytes on a blood film, as seen in hereditary spherocytosis.

Haemolysis: investigation findings	
Test	Findings
Full blood count	Anaemia
	High reticulocyte count
Blood film	Fragmented red blood cells
	Spherocytes
	Nucleated red blood cell
Others	Unconjugated hyperbilirubinaemia
	Increased lactate dehydrogenase
	Reduced or absent haptoglobin (a protein that binds haemoglobin)

Table 14.5 Investigation findings providing evidence of haemolysis

Glucose 6-phosphate dehydrogenase deficiency

This is a genetic blood disorder character-ised by the deficiency of glucose 6-phosphate dehydrogenase, an enzyme involved in red blood cell metabolism, particularly the path-way which protects the cell from oxidative damage. This increased susceptibility to oxi-dative stresses leads to haemolysis in older red blood cells.

Glucose 6-phosphate dehydrogenase de-ficiency is inherited in an X-linked recessive manner. It commonly affects individuals of Mediterranean and Asian origin.

Clinical features

Patients are usually male and are often asymptomatic. The frequency of neonatal jaundice is higher than in the general popu-lation, although the reason for this is poorly understood because it is not always secondary to an acute episode of haemolysis. Symptoms develop as a consequence of haemolysis (**Table 14.6**), which is usually acute, but is chronic in rare cases. Typical precipitants of acute haemolysis include:

■ infection

Signs and symptoms of haemolysis	
Consequence of	Signs and symptoms
Anaemia	Pallor
	Fatigue or weakness
	Breathlessness
	Tachycardia
Excess bilirubin	Jaundice
	Gallstones
	Dark urine

Table 14.6 Signs and symptoms of haemolysis. These occur either as a consequence of the resulting anaemia or the breakdown products of haemolysis, such as bilirubin. Splenomegaly is present if the haemolysis is extravascular

■ use of certain drugs, e.g. antimalarial agents and sulfonamides
■ consumption of broad beans (also known as fava beans), in which case the acute haemolysis is known as favism

During a haemolytic crisis, the patient may have symptoms of anaemia, be visibly jaun-diced and have splenomegaly.

Diagnostic approach

The blood count is usually normal in asymptomatic individuals. However, during an acute crisis there is anaemia with other evidence of haemolysis (see **Table 14.5**). Heinz bodies, i.e. denatured haemoglobin cells, are also present on blood film.

G6PD deficiency is a non-immune haemolytic process, so the direct antiglobulin test (Coombs test) result is negative. The finding of reduced activity of the glucose 6-phosphate dehydrogenase enzyme after recovery from haemolysis confirms the diagnosis (there may be a false negative result if performed during an episode of acute haemolysis).

Management

Most individuals have normal life expectancy and need only to avoid precipitants of acute haemolysis. In severe haemolysis, blood transfusion may be needed. Neonatal jaundice usually requires phototherapy. A small proportion of individuals develop chronic haemolysis, which requires folic acid supplementation.

Bleeding disorders

A bleeding disorder results in excessive bleeding. Underlying causes are:

- a coagulation factor deficiency or defect at any step of the coagulation pathway
- a platelet problem
  - thrombocytopenia (low platelets) (see **Table 14.7** for causes)
  - a platelet function defect, with normal platelet count (rarely), for example in Bernard-Soulier syndrome
- defective blood vessels, for example in Ehlers-Danlos syndrome, in which a collagen defect leads to vascular fragility

Immune thrombocytopenia

Immune thrombocytopenia, formerly known as idiopathic thrombocytopenic purpura, is an autoimmune disease in which antibodies attach to antigens on the surface of platelets, causing the platelets to be ingested by macrophages as they pass through the spleen. It results in thrombocytopenia (platelet count < 150,000/mL). In children, there is often a preceding viral illness.

The condition occurs in about 3–5 out of 100,000 children; it can present at any age, but most commonly occurs between 2 and 5 years.

Clinical features

The clinical features of immune thrombocytopenia, which include easy bruising and petechiae, are a result of the low level of platelets. There may be spontaneous nose bleeds or prolonged bleeding after sustaining a cut. There is a risk of intracranial bleed

Thrombocytopenia: causes		
Increased destruction of platelets	Decreased production of platelets	
	Congenital	Acquired
Immune thrombocytopenia (formerly known as idiopathic thrombocytopenic purpura)	TAR syndrome	TORCH infections
Thrombotic thrombocytopenic purpura	Bernard–Soulier syndrome	Malignancies affecting the blood (see page 386)
Disseminated intravascular coagulation	Wiskott–Aldrich syndrome	Chemotherapy drugs
Haemolytic uraemic syndrome		
Neonatal alloimmune thrombocytopenia		

TAR, Thrombocytopenia–Absent Radius; TORCH, Toxoplasmosis, Other (varicella-zoster virus, syphilis and parvovirus), Rubella, Cytomegalovirus and Herpes.

Table 14.7 Causes of thrombocytopenia

as a result of head trauma. A small proportion of patients are asymptomatic.

Diagnostic approach

Diagnosis is confirmed by the finding of isolated thrombocytopenia on the full blood count. A blood film is required to ensure that there is no evidence of haemolysis, or other abnormal cells which would suggest a malignancy affecting the blood.

Management

Most children with immune thrombocytopenia do not require treatment; the condition resolves spontaneously after 3–6 months, but patients are advised to avoid contact sport or situations which may lead to trauma. Platelet transfusions are unhelpful, because transfused platelets are destroyed by the spleen. However, if there is significant bleeding, intravenous immunoglobulin rapidly increases the platelet count. Chronic immune thrombocytopenia is diagnosed when the condition lasts > 1 year.

Haemophilia A

Haemophilia A is a genetic disorder inherited in an X-linked recessive manner. It affects 1 in 5000 male births. It results in low levels of the clotting factor factor VIII, and consequently the patient is at increased risk of prolonged bleeding.

Clinical features

Haemophilia A may have been diagnosed through prenatal testing or genetic testing at birth in children with a family history of haemophilia. However, up to a third of those diagnosed arise from spontaneous mutations. The clinical features and age at presentation depend on the disease severity, which is determined by factor VIII activity (**Table 14.8**). Haemarthrosis (bleeding into a joint space) can result in joint damage, leading to arthritis.

Diagnostic approach

The diagnosis of haemophilia A is suspected when activated partial thromboplastin time (APTT) is prolonged. A low level of factor VIII, along with genetic testing, confirms the diagnosis.

Management

Management depends on the severity of the condition.

- Children with severe haemophilia receive prophylactic factor VIII infusions; if an acute bleed occurs, factor VIII is administered and advice sought from the consultant haematologist
- For children with mild and moderate disease, desmopressin can be administered to boost factor VIII levels, for example before surgical or dental procedures

Haemophilia: classification of severity			
Severity	Activity of factor VIII (%)	Age at presentation	Common presenting symptoms
Mild	5–40	Any age, including adulthood	Excessive bleeding after surgery (e.g. tooth extraction)
Moderate	1–5	Usually by 2 years	Bleeding after minor trauma, e.g. venepuncture
Severe	< 1	Neonatal period or within 1st year	Spontaneous bleeding at any site and especially once the child is mobile (e.g. site of attachment to umbilical cord, joints, intracranial haemorrhage)

Table 14.8 Classification of the severity of haemophilia

Von Willebrand's disease: classification			
Type	Inheritance pattern	Type of defect	Clinical feature
1	Autosomal dominant	Quantitative	Asymptomatic Epistaxis Menorrhagia
2	Autosomal dominant	Qualitative	Bleeding of variable severity
3	Autosomal recessive	Quantitative Very low levels	Severe bleeding

Table 14.9 Classification of von Willebrand's disease. Type 2 has multiple subtypes. About 75% of cases are type 1

In addition, children with haemophilia A must avoid contact sports. With appropriate treatment, prognosis is generally good.

Haemophilia B

Haemophilia B, sometimes called Christmas disease, is an X-linked recessive disorder that results in deficiency of factor IX. It is less common than haemophilia A, affecting 1 in 30,000 males. Severity varies, and patients present similarly to patients with haemophilia A. Treatment is with factor IX concentrate.

Von Willebrand's disease

Von Willebrand's disease is a genetic disorder of the von Willebrand clotting factor, a protein with a role in platelet adhesion and stabilisation of factor VIII. Von Willebrand's disease is inherited in an autosomal dominant manner. It is the most prevalent coagulation defect, detectable in 1% of the population, but only a small number of people are symptomatic.

In von Willebrand's disease, either there are low levels of von Willebrand factor, or there are normal levels but the factor is defective. There are several different types of von Willebrand's disease, which are associated with different features (**Table 14.9**).

Coagulation studies (see page 100) show a prolonged bleeding time. APTT may also be prolonged. These findings prompt measurement of von Willebrand factor antigen in plasma, von Willebrand factor activity and factor VIII activity.

Management depends on the severity of the bleeding. Desmopressin and factor VIII (which also contains VWF) concentrate are administered in severe haemorrhages.

Answers to starter questions

1. Repeated blood transfusions increase the level of iron in the body. It deposits in organs, such as the liver and heart, causing them to fail. Chelation therapy prevents this by binding to iron in the blood.

2. Reduced platelet counts are seen in immune thrombocytopaenia. Platelet transfusions are rarely given because the spleen rapidly destroys the transfused platelets, drastically reducing the effectiveness of the transfusion.

Chapter 15
Childhood cancer

Starter questions

Answers to the following questions are on page 396.

1. Why do children with brain tumours often have restricted growth?
2. How does taking a photograph with a flash help with diagnosing a tumour in childhood?

Introduction

Childhood cancer is an emotive area of clinical practice; the diagnosis is devastating for the families affected. Treatment regimens are gruelling, and it is distressing for parents to watch their child experience unpleasant adverse effects, such as those associated with chemotherapy. Families also have to cope with uncertainty regarding the outcome and late effects of treatment. Cancer treatment often interrupts the child's schooling and interferes with friendships. Usually the child begins treatment in a tertiary centre, often far from home. Being away from family and friends, and the support they offer, makes a difficult time even harder. Most childhood cancers respond well to treatment; just over 80% of affected children are alive more than 5 years after diagnosis.

The relative incidence of cancers in childhood is shown in **Figure 15.1**. Some conditions, primarily genetic or previous treatments for cancer are associated with certain cancers (**Table 15.1**). Children with some of these conditions have screening for the malignancies during childhood, for example in hemihyperplasia the child will have 3–6 monthly abdominal US scans until they are 7 years old (when the risk of nephroblastoma developing becomes minimal). In other conditions awareness of the possibility of malignancy will prompt early investigation of non-specific symptoms.

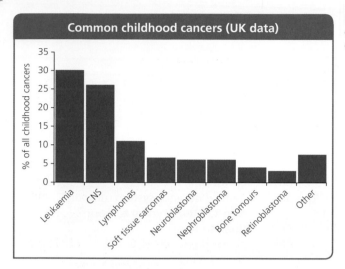

Figure 15.1 The relative incidence of the most common childhood cancers (UK data).

Conditions associated with malignancy		
Group	**Condition(s)**	**Malignancy**
Neurocutaneous syndromes	Neurofibromatosis	Brain tumours
		Neurofibrosarcomas
Hereditary cutaneous syndromes	Xeroderma pigmentosa	Malignant melanoma
		Squamous cell carcinoma
Chromosomal abnormalities	Down's syndrome	Acute leukaemia (myeloid and lymphoblastic)
Hereditary or acquired immunodeficiency	Ataxia telangiectasia	Leukaemia
		Lymphoma
Syndromes	Hemihyperplasia (formerly known as hemihypertrophy) including Beckwith-Wiedemann syndrome	Nephroblastoma
		Hepatoblastoma
Metabolic diseases	Alpha-1 antitrypsin deficiency	Hepatocellular carcinoma
Previous cancer treatment		Bone marrow malignancies, brain tumours

Table 15.1 Conditions associated with increased risk of malignancy

Case 21 Bruising in a 3-year-old

Presentation

Amelia, aged 3 years, has been brought to see her general practitioner (GP) by her mother, who is concerned that Amelia has been bruising easily after trivial bumps over the past few weeks.

Initial interpretation

There are many reasons why a child may appear to bruise easily. At this age, the most likely causes are accidental injury on playing, non-accidental injury or a problem with platelets or coagulation factors.

Case 21 *continued*

Further history

On further questioning, the GP ascertains that Amelia has recently been unwell with a viral infection, but her mother feels that she is over this now. Amelia has had some bleeding from her gums while cleaning her teeth, but her mother put this down to brushing too hard. There is no family history of bleeding problems.

Amelia's mother said that a family member who had not seen Amelia for a while commented that she was looking pale. She has lost a little weight recently, but her mother attributes this to the viral illness. Bruising could suggest that there is a child protection issue. However, the medical records indicate that the family are not known to social services, and there have not been any previous concerns.

Examination

Amelia appears pale. Examination finds several large bruises over bony prominences, including the knees and elbows. A 2-cm liver edge and 3-cm spleen are palpable, i.e. there is hepatosplenomegaly (enlargement of both organs). Blood pressure is normal, but on removing the cuff the GP notes some petechial spots at the site of application.

Interpretation of findings

Non-accidental injury is unlikely in this case with no previous concerns, and the bruising is located in a typical area for bruising in active children. The history suggests pathology with Amelia feeling unwell and suffering bleeding of her gums.

Five steps to breaking bad news

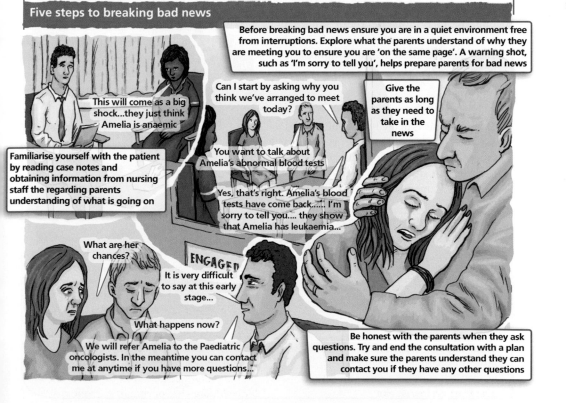

Case 21 continued

The rest of the examination with pallor and hepatosplenomegaly is concerning; at this age the liver and spleen would not normally be palpable, or occasionally with infections a spleen tip just palpable.

A new history of easy bruising in the absence of a family history of coagulation disorders suggests a diagnosis of thrombocytopenia in the first instance, particularly as applying pressure to the arm resulted in a petechial rash. However, although the history of viral infection could fit with a history of immune thrombocytopenia, the presence of hepatosplenomegaly goes against this diagnosis. This finding, in conjunction with the history of pallor and weight loss, is concerning, because they suggest malignancy affecting the blood.

Investigations

Results of the full blood count are shown in **Table 15.2**. In light of these abnormal results, a blood film is carried out, which confirms the presence of lymphoblasts (see **Figure 15.2a**).

Diagnosis

The diagnosis is acute lymphoblastic leukaemia, confirmed by the presence of lymphoblasts on the blood film along with the findings of associated anaemia and thrombocytopenia. Amelia's parents are given the difficult news. Amelia is transferred immediately to the local paediatric oncology unit for further work-up, including bone marrow biopsy, before starting chemotherapy once the results are available, i.e. within the next few days. The initial chemotherapy is to achieve bone marrow remission and will be followed by a consolidation and then maintenance phase for 2–3 years. Her prognosis at this age is good with a 5-year survival rate around 90%.

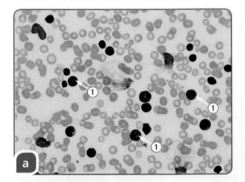

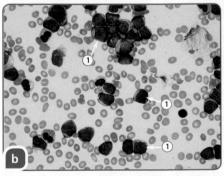

Figure 15.2 Blood films in different types of acute leukaemia. (a) Lymphoblasts ① in acute lymphoblastic leukaemia. (b) Myeloblasts ① in acute myeloid leukaemia. Compared with lymphoblasts, myeloblasts tend to have more cytoplasm, finer chromatin and more prominent nucleoli. They also often contain cytoplasmic granules and/or Auer rods.

Blood counts		
Count	Result	Reference range
Haemoglobin (g/L)	78	100–130
White blood cells (x 10⁹/L)	22.8	4–11
Platelet count (x 10⁹/L)	6	150–400

Table 15.2 Typical blood counts for a child with acute lymphoblastic leukaemia

Case 22 Abdominal pain and a mass in a 3-year-old

Presentation

Miles, who is 3 years old, is taken to see the GP by his father, who is concerned that Miles has been complaining of abdominal pain for 2 weeks. He was seen by a locum GP 10 days ago, who diagnosed mesenteric adenitis. Miles's father remains concerned and now tells the GP that Miles's tummy has become swollen.

Initial interpretation

In the presence of a viral illness, mesenteric adenitis is a reasonable initial diagnosis. However, it is unusual for mesenteric adenitis to continue to cause pain for this duration, because it normally settles once the acute illness is over.

Constipation is common in children of Miles's age and causes abdominal pain and distension. However, abdominal distension is an unusual presenting feature in children and requires investigation.

Further history

His father feels that Miles has not been himself for a few weeks. He seems to have less energy and is not eating as much as normal. Miles is opening his bowels daily, and the stool is soft. The abdominal pain is intermittent. Miles's father became aware of the abdominal swelling when Miles's T-shirts started to look tight over his belly.

Examination

Miles appears pale. His weight and height are both on the 50th centile. His personal child health record has not been brought to the consultation, so comparison with previous centiles is not possible. Miles's abdomen appears distended but is soft on palpation, with some central tenderness. A large smooth, hard mass is palpable in the right loin area; it does not cross the midline. Dipstick urinalysis is positive for blood.

Interpretation of findings

Children often present with non-specific features, such as lethargy and poor appetite. These are usually caused by a viral illness; however, in rare instances they are the presentation of more serious pathology. It is essential to plot the child's current weight and compare the centile with previous records to identify any weight loss.

Abdominal distension can be a sign of constipation, and associated masses may also be palpated. However, in constipation the mass is normally soft and in the left iliac fossa.

A hard mass in the loin area, combined with a history of non-specific symptoms and abdominal distension, should always prompt consideration of malignancy. Palpable abdominal malignancies include nephroblastoma (Wilms' tumour) and neuroblastoma. To aid differentiation, generally a nephroblastoma does not cross the midline. Haematuria can also be present in nephroblastoma.

Investigations

Miles undergoes an urgent abdominal US scan. This shows a mass in the right kidney.

Diagnosis

The impression from the US scan is that Miles has a nephroblastoma. He is referred to the paediatric oncologists, who arrange a CT scan to evaluate the tumour in further detail before discussion of the findings at a multidisciplinary meeting to decide the best course of treatment. This usually involves nephrectomy followed by chemotherapy, with or without postoperative radiotherapy. He will have a 5-year survival rate of around 90–95%, depending on the histology staging.

Leukaemia

Leukaemia is a malignant disease of the bone marrow. It is the commonest type of cancer diagnosed in childhood, responsible for one quarter of all childhood cancers worldwide.

Bone marrow contains stem cells that develop into either myeloid or lymphoid cells, which further differentiate into the various types of blood cell. These cells mature in the bone marrow before being released into the bloodstream. In leukaemia there is arrest at an early stage of hematopoietic cell development in the bone marrow and therefore early lymphoid precursors (blasts), of either the lymphoid (lymphoblasts) or myeloid (myeloblasts) lineage, proliferate, replacing the normal marrow cells and so resulting in decreased production of normal blood cells.

The symptoms and average age at presentation depend on the type of leukaemia.

> 'Acute' leukaemias develop and progress rapidly, whereas 'chronic' leukaemia has a more insidious course and may be asymptomatic for a few years.

Acute lymphoblastic leukaemia

Acute lymphoblastic leukaemia is caused by abnormal proliferation of immature lymphocytes, usually B cells, called lymphoblasts. It is the commonest type of leukaemia diagnosed in children, accounting for almost 80% of childhood cases worldwide. Acute lymphoblastic leukaemia is much more common in children than in adults: 55% of patients are children. Incidence peaks at 2–3 years of age and declines thereafter.

Aetiology

The underlying cause of acute lymphoblastic leukaemia is unclear, but it is thought to result from a combination of factors, including a genetic element. Children with certain genetic disorders, such as Down's syndrome, are at a significantly higher risk of developing acute lymphoblastic leukaemia.

Clinical features

Early symptoms of leukaemia are usually non-specific. Table 15.3 lists the most common clinical features. Bone pain may manifest as an unexplained limp in a young child. Hepatosplenomegaly may be found on examination. Headaches, cranial nerve abnormalities and neck stiffness may indicate central nervous system (CNS) involvement.

> Leukaemias usually present with non-specific symptoms. These are often caused by deficiencies in other blood cell lines rather than the presence of the leukaemic cells themselves.

Diagnostic approach

Acute lymphoblastic leukaemia is initially suspected on the results of a full blood count and peripheral blood film, although these can be normal in the early stages of the disease. Typically, there is evidence of anaemia, thrombocytopenia and lymphocytosis, but the white blood cell count can also be normal or low. Lymphoblasts are usually seen on peripheral blood film (Figure 15.3a).

A bone marrow biopsy showing lymphoblasts confirms the diagnosis. A lumbar puncture determines whether or not leukaemic cells have invaded the CNS.

Leukaemia: clinical features	
Feature	Cause
Easy bruising	Thrombocytopenia
Easy bleeding (e.g. bleeding gums when brushing teeth)	Thrombocytopenia
Lethargy	Anaemia
Frequent infections, often of a serious nature	Abnormal or dysfunctional white blood cells
Lymphadenopathy (e.g. large nodes in neck and/ or groin)	Accumulation of leukaemic cells in lymph nodes
Bone pain, especially in long bones	Leukaemic infiltration of periosteum

Table 15.3 Clinical features of leukaemia

Management

Acute lymphoblastic leukaemia is treated with chemotherapy. Chemotherapy has several phases.

- The induction phase achieves bone marrow remission, i.e. normal blood count results and no lymphoblasts visible on microscopy of bone marrow, although there may be minimal residual disease
- The consolidation phase lasts for several months; in this phase, the aim is to eliminate all leukaemic cells
- The maintenance phase lasts up to 3 years; the aim is to prevent recurrence after remission

During treatment, there is also a focus on CNS prophylaxis, i.e. prevention of the spread of leukaemia to the CNS in high risk cases or treatment for confirmed CNS disease. Cranial irradiation has a risk of subsequent neurotoxicity and brain tumours. Therefore such radiotherapy has been replaced with intensive intrathecal and systemic chemotherapy unless there is CNS disease with a very high lymphoblast count (>5/mL) in the CSF, or clinical signs of CNS involvement such as facial nerve palsy.

Relapse (lymphoblasts reappearing after complete remission) occurs in 20%, and while they often go into remission again with repeated chemotherapy, some will subsequently require a stem cell (bone marrow) transplant.

> Because of its irritant nature especially with extravasation (leakage to the surrounding tissues) and prolonged course, chemotherapy has to be administered via large veins. A central venous catheter (Hickman line, **Figure 15.3**) is sited in a child who is due to start chemotherapy. Blood can also be taken from this line, which prevents the need to subject the child to frequent venepuncture.

Prognosis

In acute lymphoblastic leukaemia in children, prognosis is good, with a 5-year survival rate of 80–90%.

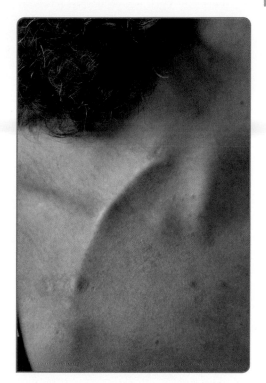

Figure 15.3 A Hickman line, used to administer chemotherapy.

Acute myeloid leukaemia

Acute myeloid leukaemia results from abnormal proliferation of myeloblasts, i.e. a cancer of the myeloid line of blood cells. These abnormal cells egress into the circulating blood to infiltrate other organs. It is the second most common leukaemia diagnosed in children, accounting for 15% of cases. Incidence is highest in children under the age of 1 year.

Aetiology

The trigger for acute myeloid leukaemia is unknown. However, the risk of developing it is increased in children with certain genetic conditions, such as Down's syndrome (see **Table 15.1**). Other risk factors include previous exposure to radiation.

Clinical features

As in other leukaemias, many symptoms of acute myeloid leukaemia occur secondary to deficiencies of blood cells other than the leu-kaemic cells (see **Table 15.3**). Bone pain and lymphadenopathy are less common than in acute lymphoblastic leukaemia, but organo-megaly and haemorrhage or disseminated intravascular coagulation, are more com-mon. In addition, the proliferation and infil-tration includes formation of mediastinal masses (which cause respiratory distress or superior vena cava syndrome) and abdomi-nal masses (which cause pain or obstruc-tion of gastrointestinal or urogenital tracts). Swollen and bleeding gums are also com-mon at presentation.

Diagnosis

As in acute myeloid leukaemia, a full blood count raises the initial suspicion. It shows a normocytic anaemia, with lower than expected reticulocyte count, and thrombo-cytopenia with a variable white blood cell count, although it is not unusual for this to be extremely high in acute myeloid leukae-mia, while the neutrophil count remains low. Myeloblasts are usually seen on the periph-eral blood film which may containe Auer rods (thin, needle-shaped, eosinophilic cytoplas-mic inclusions) (**Figure 15.2b**). Diagnosis is confirmed by bone marrow biopsy.

Management

Acute myeloid leukaemia is treated with inten-sive induction chemotherapy followed by con-solidation chemotherapy and bone marrow transplantation, if a match is available.

The 5-year survival rate for acute myeloid leukaemia is less than that for acute lympho-blastic leukaemia, at about 60%.

> **Children with Down's syndrome are at higher risk of developing acute myeloid leukaemia**. However, they have a higher survival rate than other children who develop myeloid leukaemia (80–100%).

Chronic myeloid leukaemia

Chronic myeloid leukaemia is caused by unregulated production of myeloid cells in the bone marrow, causing an excess of granulocytes, usually neutrophils. It is rare in children, accounting for only 5% of leukae-mias. Incidence peaks in children younger than 1 year of age and in teenagers.

The condition has an initial 'chronic' phase in which blood abnormalities are present but the patient is usually asymptomatic. When symptoms develop, in most cases they are non-specific, including tiredness and malaise. There follows an 'accelerated' phase, in which there is an increased number of myeloblasts in the blood, and a 'blast' phase, which can re-semble acute leukaemia.

Full blood count shows high counts of granulocytes at various stages of maturation, with normocytic anaemia and high or normal platelet count. Chemotherapy can control the disease, but the only curative option is stem cell transplantation.

Lymphoma

Lymphoma is a cancer of the lymphatic sys-tem in which there is malignant proliferation of cells derived from B or T cells. The malig-nant cells accumulate in the lymphatic system and lymph nodes, resulting in solid tumours. Lymphomas account for 11% of childhood cancers. The male to female ratio of those affected is 2:1. The two main types of lympho-ma, Hodgkin's lymphoma and non-Hodgkin's lymphoma, require different treatments.

Hodgkin's lymphoma

In Hodgkin's lymphoma, the typical malig-nant cell is the Reed-Sternberg cell. Reed-Sternberg cells are giant, multinucleated cells, usually derived from B cells. Hodgkin lymphoma is classified into five histological types: nodular sclerosing, mixed cellularity, lymphocyte depleted, lymphocyte rich, and nodular lymphocyte-predominant.

Hodgkin's lymphoma accounts for 45% of cases of lymphoma in childhood. It is rare before the age of 2 years, but incidence steadily increases until the teenage years, when there is a sharp rise. The cause of the malignant proliferation is unknown, but the Epstein–Barr virus has been linked with Hodgkin's lymphoma.

> With modern advances in cancer management, mortality from Hodgkin's lymphoma is higher from the later effects of treatment such as fibrotic lung disease, congestive heart failure and neuropathy from chemotherapy and secondary cancers in the radiation fields, than from the disease itself. Therefore the intensity of the treatment must be tailored to the histological classification and stage of the disease.

Clinical features

The commonest feature of Hodgkin's lymphoma is the presence of painless lymphadenopathy, which may be present for several months. Typically, the lymphadenopathy is above the clavicle, but it can be present anywhere along the lymphatic system. Systemic features include unexplained weight loss, fever and night sweats. Mediastinal lymphadenopathy or masses are common and may cause dyspnoea, cough or stridor.

Diagnostic approach

The diagnosis of Hodgkin's lymphoma is confirmed by the presence of Reed-Sternberg cells on lymph node biopsy. After diagnosis, CT and positron emission tomography (PET) scans, and in some children bone marrow biopsy, are required for staging the lymphoma (**Table 15.4**) and planning management.

Management

The exact management of Hodgkin's lymphoma depends on the stage of the lymphoma, but in all cases consists of a combination of chemotherapy and radiotherapy.

Hodgkin's lymphoma responds well to treatment and 5-year survival rates are as high as 95%.

Non-Hodgkin's lymphoma

Non-Hodgkin's lymphoma encompasses all lymphomas that are not Hodgkin's lymphoma. The commonest types are:

- mature B-cell lymphoma, including Burkitt's lymphoma and diffuse large B-cell lymphoma; the malignant cells are derived from B cells
- lymphoblastic lymphoma, which is similar to acute lymphoblastic leukaemia; the malignant cells are derived from T cells
- anaplastic large cell lymphoma, in which the malignant cells have a loss of distinctive cell features, but have membrane expression of the CD30 antigen which is an activation marker for B and T cells

Lymphomas are further classified into groups based on the clinical behaviour (low-grade, intermediate-grade and high-grade) depending on their speed of evolution and the severity of symptoms. As a group, non-Hodgkin's lymphoma accounts for just over half of all diagnosis of lymphoma in children. The exact cause of non-Hodgkin's lymphoma

Lymphoma staging			
Stage 1	**Stage 2**	**Stage 3**	**Stage 4**
One group of affected lymph nodes	Two or more groups of affected lymph nodes	Multiple lymph node groups	Multiple extranodal sites or lymph nodes and extranodal disease
Affected lymph nodes on one side of diaphragm	Affected lymph nodes on one side of diaphragm	Affected lymph nodes above and below diaphragm	Extra nodal disease e.g. spread to bone marrow or lungs

Table 15.4 Staging of lymphomas

is unknown, but risk factors include immunodeficiency and treatment for previous malignancy. Epstein–Barr virus is also implicated in Burkitt's lymphoma.

The incidence of non-Hodgkin's lymphoma increases sharply between the ages of 1 and 3 years, and increases gradually with age. Non-Hodgkin's lymphoma is more likely than Hodgkin's lymphoma to spread to extranodal sites, and children tend to have more aggressive forms of the disease.

> **Superior vena cava syndrome occurs when a person's superior vena cava is partially blocked or compressed, usually by a tumour.** Signs and symptoms are facial and arm oedema, dyspnoea and cough, dysphagia, stridor and congestion of the collateral veins of the anterior chest wall.

Clinical features

Signs and symptoms depend on the type of non-Hodgkin's lymphoma and the grade, which includes the rate of tumour growth, function of the organ being compromised or displaced by the lymphoma and systemic symptoms. Children generally present with enlarging, non-tender lymphadenopathy or with symptoms of compression from a mass. Symptoms of compression include:

- respiratory symptoms, such as dyspnoea due to pleural effusion or superior vena cava (SVC) syndrome, for a mass in the chest
- abdominal pain, constipation or, rarely, intestinal or urinary obstruction for a mass in the abdomen

There may be hepatosplenomegaly in up to 40% of cases at presentation. Less commonly, systemic symptoms, such as fever, weight loss, night sweats and lethargy, are present. These are called B symptoms and are more likely to occur with moderate or high grade lymphomas.

Diagnostic approach

The diagnosis is confirmed by biopsy of any mass or enlarged lymph nodes. Further cytogenetic analysis of the sample helps to identify the subtype. Once diagnosis is confirmed, a bone marrow biopsy is carried out to exclude leukaemia and assist with staging, in addition to the results of imaging with CT and PET scans.

Management

Specific management depends on the subtype, but combination chemotherapy is the standard method of treatment. Lymphoblastic lymphoma is closely related to acute lymphoblastic leukaemia, so they are treated in a very similar way.

Prognosis is good. The overall 5-year survival rate for children diagnosed with non-Hodgkin's lymphoma is about 85%.

Central nervous system tumours

Childhood central nervous system (CNS) tumours are the second most common cancer in childhood, accounting for just over 25% of all cancer diagnosed. They are almost always primary rather than metastatic from distant cancers. In children about 60% arise in the cerebellum, also referred to as infratentorial as they are below the tentorium cerebelli. The 30–40% of tumours that are in the cerebrum are referred to as supratentorial (above the tentorium cerebelli).

Some tumours occasionally originate in the spine, e.g astrocytomas, whereas others, such as medulloblastoma arise in the brain (cerebellum) but seed via cerebrospinal fluid throughout the CNS (20% of medulloblastomas have spinal metastases at diagnosis).

The incidence rate of primary CNS tumours is 3.6 cases per 100,000 children each year worldwide, and they are the main cause of deaths from childhood cancer. A few inherited conditions such as neurofibromatosis and tuberous sclerosis are associated with CNS tumours.

> **Brain tumours in children can be malignant or benign,** with 'low grade', i.e. slow-growing, tumours considered benign. However, even benign tumours can cause significant morbidity and mortality if they occur in certain areas such as the brain stem, which is responsible for basic vital life functions (breathing, heartbeat, and blood pressure) or some areas of the cortex which result in seizures

Types

Tumours of the CNS are classified according to their origin:

- Gliomas arise from glial cells in the brain or spinal cord
- Embryonal tumours are neural crest tumours that originate from neuroectoderm, which is normally present only in the embryo (see pages 4 and 8)
- Craniopharyngiomas are epithelial tumours that arise from remnants of Rathke's pouch, an embryological structure that forms the anterior pituitary

Gliomas

These tumours are categorised according to the specific type of glial cell from which they originate:

- astrocytomas originate from astrocytes
- ependymomas originate from the ependymal cells lining the ventricles of the brain and the central canal of the spinal cord
- oligodendrogliomas originate from oligodendrocytes

Astrocytomas are the largest subgroup of gliomas. They account for almost 45% of all CNS tumours. Most astrocytomas (75%) are low grade, meaning they are slow growing. Astrocytomas can be diagnosed at any time during childhood, with no preponderance for age or gender. Prognosis is good: 80% of patients are alive 5 years after diagnosis.

Ependymomas account for 10% of all CNS tumours. Peak incidence is at 1 year of age. Two thirds of patients with ependymoma are alive at 5 years.

Oligodendroglioma is mainly encountered in adults.

Embryonal tumours

These tumours account for 20% of CNS tumours. They are known as primitive neuroectoderm tumours and named according to their location. They are fast growing.

Most embryonal tumours are medulloblastomas which form in brain cells in the cerebellum (infratentorial). The incidence is up to 0.45 cases per 100,000 children per year. Other CNS primitive neuroectodermal tumours (PNETs) are rare and usually form in the cerebrum (supratentorial) but they may also form in the brain stem or spinal cord. There are four types of CNS PNETs: ganglioneuroblastomas, neuroblastomas, medulloepitheliomas and ependymoblastomas.

Primitive neuroectoderm tumours affect individuals of all ages, but their incidence decreases with age. Prognosis is poor in comparison with other CNS tumours: only 56% of patients are alive at 5 years.

Craniopharyngiomas

These account for 6-10% of brain tumours in children. They arise most frequently in the pituitary stalk and project into the hypothalamus and press on the optic chiasm.

Therefore, patients often also present with visual and endocrine problems, because of the location of these tumours near the optic chiasm and pituitary gland, respectively.

These embryonal tumours are considered histologically benign, with a very good prognosis (5-year survival is up to 99% in children). However, they can cause long-term endocrine and visual morbidity.

Clinical features

Symptoms of brain tumours vary greatly, depending on their size and location, and can be caused by increased intracranial pressure, due to the size of the mass or obstruction of CSF flow, or the effect of the mass pressing on local structures (**Table 15.5**). Spinal tumours present with back pain, peripheral weakness of arms or legs or bladder/bowel dysfunction, depending on the level of the lesion.

Clinical examination often finds papilloedema, reflecting an increase in intracranial pressure. Other common signs of brainstem and cerebellar tumours are cranial nerve palsies, ataxia, incoordination or nystagmus, whilst supratentorial tumours often produce focal or generalized neurological motor signs. Most children with craniopharyngioma present with growth failure and delayed puberty due to the endocrine effects of pituitary involvement and in addition to papilloedema there is often loss of visual acuity, constriction of visual fields or horizontal double vision.

> **Symptoms of brain tumours are usually insidious. The median time from the first symptoms to diagnosis of a brain tumour in children is 3.3 months.** Headache is the most common first symptom (40% of cases), but by diagnosis patients have a median of six signs or symptoms.

> **Although up to 70% of children with craniopharyngioma have visual disturbances on examination at presentation only 20–30% of children are aware of their visual problems.** The usual presenting features being growth failure and delayed puberty, headache and vomiting.

Brain tumours in children: symptoms	
Age < 5 years	Age > 5 years
Vomiting	Vomiting
Headache (more likely to present as irritability, because young children have difficulty localising pain)	Headache (persistent or recurrent, and worse on waking)
Abnormal gait, balance and/or coordination	Abnormal gait, balance and/or coordination
Behavioural change	Personality change
Lethargy	Lethargy
Afebrile seizures	Seizure
Abnormal eye movement or squint	Abnormal eye movement or squint
Increasing head circumference (age < 18 months)	Blurred or double vision
Developmental delay	Deterioration in schoolwork

Table 15.5 Symptoms associated with brain tumours in children

Management

Management of brain tumours in children depends on the type and location of the tumour, but the standard treatment is surgical removal. If surgery is not practical due to its location near vital centres such as the brain stem, or if the entire tumour cannot be removed, chemotherapy or radiotherapy is required. Radiotherapy is avoided in children under 3 years old, because it can damage the developing brain.

Possible complications include cognitive or endocrine problems secondary to the effects of radiotherapy on the pituitary gland.

Non-CNS embryonal tumours

Embryonal tumours are the result of malignant proliferation of tissue normally present only in the developing embryo. In addition to the primitive neuroectoderm tumours affecting the CNS, discussed in the previous section, they include:

- neuroblastoma
- retinoblastoma
- nephroblastoma (Wilms' tumour)
- rhabdomyoscarcoma

Neuroblastoma

A neuroblastoma is a tumour originating from the neural crest part of the sympathetic nervous system (neuroblasts). Neuroblastoma is rare in the general population (adults and children), but is the third most common childhood cancer and the commonest solid tumour (i.e. excluding leukaemia) in infancy (<1 year). Incidence is highest in the first year of life (40% of cases), and declines thereafter. In total it accounts for 8% of childhood cancers in developed countries. It is very rare in children older than 5 years.

Neuroblastomas occur anywhere in the sympathetic nervous system, but almost half are in the adrenal gland. Other common sites are the abdomen (25%) and chest (**Table 15.6**). By the time of diagnosis, 50% of cases have metastasised. The cause is unknown.

Clinical features

Features of neuroblastoma depend on the site affected. There are often non-specific features, such as lethargy, reduced appetite and weight loss. **Table 15.5** lists specific signs and symptoms. Some children may present with an incidental finding of an abdominal mass.

Diagnostic approach

Diagnosis of neuroblastoma requires histological confirmation from a tumour biopsy or examination of tumour cells from a bone marrow aspirate, in conjunction with the finding of increased urinary catecholamine metabolites (homovanillic acid [HVA] and vanillylmandelic acid [VMA]) due to defective catecholamine synthesis by the tumour. Scanning with the radioisotope metaiodobenzyl guanidine is a sensitive investigation for the detection of metastases; a technetium[99] bone scan evaluates bone metastases. CT and bone marrow aspiration to detect metastatic disease, assist with staging.

Management

Management of neuroblastoma depends on the risk category assigned to the individual case. Histology and molecular studies, such

Neuroblastoma: signs and symptoms	
Site affected	**Signs and symptoms**
Abdomen	Abdominal distension
	Constipation
	Abdominal pain
Thorax	Breathlessness
	Oculosympathetic palsy (Horner's syndrome)
	Signs of superior vena cava obstruction
Spinal cord	Leg weakness
	Loss of ability to walk or crawl
Orbital bone	Bruising around the eyes
Endocrine effects	Hypertension (from effects of catecholamines)
	Diarrhoea (from effects of vasoactive intestinal peptide)
Skin	'Blueberry muffin' appearance (purple or blue rash)
Eyes	Opsoclonus myoclonus (i.e. jerking of limbs and rapid eye movements)

Table 15.6 Signs and symptoms of neuroblastoma

as fluorescent in situ hybridization (FISH), on tissue samples from a biopsy or resection of the primary tumour, enable assignment of risk to each case. This is combined with the stage, which ranges from a local tumour not involving vital structures through to distant metastatic disease, to determine the intensity of the treatment.

- Low-risk group treatment strategy: surgical excision of tumour only. Some very low risk spontaneously regress and so may have observation only as initial management with no intervention
- Intermediate-risk group treatment strategy: surgery and multi-agent chemotherapy
- High-risk group treatment strategy: surgery, multi-agent chemotherapy and radiotherapy, followed by high-dose chemotherapy and peripheral blood stem cell rescue

The prognosis for neuroblastoma varies greatly. The overall childhood 5-year survival rate is about 70%, but this figure is much higher in children under 1 year of age (up to 95%) and much lower in adolescents.

Retinoblastoma

Retinoblastoma is an embryonal tumour of retinal cells. It accounts for 3% of all childhood tumours. In about 40% of cases, there is a genetic mutation at the *RB1* gene on chromosome 13, which may be sporadic or inherited. Only about 5% of cases have a positive family history. If the mutation is present, the tumour is more likely to be bilateral. Cases in which no *RB1* gene mutation is present are usually unilateral.

Average age at diagnosis is 18 months. Incidence decreases with age, and retinoblastoma is extremely rare in children older than 5 years.

Clinical features

Leukocoria (white pupil) is usually the first sign of retinoblastoma. It is often noted in flash photographs of the child (**Figure 15.4**) or during routine examination with an ophthalmoscope, with the finding of a white pupillary reflex rather than the normal red reflex.

> **A false positive leukocoria**, rather than the normal 'red eye', can be obtained with flash photography if the optic nerve is in the axis of the camera lens.

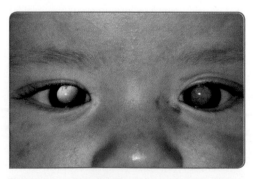

Figure 15.4 Bilateral leukocoria: a white pupillary reflex in a child with bilateral retinoblastoma. The reflex is less obvious in the left eye, because the tumour in the left eye is slightly off the photographic axis, so the reflex is not as white as it is on the right.

Another common presenting symptom is squint. If there is a known family history of retinoblastoma, the diagnosis may be made by routine screening, which should be carried out at regular intervals (every 3–4 months until age 4 years, and then 6 monthly until age 6 years and annually thereafter).

Diagnostic approach

Unlike many other cancers, a retinoblastoma is diagnosed on its clinical appearance, therefore examination under anaesthesia (due the young age and therefore lack of cooperation of the child) is carried out. Biopsy of tissue from the abnormal area is not required. Additional imaging, including US and MRI, may be required to stage the disease.

Management

The aim of management is to treat the tumour while preserving vision. Small tumours are treated with local therapy, such as cryotherapy or laser therapy. Local radiotherapy can also be applied to the eye. Larger tumours may necessitate removal of the eye itself or chemotherapy.

Prognosis is excellent, with a 5-year survival rate of 99%. However, some patients may have long-term problems with vision, especially when the condition is bilateral.

Nephroblastoma (Wilms' tumour)

Nephroblastomas are embryonal tumours of the kidney. They account for 90% of all renal tumours.

Although nephroblastoma is rare, it accounts for about 6% of all childhood cancers. Incidence peaks between 1 and 3 years of age, and 5% of cases are bilateral. Most cases are sporadic, but nephroblastoma can also be familial. About 10% of cases of nephroblastoma are associated with other syndromes such as Beckwith–Wiedemann syndrome and hemihyperplasia (see page 382):

Clinical features

Nephroblastoma usually presents with an asymptomatic abdominal mass, which is sometimes associated with abdominal pain. The abdomen may appear distended. Haematuria, fever or hypertension may also be present.

Diagnostic approach

The initial investigation in a child found on examination to have an abdominal mass is US, which identifies a renal tumour. Further imaging, for example with CT or MRI, is carried out to determine the stage of the disease. However, the conclusive diagnosis is reached only by histological examination after nephrectomy. Transcutaneous biopsy is not recommended, because it may cause the tumour to metastasise.

Regular abdominal US scans are used to screen children at high risk of developing nephroblastoma (see page 382).

Management

Nephrectomy is the first-line treatment in unilateral tumours, followed by chemotherapy. In children with bilateral tumours, preoperative chemotherapy is often given, followed by excision of the masses in an attempt to spare some functioning renal tissue.

Prognosis depends on stage, but overall 5-year survival is about 85%.

Rhabdomyosarcoma

Rhabdomyosarcoma is a type of sarcoma (tumour of connective tissue) arising from primitive muscle cells. Although it is rare, 50% of all paediatric sarcomas are rhabdomyosarcomas with an incidence of 6 cases per million children <15 years, annually. Incidence peaks at 3 years, after which it gradually decreases. Most tumours are sporadic. It presents as a hard swelling that is growing; it typically affects the head and neck, and chest or abdominal wall. Diagnosis is confirmed by biopsy, with radiological imaging used to stage the disease.

Rhabdomyosarcoma is treated by surgical excision followed by chemotherapy and radiotherapy. However, this approach is difficult if the tumour is infiltrating surrounding tissues. Rhabdomyosarcoma has one of the worst prognoses of all childhood cancers. Overall 5-year survival is about 70%, and only 50% in adolescents.

Bone tumours

Most bone tumours in children are benign: simple cysts or osteoid osteomas. Although they may present with pain or swelling, most are discovered as incidental findings during imaging for another reason, for example after injury.

Malignant bone tumours present with persistent bone pain, local swelling or a limp. The most common paediatric malignant bone tumours are osteosarcoma and Ewing's sarcoma; both have a poor prognosis.

Osteosarcoma

Osteosarcoma is the commonest bone tumour occurring in children. It is thought to arise from primitive mesenchymal bone-forming cells. Incidence increases with the age of the child, peaking during the adolescent growth spurt. The incidence is 4.8 cases per million persons <20 years of age each year. It is rare <5 years of age, and the annual incidence age 10–19 years is 8 cases per million. The tumour is commonly located at the metaphyses of long bones, usually in the distal femur (40% of cases). The child may be asymptomatic, or they may have associated pain, swelling or both at the site of the tumour. They may also present with a pathological fracture.

> **A pathological fracture is a fracture that occurs as a result of normal force being applied to abnormal bone.** A history of minimal trauma causing a fracture alerts the clinician to the possibility of an abnormality of the underlying bone.

Diagnosis is based on imaging and biopsy. Treatment is surgical resection followed by chemotherapy. Amputation may be required. Osteosarcoma is rapidly and locally destructive, and metastasises easily.

Prognosis is poor: the 5-year survival of individuals with localised disease is about 70%; this decreases to < 30% in those with metastatic disease at diagnosis.

Ewing's sarcoma

Ewing's sarcoma is a primitive neuroectoderm tumour of connective tissue. It is rare; the incidence from birth to age 20 years is 2.9 cases per million population. Ewing's sarcomas are most often located in bones of the leg and pelvis (**Figure 15.5**), but they can occur in any bone. Peak incidence is in late adolescence with approximately half of all patients aged 10–20 years. The presentation and diagnostic approach is similar to that for an osteosarcoma. The associated periosteal reaction can cause an onion skin appearance on plain radiography. Chemotherapy is the first-line treatment, and surgery may be required. Prognosis is variable dependent on the presence or absence of metastatic disease; the location of the primary site of the tumour, with distal extremities being more favourable than central or pelvic sites, and an age <15 years having a more favourable prognosis. Two thirds of patients are alive at 5 years.

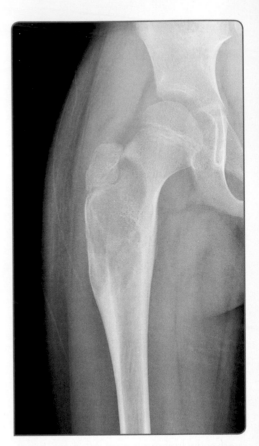

Figure 15.5 Radiograph showing a Ewing's sarcoma. Although the typical onion layer appearance is not seen in this example, it shows the cortical destruction and periosteal reaction typical of such lesions.

Answers to starter questions

1. Children with brain tumours may have direct or indirect involvement of the pituitary gland, which leads to endocrine disturbances (hypopituitarism) that growth and puberty. In addition, children with brain tumours or leukaemia often have radiotherapy to the brain as part of their treatment. The radiation affects healthy tissue in the pituitary gland and hypothalamus causing hypopituitarism. Growth is closely monitored in these patients.

2. Retinoblastomas are often detected by parents when a photograph taken with a flash (not using the anti-red eye function) of their baby or young child shows a red reflex from the normal eye, and a white pupil (leukocoria) from the eye affected with a retinoblastoma. This is more difficult to detect if the tumours are bilateral as there is not a red reflex for comparison.

Chapter 16
Emergencies

Introduction

Both infant and child mortality rates have steadily decreased in developed countries over the past 30 years. More than half the deaths occur during the first year of life (**Table 16.1**) and most are attributed to prematurity, congenital anomalies and sudden infant death syndrome. The predominant cause changes with age. For example the most common cause of death in British children aged 10–18 years is injury, and > 75% of these deaths are the result of road traffic accidents. Common childhood conditions also have the potential to cause death; for example, asthma, epilepsy and diabetes all cause life-threatening episodes.

Recognition of serious illness in a child requires knowledge of the normal physiological values in children (see page 68). Resuscitation and treatment must be started promptly. Sick children can deteriorate quickly. Unlike adults, children rarely suffer cardiac arrest from a primary cardiac cause. Instead, cardiac arrest is usually preceded by respiratory arrest

Childhood deaths by age group (UK data)		
Age (years)	Percentage of total	Approximate number
< 1	60	3220
1–4	10	525
5–9	6	325
10–14	6	340
15–19	18	959

Table 16.1 Childhood deaths by age group (UK data). The overall death rate for 0–19 year olds in developing countries varies between 30 and 84 per 100,000, with similar proportions in each age group

as a consequence of prolonged hypoxia and acidosis, or circulatory failure. Whatever the underlying cause, progression to cardiac arrest has a poor prognosis.

Case 23 Septic shock

Presentation

Rosie, who is 8 months old, presents with a 24-h history of being unwell, with a high temperature, poor feeding and lethargy. Today, she started developing a rash and has been vomiting. Rosie's observations on admission show a temperature of 39.4°C, a heart rate of 180 beats/min and a capillary refill time of 3 s.

Initial interpretation

Rosie's history is very non-specific, and taken in isolation could indicate just a minor viral illness; however, her observations are worrying. She is showing signs of shock (tachycardia and decreased perfusion), which in view of her high temperature is likely to be septic shock.

Further history and examination

Rosie's mother reports that Rosie has been increasingly irritable and drowsy throughout the day, and started vomiting and having diarrhoea over the past few hours. On examination, Rosie is drowsy but rousable. She looks unwell. Her skin is mottled and her peripheries are cold. There is a widespread maculopapular rash, with petechiae appearing in some areas (**Figure 16.1**).

Working diagnosis

Based on the presence of high temperature and shock, the working diagnosis is sepsis. The specific causative organism is unimportant at this time, because the principles of management are the same for different causes of sepsis.

Immediate intervention

Sepsis requires prompt management. Vascular access is gained and blood samples are taken for culture, full blood count, C-reactive protein and blood gas analysis. A blood gas shows a metabolic acidosis with high lactate level.

Rosie is given IV cefotaxime (a broad-spectrum antibiotic) and a fluid bolus. Her tachycardia improves briefly, but then returns. Therefore she is given another fluid bolus, with a good response. Rosie is transferred to high-dependency unit, where she will be closely monitored during ongoing treatment.

Shock and sepsis

Shock is defined as a clinical condition in which there is failure to deliver adequate oxygen and nutrients to meet the metabolic demands of tissues and organs, or failure to remove the waste metabolites as a result of circulatory failure. Shock has many causes (**Table 16.2**), but in all patients early recognition and treatment in the 'compensated' phase, i.e. when essential tissues and organs are still being perfused, is the key to a successful outcome.

Signs of shock include tachycardia, prolonged capillary refill time, skin pallor or mottling, cool peripheries and mild agitation. If untreated, respiratory and cardiac arrest will follow.

> **Meningococcal sepsis does not always present with the classic purpuric rash.** In about 15% of patients, the rash is maculopapular and blanching (see **Figure 16.1**).

Sepsis in children has a mortality of about 10% and causes significant morbidity in a minority of survivors. Shock in sepsis occurs partly because of hypovolaemia as a result of poor intake and losses (e.g. from vomiting), but it is caused primarily by maldistribution of fluid secondary to the inflammatory response and subsequent capillary leak.

Shock: classification and causes		
Type of shock	Pathophysiology	Examples of underlying causes
Hypovolaemic	Intra- and extravascular fluid depletion	Haemorrhage (e.g. from trauma)
		Severe gastroenteritis
		Intussusception
		Burns
Distributive	Intravascular fluid depletion as a consequence of peripheral vasodilation and maldistribution of fluid because of capillary leak	Septicaemia
		Anaphylaxis
Cardiogenic	Insufficient cardiac output to maintain perfusion, secondary to inefficient pumping action of the heart	Arrhythmias
		Cardiomyopathy
		Heart failure
Obstructive	Insufficient cardiac output secondary to an obstruction hindering the filling or emptying of the heart	Congenital heart disease (e.g. coarctation of the aorta, or aortic stenosis)
		Tension pneumothorax
		Cardiac tamponade
Dissociative	Inadequate tissue perfusion because of a left shift in the oxygen–haemoglobin dissociation curve	Anaemia
		Carbon monoxide poisoning

Table 16.2 Classification and causes of shock

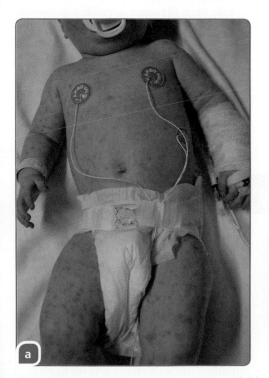

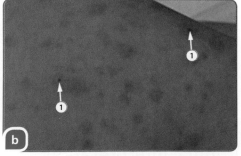

Figure 16.1 Meningococcal sepsis presenting with (a) atypical maculopapular rash and (b) developing petechiae ①.

Remember the 4 H's and the 4 T's as reversible causes of cardiac arrest:

- Hypoxia, Hypovolaemia, Hyperkalaemia and Hypothermia
- Toxic substances, Tension pneumothorax, cardiac Tamponade and Thromboembolism

The commonest causative organism for sepsis in infants and older children is *Neisseria meningitidis*, and in neonates group B streptococci. In both instances, there may be concomitant meningitis (see page 251). Group A streptococci may be the cause of sepsis in older children. Infections with other organisms may begin as a localised infection before systemic spread, for example in children with infection with Gram-negative organisms from the urinary or gastrointestinal tract.

Toxic shock syndrome is a specific kind of sepsis caused by superantigen toxins from *Staphylococcus aureus* or *Streptococcus pyogenes* bacteria. There may be a history of preceding minor injury or illness. Toxic shock syndrome is characterised by a high fever, diffuse erythematous rash and multiorgan failure. It is rare, affecting 3 per 100,000 people globally, and less common in children than in adults.

Other causes of shock are often apparent from the history and examination.

Management

Management of shock follows the ABC approach (see page 113). Effective oxygenation prevents tissue hypoxia. Ensuring an adequate circulating volume, with 20 mL/kg boluses of crystalloid fluids (usually 0.9% saline, unless there is a severe haemorrhage in which case packed red cells would be appropriate), is crucial to prevent worsening acidosis. Repeat boluses may be required, but caution must be exercised in children with suspected increased intracranial pressure or cardiac disease as excess fluid can worsen these problems.

Further management depends on the underlying cause. In all children diagnosed, the blood glucose is checked and any hypoglycaemia treated. If sepsis is likely, a third-generation cephalosporin antibiotic is given intravenously, with flucloxacillin added to cover *Staph. aureus* if toxic shock syndrome is suspected.

The child is constantly reassessed. If the child remains unstable once 40 mL/kg of fluid has been given, urgent intubation is considered; they are likely to require inotropic support and transfer to the paediatric intensive care unit.

Remember that the **intraosseous route** is an alternative for administration of fluids and drugs in an emergency situation if IV access is not possible.

Case 24 Upper airway obstruction

Presentation

Adi, aged 2 years, presents at 5 a.m. after waking in the night with a cough and noisy breathing. He now appears to be having difficulty breathing. During triage, there is obvious inspiratory stridor and a loud barking cough.

Initial interpretation

Breathing difficulties associated with stridor suggest an upper airway problem.

At Adi's age, the most likely diagnosis is viral croup. However further history and examination is required to assess the severity and exclude a more serious pathology.

Further history and examination

Adi had been 'snuffly' the previous day, but otherwise well. There was no history of fever and no history of any choking episode. Adi is examined while he is sitting

Case 24 continued

on his mother's lap. He has some chest recessions and tracheal tug. He is upset by the oxygen saturation probe on his finger (reading 97%) and having his temperature taken (result, 37.7°C). As a consequence of his distress, his stridor becomes even louder but he otherwise looks well.

Working diagnosis

The short history of coryza and stridor in a child who is not systemically unwell, are consistent with viral croup.

Immediate intervention

Any distress will worsen Adi's airway obstruction, so all unnecessary medical examination and monitoring is avoided. His mother is encouraged to reassure and soothe him. He is given oral dexamethasone and allowed to settle. When reviewed an hour later, Adi is much improved.

Upper airway obstruction

The most common cause for upper airway obstruction (manifesting as stridor with breathing difficulties) is viral croup (laryngotracheobronchitis). Croup is common and accounts for 5% of emergency hospital admissions in children under 6 years.

Croup usually occurs between the ages of 6 months and 3 years, but it can present in children up to 6 years old. It is caused by a virus, most commonly parainfluenza viruses (75% of cases), and presents in the autumn and winter. Croup is usually mild and self-limiting but may present with a wide spectrum of severity, however in rare cases it is life-threatening.

The severity of croup is assessed by the modified Westley Score. Points are awarded in five areas. Those features scoring the most points, and likely to indicate severe croup, include:

- Stridor at rest
- Severe intercostal recessions
- Severly decreased air entry
- Cyanosis at rest
- Altered conscious level

Do not be falsely reassured by normal oxygen saturation in children with upper airway obstruction. In contrast to lower airway conditions, a reduction in saturation indicates severe disease and is a late sign.

In young children, foreign body inhalation should always be considered, even in the absence of a history of choking. Objects can also be aspirated by older children, if they have learning disabilities.

Table 16.3 compares the different causes of stridor, both common and rare, along with the history and presentation of each. Chronic stridor is discussed in Chapter 4 (see page 171).

Before the advent of routine immunisation, epiglottitis was usually caused by *Haemophilus influenzae* type b (Hib). In vaccinated populations, the annual incidence is < 1 case per 100,000 children, and it is usually caused by other bacteria. However, Hib can occur in unvaccinated children and because of vaccine failure.

Acute stridor: causes			
Diagnosis	Quality of stridor	Appearance of child	Significant history
Foreign body	Sudden onset	Well but struggling to breathe	Usually a younger child with a history of choking (or an older child with learning disability)
Viral croup	Harsh	'Viral' (e.g. coryza and low-grade temperature), but otherwise well	Typically occurs at night Preceding coryza 'Barking' cough
Laryngomalacia	Variable, intermittent	Well	Usually intermittently apparent since birth May be worse when feeding or with upper respiratory tract infection
Epiglottitis	Soft	'Toxic' (miserable, flushed or pale, sitting upright, drooling saliva) and unwell	High temperatures Drooling (due to difficulty with swallowing saliva) Low-pitched expiratory sound No cough May be unvaccinated
Bacterial tracheitis	Harsh	Unwell	High temperatures Barking cough, similar to that of croup

Table 16.3 Causes of acute stridor

Management

The most important principle in treating a child with upper airway obstruction is not to upset them, because distress may precipitate complete obstruction of the airway and respiratory arrest. Standard treatment is with oral dexamethasone or nebulised budesonide (both steroids), which relieve the obstruction by reducing inflammation and swelling. Some children with a severe episode need further treatments, including nebulised adrenaline (epinephrine) and intubation. Nebulised adrenaline is thought to work by causing vasoconstriction in the upper airway, thereby relieving the obstruction by decreasing mucosal oedema. However, the effects are short lived and therefore it should only be used to 'buy time' while arranging intubation.

Treatment for bacterial causes, i.e. epiglottitis and bacterial tracheitis, requires IV antibiotics, usually third-generation cephalosporins. However, any intervention should only be attempted once the airway is secure, because there is a high risk of complete airway obstruction if the child becomes more distressed, for example during venepuncture to gain IV access.

Case 25 Anaphylaxis

Presentation

Maisie is 8 years old. She is en route to the hospital from her friend's birthday party. Maisie had been eating party food with the other children when she suddenly started complaining that her tongue 'felt funny'. One of the parents noticed that she was developing a rash, and her face became swollen. When her breathing became noisy they called an ambulance.

Initial interpretation

The initial history (sudden-onset rash and oropharyngeal and facial swelling) suggests that Maisie is having an allergic reaction, which along with the airway involvement suggests anaphylaxis. On arrival, she will need immediate assessment of her ABC, including for signs of shock.

Further history and examination

Maisie has asthma, which is well controlled on inhaled steroids. She is otherwise normally fit and well. She previously had a rash after eating a cereal bar, and has avoided eating nuts since then.

On assessment of her airway, she is breathing independently but has a stridor. She has increased work of breathing, is tachypnoeic and has an oxygen saturation of 92% in air. There is air entry throughout her chest, but with widespread wheeze bilaterally. Cardiovascular assessment shows tachycardia with a normal capillary refill time and blood pressure (99/60 mmHg). Further examination finds a widespread urticarial rash with swelling of the face, lips and tongue.

Working diagnosis

Although at present Maisie is well perfused and maintaining a blood pressure appropriate for her age, the signs described above indicate she has anaphylactic shock, and without treatment, decompensation may occur.

Immediate intervention

High-flow oxygen is administered via a non-rebreathing mask. This is immediately followed by a dose of intramuscular adrenaline (epinephrine). Maisie then receives nebulised salbutamol (a bronchodilator), IV hydrocortisone (a steroid) and IV chlorphenamine (an antihistamine).

Maisie shows no initial response to treatment, so after 5 minutes she is given a second dose of intramuscular adrenaline and a bolus of 0.9% saline. Subsequently her tachycardia and symptoms improve. Maisie is taken to the paediatric ward for close observation to monitor for any signs of a biphasic reaction (return of symptoms).

Anaphylaxis

Anaphylaxis is a severe and often life-threatening allergic reaction with multisystem involvement. Because of inconsistencies in its definition and diagnosis, the true incidence is difficult to determine. However, it is clear that the incidence of anaphylaxis in children is increasing worldwide, especially in children under 5 years.

It is an immunoglobulin E (IgE)-mediated hypersensitivity reaction (**Figure 16.2**), so individuals with a background of other IgE-mediated conditions such as asthma or other atopic conditions are more susceptible. The most common triggers in children are foods, especially nuts. Other relatively common triggers are:

- drugs, particularly β-lactam antibiotics (e.g. penicillin), non-steroidal anti-inflammatory drugs and aspirin
- insect stings or bites

Multisystem involvement means that the symptoms of anaphylaxis are varied (**Table 16.4**). Some individuals may experience a biphasic reaction, in which the symptoms return 8–12 h later in the absence of re-exposure to the allergen.

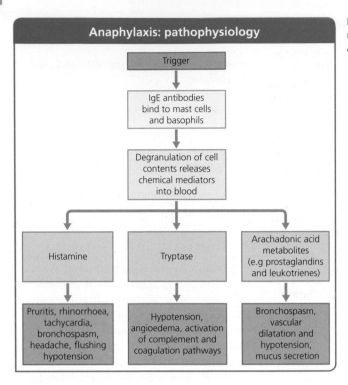

Anaphylaxis: pathophysiology

Trigger

IgE antibodies bind to mast cells and basophils

Degranulation of cell contents releases chemical mediators into blood

| Histamine | Tryptase | Arachadonic acid metabolites (e.g prostaglandins and leukotrienes) |

Pruritis, rhinorrhoea, tachycardia, bronchospasm, headache, flushing hypotension

Hypotension, angioedema, activation of complement and coagulation pathways

Bronchospasm, vascular dilatation and hypotension, mucus secretion

Figure 16.2 The chemical mediators of the symptoms of anaphylaxis. Ig, immunoglobulin.

Allergy and anaphylaxis: signs and symptoms

System affected	Allergy	Anaphylaxis
General	Urticarial rash	Swelling of tongue and/or throat
	Itching	
	Burning or tingling of lips and/or mouth	Agitation
		Collapse
	Angioedema	
	Sweating	
Respiratory	Cough	Shortness of breath
		Wheeze or stridor
Gastrointestinal	Nausea	Cramping abdominal pain
	Abdominal pain	Nausea
	Loose stools	Vomiting, loose stools
Cardiovascular	None	Palpitations and tachycardia
		Hypotension

Table 16.4 Comparison of signs and symptoms of an allergic reaction and those of anaphylaxis

Although the principles of management of shock apply in all cases, additional treatments may depend on the underlying cause, e.g. antibiotics for septic shock or adrenaline for anaphylactic shock.

If a diagnosis of anaphylaxis is uncertain, measurement of serum tryptase at the time of presentation may be useful, because in anaphylaxis mast cell degranulation markedly increases the level of tryptase in the blood.

Management

Management of anaphylaxis follows ABC principles. The priority is administration of intramuscular adrenaline, because this is the only treatment targeting the life-threatening features. Adrenaline works in two ways: by causing peripheral vasoconstriction and improving contractility of the heart which raises the blood pressure; and by causing bronchodilation to relieve life-threatening airway obstruction

Steroids and antihistamines are not effective acutely, because of their slower onset of action. However, they help provide symptomatic relief later.

A child who has had anaphylaxis should avoid the trigger, if one has been identified.

The child is also supplied with and taught to use an adrenaline pen injector for any future episodes.

Case 26 Severe breathlessness

Presentation

Scott, aged 12 years, has just arrived at the emergency department via ambulance from school. He has asthma and became breathless during a physical education class, despite using his salbutamol inhaler. Paramedics administered nebulised salbutamol and ipratropium bromide in the ambulance, with minimal improvement in Scott's condition. He is too breathless to talk.

Initial interpretation

Scott is having an acute exacerbation of asthma. He needs further urgent assessment. It is worrying that he is severely breathless and unable to talk despite treatment.

Further history and examination

Scott's mother arrives and reports that his asthma has been difficult to manage.

He is on a high dose of inhaled steroid and a long-acting β_2 adrenergic receptor agonist, but still needs to use salbutamol a few times a week. He has had one previous admission to the high-dependency unit, but never to intensive care.

On examination, Scott has a respiratory rate of 32 breaths/min, an oxygen saturation of 90% in air and a heart rate of 130 bpm. He is using his accessory muscles to breathe and remains too breathless to talk. Auscultation of his chest finds widespread wheeze bilaterally, with decreased air entry towards the bases.

Working diagnosis

Although the exacerbation is severe, at present it does not display features of a life-threatening exacerbation (**Table 16.5**). Scott requires close monitoring and treatment needs to be aggressive.

Acute exacerbation of asthma: assessment of severity			
Acute severe asthma			**Life-threatening asthma**
	2–5 years old	>5 years old	
General condition	Too breathless to feed or talk	Unable to complete sentences	Features of acute severe asthma plus:
Heart rate	>140 bpm	>125 bpm	
Oxygen saturation	<92%	<92%	■ exhaustion or poor respiratory effort
Respiratory rate	>40 breaths/min	>30 breaths/min	■ silent chest
Peak flow	N/A	33–35% of usual best or predicted value	■ cyanosis ■ hypotension ■ confusion ■ coma

Table 16.5 Assessment of severity in acute exacerbation of asthma

Case 26 *continued*

Immediate intervention

Further nebulisers including a combination of salbutamol, ipratropium bromide and magnesium sulphate are given, driven by high-flow oxygen due to his low saturations. There is minimal improvement therefore Scott receives IV hydrocortisone (a steroid) and a loading dose of IV salbutamol, followed by a continuous salbutamol infusion. His cardiac activity is monitored closely, and he is transferred to the paediatric high-dependency unit.

Scott shows some improvement, but his condition remains unstable. Therefore he is given a bolus of IV magnesium sulfate (which works by causing smooth muscle relaxation) after which Scott starts to show a response. His breathing rate slows and his work of breathing and air entry improve.

Acute severe asthma

Acute severe asthma remains a significant problem, for example it causes the death of up to 16 children per year in the UK. A severe exacerbation can quickly progress to a life-threatening exacerbation if managed inadequately (see **Table 16.5**). Risk factors for a life-threatening episode include previous admission to a high-dependency or intensive therapy unit, 'brittle' (i.e. unpredictable and difficult to control asthma) and frequent use of β_2 agonists (bronchodilators). Chronic asthma is discussed in Chapter 4 (see page 160).

The likely possible causes of wheeze depend on the child's age. They are similar to those for chronic cough and wheeze.

> **Do not rely on severity of wheeze as an indicator of the severity of an acute asthma exacerbation**. Very tight wheeze can be quiet and may become much louder after bronchodilation. Therefore a silent chest can be a sign of impending respiratory failure.

It should be borne in mind that acute difficulty in breathing and wheeze, even in children with known asthma, may be caused by anaphylaxis.

Management

The management of an acute asthma exacerbation is shown in **Figure 16.3**. A β_2 agonist for bronchodilation is preferably given via spacer, with or without a face mask, to ensure maximal delivery of drug particles into the lungs. It is administered one puff at a time, with each puff inhaled separately using tidal breathing. Nebulisers are used in severe exacerbations if saturations are low and administration of oxygen is required. Steroids are as effective orally as intravenously, but the IV route is used if there is vomiting.

Intubation and mechanical ventilation is the last resort, because ventilation can be very difficult in patients with asthma: it requires high pressures due to the airway resistance. A chest radiograph or blood gas is rarely indicated in children with an acute asthma exacerbation, unless ventilation is being considered or there are atypical features, such as clinical features of a pneumothorax.

A discharge plan consists of:

- a written asthma action plan for future exacerbations
- a check of inhaler technique
- review of the regular treatment and adherence
- arrangements for follow-up with the patient's general practitioner (GP)

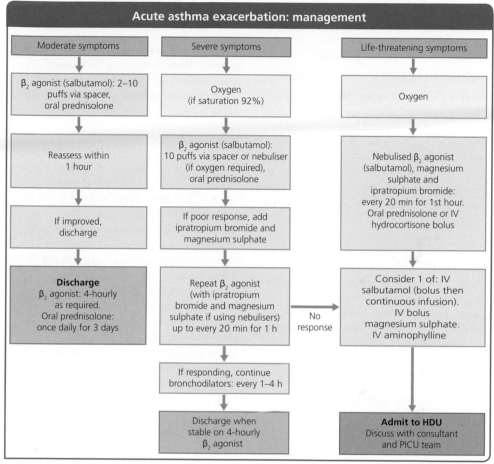

Acute asthma exacerbation: management

Moderate symptoms	Severe symptoms	Life-threatening symptoms
β₂ agonist (salbutamol): 2–10 puffs via spacer, oral prednisolone	Oxygen (if saturation 92%)	Oxygen
Reassess within 1 hour	β₂ agonist (salbutamol): 10 puffs via spacer or nebuliser (if oxygen required), oral prednisolone	Nebulised β₂ agonist (salbutamol), magnesium sulphate and ipratropium bromide: every 20 min for 1st hour. Oral prednisolone or IV hydrocortisone bolus
If improved, discharge	If poor response, add ipratropium bromide and magnesium sulphate	
Discharge β₂ agonist: 4-hourly as required. Oral prednisolone: once daily for 3 days	Repeat β₂ agonist (with ipratropium bromide and magnesium sulphate if using nebulisers) up to every 20 min for 1 h → No response	Consider 1 of: IV salbutamol (bolus then continuous infusion). IV bolus magnesium sulphate. IV aminophylline
	If responding, continue bronchodilators: every 1–4 h	
	Discharge when stable on 4-hourly β₂ agonist	**Admit to HDU** Discuss with consultant and PICU team

Figure 16.3 Management of an acute asthma exacerbation in a child. Reassess regularly. For life-threatening episodes, the additional infusions are given only if there is no response to the earlier treatment. A loading dose of aminophylline is given as a bolus (unless the child is on maintenance theophylline therapy), followed by an infusion. HDU, high-dependency unit; PICU, paediatric intensive care unit.

Case 27 Status epilepticus

Presentation

Harvey is 7 years old. His parents report that he was playing when he suddenly collapsed and started shaking all over. They called an ambulance, which arrived after 6 minutes. The paramedics have given him buccal midazolam, but the seizure is ongoing on arrival to hospital.

Initial interpretation

Harvey is having a seizure, and having lasted over 5 min it is now unlikely to stop spontaneously and may develop into status epilepticus. The cause of the seizure is unclear at present, so further assessment is required.

Case 27 *continued*

Further history and examination

Harvey's parents report that he is awaiting an appointment to see a paediatrician because of recurrent 'blank' episodes, but he has no other medical problems. He has been developing normally, and his parents describe him as 'average' at school. He has been well, with no history of high temperatures or recent injuries, and he has not complained of headaches.

On examination, Harvey's airway is patent and he is breathing spontaneously. He is mildly tachycardic but well perfused, with a blood pressure of 124/86 mmHg. Harvey is unresponsive; he has fixed, dilated pupils and his body and limbs are jerking rhythmically. His blood glucose concentration is 5.2 mmol/L.

Working diagnosis

Harvey is having a generalised tonic–clonic seizure, most likely epileptic in origin. At present, there is nothing to suggest any other underlying cause for a seizure, such as intracranial infection or a space-occupying lesion.

Immediate intervention

Harvey is given high-flow oxygen via a face mask, and his airway is monitored. A cannula has been sited, so he is given IV lorazepam to try and terminate the seizure. Observations of vital signs continue.

A phenytoin infusion is prepared and then started because the seizure is still ongoing. An anaesthetist is called to prepare for rapid sequence induction (rapid induction of general anaesthesia) with thiopental; however, the seizure stops 5 min after starting phenytoin. The phenytoin infusion is completed and Harvey is taken to the paediatric high-dependency unit for observation until he has recovered fully.

Status epilepticus

Status epilepticus is defined as either of the following:

- a generalised seizure lasting ≥ 30 min
- a series of seizures over a period of ≥ 30 min, occurring without full recovery of consciousness between seizures

It occurs in 10–20% of children with epilepsy and in 5% of children presenting with a febrile seizure (febrile convulsion). The mortality rate during status epilepticus is about 4%. Subsequent morbidity such as focal neurological deficits and learning disabilities depends on the age of the child and any underlying condition.

There are several diagnoses to consider for the underlying cause of a prolonged seizure (**Table 16.6**).

Seizure: causes	
Condition	Comments
Epilepsy	Increased incidence in children with neurodevelopmental problems
Febrile seizure (febrile convulsion)	Seizure that is triggered by fever usually in children aged < 5 years
Meningitis	Neck rigidity may be present, may also have rash and sepsis
Hypoglycaemia	Consider metabolic conditions
Increased intracranial pressure	Secondary to trauma or space-occupying lesion
Poisoning	For example from tricyclic antidepressants

Table 16.6 Causes of seizure

Management

Management of prolonged seizures, with the aim of preventing status epilepticus is shown in **Figure 16.4**. High-flow oxygen and maintenance of a patent airway are vital to prevent hypoxic brain injury, especially due to increased brain oxygen consumption during a seizure. Blood glucose concentration should always be checked for hypoglycaemia, which can be a primary cause and is also a consequence of status epilepticus (there is also increased consumption of glucose by the brain during a seizure).

The use of drugs to try and terminate a seizure uses a stepwise approach at timed intervals (see **Figure 16.5**). IV lorazepam is the benzodiazepine of choice due to its efficacy and longer duration of action, but buccal midazolam or rectal diazepam is useful outside hospital or when there is no IV access. Thiopental is a general anaesthetic.

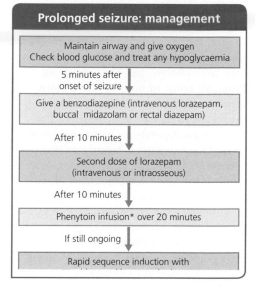

Prolonged seizure: management

Maintain airway and give oxygen
Check blood glucose and treat any hypoglycaemia

5 minutes after
onset of seizure

Give a benzodiazepine (intravenous lorazepam,
buccal midazolam or rectal diazepam)

After 10 minutes

Second dose of lorazepam
(intravenous or intraosseous)

After 10 minutes

Phenytoin infusion* over 20 minutes

If still ongoing

Rapid sequence induction with

Figure 16.4 Management of a prolonged seizure (medications are given if the seizure has been ongoing for greater than 5 minutes). *If the child is already on phenytoin, phenobarbital (phenobarbitone) is given at this point instead.

> **Early preparation for the next step in the prolonged seizure pathway is recommended.** This is because any time spent preparing drugs and infusions delays treatment, if the need for them is not anticipated.

Once the seizure has been stopped, the child requires close observation. This includes monitoring for adverse effects of the medication, such as respiratory depression from benzodiazepine use and hypotension or arrhythmias from phenytoin use.

Case 28 Diabetic ketoacidosis

Presentation

Lacey is 11 years old. She has been sent urgently to the paediatric assessment unit by her GP. Lacey originally attended the GP's clinic 2 weeks ago, complaining of lethargy. Today she started vomiting and complaining of abdominal pain.

On questioning, Lacey reports that she had been needing to go to the toilet to pass urine more often than usual, and says that she has been thirsty and drinking a lot more fluid recently. A measurement of capillary blood glucose carried out by the GP has shown a concentration of 26.7 mmol/L.

Initial interpretation

The combination of increased thirst, frequent urination and high blood glucose confirm that Lacey has developed diabetes mellitus. Symptoms of abdominal pain and vomiting suggest that she has also developed ketoacidosis, which needs urgent diagnosis and treatment.

Case 28 continued

Further history and examination

Lacey looks unwell, with sunken eyes. Her breathing is fast, deep and sighing. Her breath has a slightly fruity smell, and she has a dry mouth. She is tachycardic, with a capillary refill time of 3 s. Dipstick analysis shows a +++ result for ketones and glucose. A bedside blood test shows an increased ketone concentration (4 mmol/L). A blood gas shows a pH of 7.18, with P_{CO_2} of 3.1 kPa, bicarbonate concentration of 14.3 mmol/L and base excess of -12.

Working diagnosis

Lacey has a high blood glucose concentration, diagnostic of diabetes mellitus. She is clinically acidotic (shown by the abnormal breathing and low blood pH) and has an increased blood ketone level, which altogether indicates diabetic ketoacidosis.

She is dehydrated and also in shock, as indicated by the tachycardia and poor perfusion.

Immediate intervention

Intravenous access is gained and blood is sent for laboratory measurement of glucose concentration, and a check of urea and electrolytes. Lacey is given a 10 mL/kg bolus of normal (0.9%) saline, which leads to improvement of her tachycardia. She is then transferred to the paediatric high-dependency unit and started on an IV 0.9% saline infusion containing potassium, to cover normal maintenance requirements and to replace her estimated fluid deficit, given over 48 h.

An hour later, IV insulin is started. Lacey's blood glucose, ketones, blood gas values and electrolytes are closely monitored; dextrose is added to the fluids once the blood glucose decreases to < 14 mmol/L.

Diabetic ketoacidosis

Type 1 diabetes is discussed in Chapter 12 (see page 327). An estimated 25% of children will have diabetic ketoacidosis on their first presentation with diabetes (35% in children under 5 years old). Alternatively, diabetic ketoacidosis may occur in children with known diabetes associated with an intercurrent illness or non-adherence with insulin therapy.

Diabetic ketoacidosis is a serious life-threatening condition, with a mortality rate of less than 1% in developed countries. The main cause of death and morbidity in diabetic ketoacidosis is cerebral oedema. Diabetic ketoacidosis is the consequence of a lack of insulin and therefore an inability to metabolise glucose, so the body metabolises fat (lipolysis leading to ketogenesis) for energy instead. This leads to the acidosis, while hyperglycaemia causes an osmotic diuresis and subsequent dehydration (**Figure 16.5**).

In addition to its effect on uptake of glucose into cells, insulin also has a role in potassium regulation by driving it from the extracellular to the intracellular space. This is why insulin (with dextrose to prevent hypoglycaemia) is used as a treatment for hyperkalaemia. It is important, therefore, to anticipate that initiation of insulin therapy in DKA may lead to hypokalaemia, and prevent it with early addition of potassium into the rehydration fluids.

Acidosis in the presence of ketones and hyperglycaemia always indicates diabetic ketoacidosis. Salicylate poisoning should be considered in young children presenting with vomiting, dehydration, rapid breathing and metabolic acidosis, but their blood glucose and ketones will be normal.

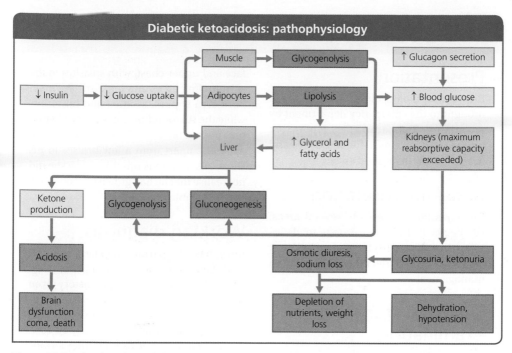

Diabetic ketoacidosis: pathophysiology

Figure 16.5 Pathophysiology of diabetic ketoacidosis.

> **Ketones on the breath** smell like nail varnish or 'pear drops' sweets.

Management

Management of a child with newly diagnosed diabetes but without diabetic ketoacidosis is discussed in Chapter 12 (see page 328). In diabetic children with diabetic ketoacidosis careful fluid management is important to correct the dehydration and electrolyte disturbance. Small boluses of 10mL/kg of normal saline can be given if the child is in shock, but any bolus should be given with caution as rapid changes increase the risk of cerebral oedema. Ideally the fluid deficit should be corrected slowly over 48 h. Careful attention should also be paid to maintaining normal electrolyte balance, particularly early addition of potassium to the fluids to prevent hypokalaemia.

Rehydration will start to normalise glucose levels by starting to restore intravascular volume, but insulin is required to 'switch off' ketogenesis. Therefore IV insulin is started an hour after commencing IV fluids, with the aim of producing a gradual decrease in glucose levels. Because insulin stops ketogenesis, it should not be stopped, even when the blood glucose normalises. Instead, dextrose is added to the fluids to prevent hypoglycaemia.

Once the blood biochemistry has normalised and the child is tolerating oral intake, IV insulin is changed to subcutaneous insulin.

> **In diabetic ketoacidosis in children, the metabolic acidosis is corrected with rehydration.** There is rarely a role for sodium bicarbonate, which should always be a senior decision.

Case 29 Burns

Presentation

Riley is a 20-month-old boy who has been brought to the emergency department by ambulance. The paramedics report that he has scald injuries to his chest, face and left arm. He is distressed and crying.

Initial interpretation

Riley has burn injuries to several areas. He needs further assessment to determine the extent of his burns, i.e. the depth and coverage, and decide on the optimum management.

Further history and examination

Riley's mother explains that she was tidying the house while Riley was playing. She had just made a cup of coffee when the telephone rang. She left her coffee on the dining table while she talked to her friend. She heard Riley cry out and saw that he had spilt her coffee all over himself. She called an ambulance, stripped off Riley's clothes and ran cold water over his burns.

On examination, Riley is distressed. He has burn injuries mainly affecting his face and upper chest, with splashes to the surrounding areas and left arm. The main burn area is pink, mottled and blistering, while the surrounding areas are erythematous but not blistered. No other injuries are apparent, apart from a few bruises to his shins. His mother is upset because she did not realise that he had grown tall enough to reach the table.

Working diagnosis

Riley has 6% partial thickness and 3% superficial burns affecting his face, neck, upper chest and left arm. The history given by his mother is consistent with the clinical findings and there has been no delay in presentation, so this is most likely an accidental injury. The bruises on Riley's shins are usual in a mobile child of his age.

Immediate intervention

Riley is given opioid analgesia to keep him comfortable. His burns are dressed, and because of the burns affecting his face, he is transferred to the local burns centre for further management.

Burns

About 30% of all burn injuries occur in children, and two-thirds of these are in the under-5s. About 70% of burns in this age group are scald injuries from hot liquids; each week, more than 300 children attend accident and emergency departments with hot drink scalds. In addition, about 400 children younger than 14 years are admitted per year with bath water scalds. Most other burns are flame injuries.

It is important, especially in younger children, that non-accidental injury is considered. In addition to the possibility of physical abuse, burns may raise concerns of neglect (e.g. lack of appropriate supervision leading to a burn), especially if the history is not consistent with the pattern of injury.

> Each year, more than 3750 children under 5 years old are admitted to hospital in England and Wales because of burns and scalds.

Management

Once ABC have been assessed as stable, adequate analgesia is the priority. Opioid analgesia is used; it can be administered intranasally until IV access is available. Cold compresses reduce pain until other analgesia is available, for example in the home and during transfer to hospital.

The whole burn area must be exposed to assess the total surface area affected, as well as the depth of the burns (**Table 16.7**). The most accurate way of evaluating the surface area involved is by using the Lund-Browder burns chart (**Figure 16.6**). Surface area can also be estimated by considering the patient's palm roughly equal to 1% of the body surface area.

Children with burns covering > 10% of their body surface area require IV fluids. The volume required is the child's usual maintenance requirements plus an additional volume based on the percentage burn area (e.g. the Parkland's formula of 4 mL × %burn × body weight in kg over 24 hours).

The burns themselves are dressed with special sterile, non-adhesive dressings. Antibiotics are not routinely required, but signs of developing infection are actively sought and treated. Some full-thickness burns require surgical excision and skin grafting.

> **In the case of burns sustained in a house fire, careful attention must be paid to the airway**. The airway may initially appear patent, but it can rapidly become obstructed by oedema from thermal inhalation injury. Early elective intubation should be considered.

Children with extensive burns, or burns affecting important areas such as the face, hands or perineum, are treated in a specialist burns centre.

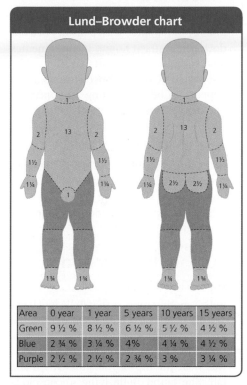

Lund–Browder chart

Area	0 year	1 year	5 years	10 years	15 years
Green	9 ½ %	8 ½ %	6 ½ %	5 ½ %	4 ½ %
Blue	2 ¾ %	3 ¼ %	4%	4 ¼ %	4 ½ %
Purple	2 ½ %	2 ½ %	2 ¾ %	3 %	3 ¼ %

Figure 16.6 The Lund–Browder chart is used to calculate percentage total body surface area of burns in children. Different percentages are used in children of different ages. The ratio of the surface area of the head and neck to the surface area of the limbs, is larger in a child than an adult.

Burns: assessment of thickness

Feature	Superficial	Partial thickness	Full thickness
Structures affected	Epidermis only	Epidermis, with some damage to dermis	Epidermis, dermis and deeper structures (e.g. nerves)
Skin appearance	Erythematous	Pale pink or mottled	White or charred
Blistering?	No	Yes	No
Pain	Yes	Yes, hypersensitive	No
Reduced/absent sensation	No	Hypersensitive	Yes
Capillary refill time	Brisk	Brisk	Absent

Table 16.7 Assessment of thickness of burns injuries

Case 30 Head injury

Presentation

Bella is 8 years old. She is en route to hospital by ambulance with a history of a fall down the stairs at home. The paramedics have rung ahead to report that after an initial period of loss of consciousness, Bella appears to be responding appropriately and her observations are satisfactory.

Initial interpretation

Bella appears to be stable at present; however, she has had a substantial fall, with potential for significant head and neck injuries. Therefore she requires thorough assessment.

Further history and examination

Bella's mother reports that Bella had been getting ready for school when she slipped and fell down the stairs. The fall was unwitnessed, but her mother thinks Bella was near the top of the stairs when she fell. She found Bella lying unconscious at the bottom of the stairs. Bella regained consciousness after about 3 minutes. She vomited once in the ambulance and is complaining of a headache.

Bella's ABC are assessed and are within normal limits. Her cervical spine has been triple immobilised. On arrival, Bella's Glasgow coma scale was 15/15, but it is now fluctuating between 9 and 14. Her left pupil is dilated and poorly reactive to light.

Working diagnosis

Bella's fluctuating Glasgow coma scale score and abnormal pupil reactions raises concerns of a brain injury with increased intracranial pressure.

Immediate intervention

Although Bella's ABC are currently satisfactory, she is electively intubated because of her deteriorating Glasgow coma scale score. Intravenous fluids are started to optimise cerebral perfusion, and she is nursed in a head-up position. She is sent for an urgent CT scan of her head, which shows left frontal and temporal extradural haemorrhages (**Figure 16.7**). Therefore Bella is referred for an urgent neurosurgical opinion.

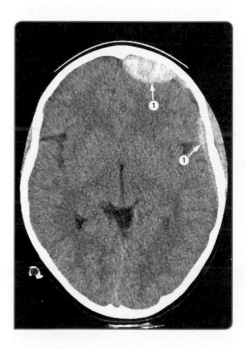

Figure 16.7 A CT scan showing left frontal and temporal extradural haemorrhages, with some mass effect ①.

Head injuries

These are common. For example, about 4011 per 100,000 children in England and Wales attend the emergency department with a head injury every year. Of these, 280 per 100,000 require admission for > 24 h. In most children the injury is mild, but 5.6 per 100,000 have an injury serious enough to require admission to the paediatric intensive care unit.

The causes of head injury vary across age groups. The commonest cause in older children is road traffic accidents, mainly as pedestrians. In younger children it is falls, and in the under-1s, being dropped or non-accidental injury. If a 'fall' is unwitnessed, the injury could have been sustained from a collapse caused by an underlying condition.

Brain injury is classified as primary or secondary.

- A primary brain injury occurs at the time of impact, with damage to neurones, blood vessels and brain cells
- A secondary brain injury results from the later consequences of the initial injury, and includes hypoxia, hypotension and increased intracranial pressure from cerebral oedema or an expanding bleed

Management

Management of a head injury depends on its mode and severity. Assessment of ABC takes priority and includes the cervical spine when trauma is evident. Particular attention is given to adequate analgesia and to treatment of hypoxia or hypotension to minimise secondary brain injury. Urgent CT scanning of the head is required if there are features of a significant head injury (**Table 16.8**). A skull radiograph is not indicated, unless non-accidental injury is suspected and is therefore performed as part of the skeletal survey.

Head injury: indications for head CT scan	
Features in the history	Signs
Witnessed loss of consciousness lasting > 5 min	Paediatric GCS score < 14 on arrival at the accident and emergency department (or < 15 in the under 1 age group)
Amnesia (antegrade or retrograde) lasting > 5 min	Paediatric GCS score < 15 by 2 h after the injury
Clinical suspicion of non-accidental injury	Abnormal drowsiness
Three or more discrete episodes of vomiting	A bruise, swelling or laceration > 5 cm in size on head (in children under 1 year)
Dangerous mechanism of injury (e.g. high-speed road traffic accident, fall from > 3 m)	Suspicion of open or depressed skull injury or tense fontanelle
	Focal neurological deficit
Post-traumatic seizure with no history of epilepsy	Any sign of basal skull fracture, e.g. haemotympanum (blood behind the ear drum), 'panda' eyes (bilateral 'black eye'), cerebrospinal fluid leakage from ears or nose, Battle's sign*

*Battle's sign: discoloration behind the ear, associated with a basilar skull fracture.

Table 16.8 Indications for CT scanning in a child with a head injury. GCS, Glasgow coma scale

Neurosurgical referral is indicated if intracranial bleeding is identified, although intervention may not always be required.

Admission for a period of observation should be considered. However, patients who are asymptomatic, with a low-risk mechanism of injury, can usually be discharged home with advice on the signs and symptoms of increased intracranial pressure.

> **Promotion of head injury prevention,** such as use of bicycle helmets, is vital to help reduce the number of significant head injuries in children.

Chapter 17
Community paediatrics and integrated care

Starter questions

Answers to the following questions are on page 441.

1. Why are chest X-rays always repeated a week later in child protection cases?
2. What is 'fever phobia'?
3. Why do the palliative care team care for children who are not dying?

Introduction

The structure of paediatric healthcare networks varies from country to country. However, it always consists of a multidisciplinary team with specialists managing different aspects of paediatric health, such as health promotion, disease prevention, and management of acute illnesses, chronic conditions and neurodisabilities. This chapter will use the UK service structure as basis for demonstrating the general principles of community and integrated paediatric care. In the UK most community-based care for healthy children is delivered by general practitioners (GPs) and health visitors, sometimes with input from community paediatricians supported by a multidisciplinary team:

- General practitioners carry out routine examination of babies as part of child health surveillance programmes, and they are also the first contact during acute illness

- Health visitors offer general support and advice to families with children under the age of 5 years, for example in the areas of parenting skills, health, nutrition and child development; they also offer additional support for vulnerable children
- Community paediatricians oversee care for children with significant problems or more complex needs, for example long-term physical disabilities and learning disabilities (or difficulties). They usually take the lead in child protection cases;

they also have a key role in monitoring the health of children in foster care
- Good communication between the multidisciplinary team is essential to ensure the best care for the child
- Hospital paediatricians (who may be general paediatricians or specialists in a particular field, e.g. paediatric cardiology) treat acute illnesses that cannot be managed in primary care and paediatric conditions outside the scope of general practice

Case 31 Unexplained bruising in a baby

Presentation

Logan is a 4-month-old baby who has been referred to the community paediatrician by his GP from the routine vaccination clinic. When Logan was undressed, she noted a bruise on his right thigh. When questioned, his mother, Jessie, said she was unaware of the bruise and could not offer an explanation as to its cause.

Initial interpretation

Any unexplained bruise in a child, especially in a baby who has yet to start crawling, requires thorough evaluation. Although Logan's mother cannot provide a reason as to the origin of the bruise, there may be an innocent explanation. However, non-accidental injury must be considered, as well as other underlying pathology.

Further history

Jessie recalls that when she came home from the shop the previous night, Logan was crying. He was on the floor with his 2-year-old brother, playing with some toys. Joe, Jessie's partner, thought Logan was just hungry, and when he gave Logan a bottle he soon settled. She cannot recall any other unusual incident. Logan is otherwise a well baby, who is happy and has

a good appetite. Jessie has no concerns regarding Logan's development.

Examination

Logan is happy and smiling, and is sat in his mother's arms. He appears clean and well cared for, and his weight is at about the 75th centile. Examination of Logan's skin finds a 1 cm × 2 cm oval bruise on his right thigh, but no other bruising or marks. The rest of the examination is normal.

Interpretation of findings

Logan's bruise is in an unusual location for accidental injury, even if he were mobile. It may have been caused accidentally by his toddler brother during some rough play, but this should not be assumed. The bruise may have been caused by pressure from a thumb, but this explanation cannot be considered certain.

Bruises cannot be accurately aged by their appearance and attempts to do this should be avoided. Logan's bruise remains an unexplained injury, and although the rest of the examination is normal, he requires further investigations to look for any additional injuries which may be hidden.

Investigations

A skeletal survey (radiographs of the whole body), CT scan of the head

Case 31 continued

Non-accidental injury: management

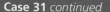

Dr Lowry, Logan's paediatrician, explores the family structure then explains why further investigations are needed

Investigation results and Logan's social situation are discussed at a strategy meeting with Dr Lowry, a social worker, a health visitor and police officer

Your GP was worried about the bruise on Logan's thigh. Do you know what happened?

This is a nightmare! How can they think I'd ever hurt him?!

I'm not sure. I only noticed it today. He was crying last night, playing with his brother, but calmed down with his bottle

Logan appears healthy and well cared for. His investigations are normal, apart from an old posterior rib fracture

They have no history with social services. Logan lives with his mum, Jessie, her boyfriend, Joe, and a 2-year-old brother

The house seemed a little chaotic but Jessie engages well with the children. She had a black eye once, but blamed a door

I'm sure you understand we always look carefully at bruises in children, especially babies. We're not accusing you of anything, but it's routine for us to perform some investigations. Logan will be admitted while they're done

The group agrees there is a concern of non-accidental injury, but that it is safe to discharge Logan under Jessie's care and his grandmother's supervision while investigations are ongoing

We have concerns that Logan has some unexplained injuries. Does Joe look after the children often?

Sometimes, when I work, but he wouldn't hurt them...he hit me once, but he was drunk and really sorry about it...

We need to investigate further, but you and the children must stay with your mother

Logan is fully examined and investigations are arranged to identify any other injuries, old or new, or other underlying medical problems

and ophthalmological examination are carried out to look for bony injuries, intracranial haemorrhages and retinal haemorrhages. Screening blood tests are also done to rule out bleeding tendency, such as that caused by a clotting abnormality, or vitamin D deficiency. A healing posterior rib fracture is discovered on radiography. The rest of the investigation results are normal.

Diagnosis

Once investigations have been completed a strategy meeting is arranged. It is attended by a paediatrician, a social worker, Logan's health visitor and the police.

It is established that the family have had no previous contact with social services. The health visitor reports that Jessie has always engaged appropriately with health care professionals, but the house appears chaotic at times. On one home visit, Jessie was noted to have a black eye, which she said was caused by walking into a door. The police report having attended two episodes of domestic disturbance at Logan's home address.

Looking at all the available evidence, a diagnosis of non-accidental injury is strongly suspected as the cause of the bruising and posterior rib fracture. With a history of violence, Jessie's partner Joe is a key suspect, but no definitive evidence is available. The social services department decide that Logan can be safely discharged into Jessie's care provided that the family are accompanied by Logan's grandmother (who is deemed capable of providing support and supervision) while further enquiries are carried out.

Case 32 Delayed speech in a 3-year-old

Presentation

Sam is 3 years old. He has been referred to the community paediatric outpatients' clinic. Sam's parents and health visitor are concerned that his speech is limited to about 50 words. He does not yet join any words together, and he does not seem to be making any further progress with his language development.

Initial interpretation

A 3-year-old is expected to have a vocabulary comprising a few hundred words, as well as the ability to form basic two- or three-word sentences. Therefore Sam has delayed speech. There are many possible causes for this. Further history is required to establish whether he has an isolated communication delay or whether he is also delayed in other developmental domains. The latter would indicate a global developmental delay.

Further history

Sam's gross and fine motor development appears to be normal. His mother reports that when he does speak, he is difficult to understand, and that he will sometimes repeat words over and over again. He does not ask for objects directly or point to indicate what he wants.

At home, Sam likes to play with his trains and spends hours lining them up in order of size. He gets very upset if his older brother moves his trains. Sometimes, he spends a long time just opening and closing the kitchen door. At nursery Sam tends to play by himself, showing no interest in the other children.

Examination

Physical examination is normal; Sam has no dysmorphic features or signs of any neurodevelopmental condition, such as tuberous sclerosis. During the consultation, Sam avoids all eye contact and does not smile socially. However, he appears happy playing with some bricks, arranging them in colour order.

Interpretation of findings

Sam is showing many features typically seen in autism (see **Table 17.6**). However, a diagnosis cannot be made on the basis of one consultation alone.

Investigations

A hearing test is arranged, the results of which rule out hearing loss as a cause for Sam's speech delay. There is no single test to confirm a diagnosis of autism, but a report from Sam's nursery is requested, along with a formal speech and language assessment.

Diagnosis

A detailed diagnostic assessment by an autism specialist is arranged (see page 431). Should a diagnosis of autism be confirmed, Sam's family will be provided with sources of information and support. They will be taught strategies to help develop Sam's communication skills and for dealing with any difficult behaviour. Sam will require an educational assessment before starting school, because children with autism respond best to specialised teaching styles.

Immunisation

Immunisation activates the immune system to mount a protective response to an infectious disease. The two types of immunisation are:

■ Active immunity, produced by an individual's own immune system in response to inoculation with a vaccine that comprises an attenuated (weakened) strain or inactivated components of a bacteria or virus; it is usually long-lasting

■ Passive immunity, in which protection is conferred by the transfer of antibodies from immune individuals, for example respiratory syncytial virus immunoglobulin; it is usually temporary, often only lasting a few weeks

Immunisations are usually provided in primary care settings or schools, delivered as part of a wider child health promotion programme.

Vaccination saves an estimated 2–3 million lives per year worldwide. The smallpox vaccine was the first to be discovered and its use in children became widespread by the late 1800s in developed countries. Smallpox was declared eradicated in 1980.

In most countries there is a comprehensive childhood immunisation programme for all children available (**Figure 17.1**). Additional vaccinations are offered when children are at higher risk of particular diseases (**Table 17.1**).

Vaccination schedules change with time, to match changing disease prevalence. For example, following introduction of the meningitis C vaccine to the UK in 1999 the overall level of invasive meningococcal disease decreased, with group B strains accounting for > 80% of cases and an increase in meningitis W

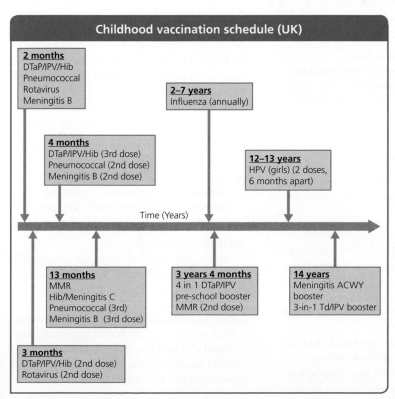

Figure 17.1 A typical childhood vaccination schedule (this is the UK schedule). DTaP/IPV, four-in-one diphtheria, tetanus, acellular pertussis and polio vaccine; DtaP/IPV/Hib, five-in-one diphtheria, tetanus, acellular pertussis, polio and *Haemophilus influenzae* type B vaccine; HPV, human papilloma virus vaccine (cervical cancer vaccine); MMR, measles, mumps and rubella vaccine; Td/IPV, three-in-one tetanus, diphtheria and polio.

Childhood vaccination schedule (UK)

2 months
DTaP/IPV/Hib
Pneumococcal
Rotavirus
Meningitis B

2–7 years
Influenza (annually)

4 months
DTaP/IPV/Hib (3rd dose)
Pneumococcal (2nd dose)
Meningitis B (2nd dose)

12–13 years
HPV (girls) (2 doses, 6 months apart)

Time (Years)

13 months
MMR
Hib/Meningitis C
Pneumococcal (3rd)
Meningitis B (3rd dose)

3 years 4 months
4 in 1 DTaP/IPV
pre-school booster
MMR (2nd dose)

14 years
Meningitis ACWY
booster
3-in-1 Td/IPV booster

3 months
DTaP/IPV/Hib (2nd dose)
Rotavirus (2nd dose)

Indications for additional vaccinations

Vaccine	Time of administration	Subjects who require vaccine
Bacillus Calmette–Guérin (BCG) vaccine	At birth (or up to 16 years if at risk and the vaccine has not previously been given)	Baby born to household originating from a country with a high rate of tuberculosis (prevalence > 40 per 100,000)
		Baby born in locality with a high rate of tuberculosis in a low-rate country (e.g. some areas of London)
Hepatitis B vaccine	At birth, 1 month, 2 months and 1 year	Child whose mothers or close contacts are hepatitis B–positive (with acute or chronic infection)
		(Hepatitis B immunoglobulin is also given to provide passive protection for children of highly infectious mothers)
Chickenpox vaccine	When indicated	Close contacts of immunocompromised child if they have not been previously exposed (it is a live vaccine so cannot be given directly to an immunocompromised child)
Influenza vaccine	During influenza season annually (all 2- to 7-year-olds routinely vaccinated)	Child with chronic conditions, such as asthma, diabetes and congenital heart disease

Table 17.1 Indications for additional vaccinations that are not on the typical schedule shown in **Figure 17.1**.

infections. Therefore, in 2014, the A, W and Y strains were added to the vaccine containing the adolescent meningitis C dose, and in 2015, immunisation against meningitis B was added to the vaccination schedule for infants.

> **For infants who were born prematurely, follow the immunisation schedule according to their chronological age rather than their corrected gestational age.**

Vaccine failure

No vaccine offers 100% protection against a particular disease. Vaccine failure is primary or secondary.

- In primary failure, there is no initial immune response to the vaccine. The rate this occurs varies between vaccinations and their components, e.g. 5–10% of children do not respond to the measles component of the first dose of the MMR vaccine
- In secondary failure, the initial immune response is good but the resulting protection wanes over time (this is the reason why a preschool booster against pertussis is required)

Vaccine controversies

Scientific evidence for the benefits of vaccination is strong. Nevertheless, media scares have led some parents to believe that vaccines cause frequent and significant harm, as happened with respect to the MMR vaccine in the late 1990s and early 2000s (see Box on page 423). Religious belief is another reason for objecting to vaccines.

Minor adverse effects and adverse reactions do occur. Most commonly these are:

- local reaction, in the form of pain, redness or swelling at the site of injection
- mild non-specific illness starting up to 10 days after vaccination (e.g. for the measles, mumps and rubella vaccine)

These minor adverse effects do not preclude further vaccinations.

There are very few absolute contraindications to vaccination. Examples include anaphylactic reaction (an estimated 0.2–1 cases per million vaccinations) and severe reaction to a previous similar vaccine. Live vaccinations are contraindicated in immunosuppressed children (see page 294). Vaccinations should be deferred during a febrile or severe illness, but not for a mild illness.

Children who cannot be vaccinated for medical reasons, or who are too young to have been vaccinated, are protected by 'herd immunity'. This is the immunity provided when a sufficient proportion of a population is immune to a disease, which effectively prevents its transmission. If vaccine uptake in a population falls below the level required for herd immunity, an epidemic can occur, as demonstrated by a measles outbreak in Wales in 2013.

When parents have concerns about vaccination, the best approach is process. Listen carefully to their concerns, and try to correct misinformation and misunderstanding of the evidence. It is helpful to put adverse effects in perspective; for example, a child's risk of encephalopathy is 1 in 1000 in measles but 1 in 1,000,000 after measles vaccination.

Child health surveillance

Child health surveillance is a formalised programme to overview the physical, social and emotional health and development of every child. It aim is to improve health and wellbeing during childhood and beyond – health in childhood and adolescence has an influence into adult life. Surveillance starts at birth and continues into the late teens, though it focuses on the early years.

The composition of child health surveillance programmes differs from country to country, but usually includes:

- Monitoring physical growth (see pages 20–22)
- Monitoring intellectual and social development (see pages 31–37)
- Screening for certain conditions (see below)
- Immunisation for disease prevention (see pages 421–423)
- Health promotion, including provision of information and support for parents (see below)

These are delivered by a range of health care professionals, mainly GPs, health visitors, school nurses and midwives, in an integrated programme that is usually dictated by a regional or national framework. Examples include the Healthy Child Programme in England which covers pregnancy and the first 5 years of life, the Healthy School Child Programme covering children aged 5–12, and the Adolescent Health Programme covering young people up to the age of 18. Child health surveillance may commence prenatally, as the English programme does, then specific assessments are carried out at defined ages (**Figure 17.2**), with additional interventions targeted at children considered to be at risk of poorer outcomes, such as those with chronic illness or subject to social deprivation.

Child health surveillance programmes use standardised documentation to record information collected over time, for example the 'red book' used in England, Scotland, Wales and Northern Ireland. Parents are given the 'red book' at the time of birth. It is the child's personal child health record and functions as a method of communication between health care professionals coming into contact with the child up to the age of 5 years. It records growth and vaccination status, and provides information for parents on normal development and common childhood problems. In tandem, the health care professionals use a 'Green Book', a government-produced reference on all available vaccinations and the diseases which they prevent.

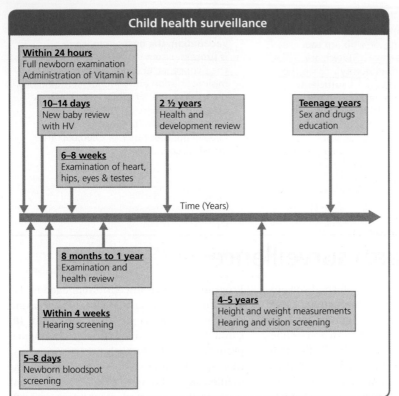

Figure 17.2 A typical timeline for child health surveillance.

Child health surveillance

Within 24 hours
Full newborn examination
Administration of Vitamin K

10–14 days
New baby review with HV

2 ½ years
Health and development review

Teenage years
Sex and drugs education

6–8 weeks
Examination of heart, hips, eyes & testes

Time (Years)

8 months to 1 year
Examination and health review

4–5 years
Height and weight measurements
Hearing and vision screening

Within 4 weeks
Hearing screening

5–8 days
Newborn bloodspot screening

Child health promotion strategies

Strategy	Examples
General health promotion	Diet and exercise advice to prevent obesity
	Promotion of benefits of breastfeeding
	Smoking cessation advice to improve parental health and minimise effects on children
	Accident prevention advice (at home and on the road)
Disease prevention	Folic acid supplementation in early pregnancy to prevent neural tube defects
	Vitamin K for all newborns to prevent haemorrhagic disease of the newborn
	Childhood immunisation programme
	Vitamin D supplementation for all pregnant and breastfeeding women, and all children aged 6 months to 5 years, to prevent vitamin D deficiency and its complications
	Sleeping advice to prevent sudden unexpected infant death
Screening	Antenatal screening of mothers for HIV and hepatitis B, to reduce risk of vertical transmission
	Newborn hearing screening
	Newborn blood spot screening (see page 425)
	Physical examination at birth, 6 weeks and 8 months to identify congenital anomalies, including heart or hip problems and cataracts
Safeguarding	Identification and prevention of child abuse (see page 432)

Table 17.2 Strategies used in child health promotion

Various child health promotion strategies are employed during the scheduled assessments, as listed in **Table 17.2** and described in Chapter 1. Emotional and psychological wellbeing are also considered: strong parent–child attachment, aiming for a stable relationship with loving yet authoritative parenting, provides the best environment to nurture a child.

> **Smoking cessation advice is an example of prenatal commencement of child health promotion.** Smoking during pregnancy has effects on the fetus that persist into childhood. Children are affected further by second-hand cigarette smoke in the home (see page 426).

Screening

The aim of screening is to identify serious conditions before symptoms arise. Early diagnosis and treatment increase the likelihood of survival and prevent secondary complications. In most health surveillance programmes, screening is offered to all children for:

- A number of inherited disorders (newborn blood spot screening)
- Hearing
- Vision

> **The principles underlying screening are:**
>
> - The condition has a significant impact on health, an asymptomatic early stage and a well-understood natural history
> - The test is simple, safe and valid, with good sensitivity and specificity
> - There is an effective treatment or intervention that improves the outcome
> - The screening programme is cost-effective and acceptable to the population

Newborn blood spot screening

The newborn blood spot screening ('heel prick test') is offered in the first days of life (e.g. days 5–8 in England). A heel prick blood sample is obtained and placed onto a sampling area on a pre-printed card that is sent to the laboratory. The list of conditions screened by the test differs from country to country; many are inherited metabolic diseases. In England the list comprises:

- Inherited metabolic diseases:
  - phenylketonuria
  - medium-chain acyl-coenzyme A dehydrogenase deficiency (MCADD)
  - maple syrup urine disease
  - isovaleric acidaemia

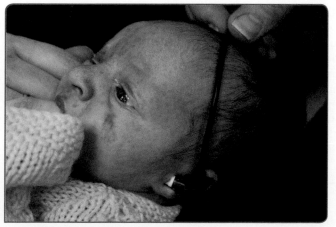

Figure 17.3 A baby undergoing newborn hearing screening.

- glutaric aciduria type 1
- homocystinuria

- Other inherited diseases:
  - congenital hypothyroidism
  - cystic fibrosis
  - sickle cell disease

Early identification of such diseases helps prevent severe disability or death by enabling early treatment, for example by instigating dietary adjustment for babies with phenylketonuria or MCADD, or thyroxine replacement for those with congenital hypothyroidism.

> **Screening for phenylketonuria was introduced in the early 1960s and became the prototype for universal newborn screening programmes.** If phenylketonuria is detected at birth and a specialised diet started, the profound cognitive impairment it would otherwise cause is averted.

Hearing

All newborn babies undergo hearing screening soon after birth, using one of the following techniques:

- an otoacoustic emission test, which records the response of the cochlea to sound (**Figure 17.3**)
- an automated auditory brainstem response test, which records brain activity in response to sound

Some countries use the latter test as their primary screening method. Others, such as the UK, uses the otoacoustic emission test for most babies, although it also checks automated auditory brainstem response in those at increased risk of hearing impairment, for example those born before term.

Early identification of hearing impairment enables early interventions to begin, to help with language and communication. In the UK all children have a further hearing test on entry to primary school.

Monitoring

Growth and development are regularly monitored, with more frequent checks for

Child development 'red flags'	
Developmental domain	Red flags
Gross motor skills	Excessive head lag past the age of 6 weeks
	Inability to sit or weight-bear at 12 months
	Not standing or walking by 18 months
	Asymmetry of gait or unsteadiness at 2–3 years
Fine motor skills and vision	Not staring or fixing on face by 6 weeks
	No pincer grip by 12–18 months
	Hand preference before 18 months
	Unable to build a three-brick tower at 2 years
Hearing, speech and language	Failure to respond to sound at any age
	No babbling by 9–12 months
	No words with meaning, or no recognition of own name, by 18 months
	Fewer than 50 words by 2 years
	No plurals or asking questions by 3 years
Personal and social skills	No social smile by 6 weeks
	Not playing with other children at 3 years

Table 17.3 'Red flags' in child development

children considered at higher risk of growth problems, for example infants who were born prematurely.

Advice on smoking cessation

Parents are provided with advice on smoking cessation as part of general health promotion strategies. Both maternal cigarette smoking during pregnancy and inhalation of secondhand cigarette smoke (passive smoking) during childhood are detrimental to a child's health.

- Smoking during pregnancy increases the likelihood of stillbirth and preterm birth, low birth weight and reduced lung function in the child

- The effects of secondhand smoke on children include more frequent and severe asthma attacks, respiratory infections, ear infections and otitis media with effusion (glue ear) and sudden unexpected death in infancy (SUDI)

Advice on smoking cessation is also necessary because children whose parents or other family members smoke are more likely to start smoking. Most adults who smoke started doing so during their teenage years.

Developmental delay and learning difficulties

Normal development follows a set pathway in which motor, proprioceptive and social skills are acquired sequentially (see Chapter 1). Developmental delay is defined as being present when a child has not acquired a particular skill by an age more than two standard deviations from the average age at which the skill is usually acquired. It is a spectrum, with symptoms varying from mild learning difficulties to global developmental delay.

Global developmental delay is defined as significant delay in at least two of the four standard developmental domains:

- gross motor skills
- fine motor skills and vision
- hearing and language
- personal and social skills

> **Intellectual disability** describes an impairment in learning new information or skills, which affects the ability to live independently. Although there is a spectrum from mild to severe, an individual's IQ is generally low (<70). Individuals with **learning difficulties** generally have an IQ >70, but problems with specific types of learning (e.g. dyslexia).

Epidemiology and aetiology

About 2% of the general population have some degree of developmental delay or learning difficulty or disability, with more boys affected than girls. In most cases, no underlying cause is found, but common causes are discussed in the following sections.

Gross motor skills

Cerebral palsy (see page 257) and muscular dystrophy (see page 261) usually present with delayed gross motor milestones. However, delayed gross motor skills are often components of global developmental delay.

Fine motor skills and vision

Fine motor skills rely on good vision. Strabismus ('squint'), i.e. abnormal alignment of the eyes, and refractory errors are common. Congenital cataract and glaucoma are rare (4 per 10,000 and 1 per 10,000 births, respectively, in the UK). Severe visual impairment or blindness is also rare, affecting 0.4 per 1,000 babies, 25% of whom have low birthweight. Causes include optic nerve hypoplasia and retinopathy of prematurity. Some babies have cortical blindness, i.e. the structure of the eye is normal but the cortex is unable to interpret the nerve signals it receives from the eye; this condition can improve with time.

In children with normal vision, delayed fine motor skills are associated with global developmental delay or cerebellar signs.

> **Congenital cataract requires** early surgery, i.e. within the first 3 months of life, for the baby to develop fixation and binocular reflexes.

Speech and language

Delay in the development of speech and communication is caused by:

- hearing impairment, either sensorineural (nerve deafness) or conductive (middle ear dysfunction)

- developmental language problems, i.e. global developmental delay or autism spectrum disorder (see page 430)

Conductive deafness affects 5–10% children and is usually temporary, caused by glue ear. However, if it is of significant duration it can affect speech and education.

The incidence of bilateral profound deafness is 1.5 per 1000 children under 5 years of age. Mostly, it is sensorineural, caused by genetic abnormalities of the hair cells in the cochlea or the result of maternal factors in pregnancy (e.g. CMV infection, drugs, toxins, alcohol).

Personal and social skills

A delay or impairment in the development of personal and social skills can be related to a condition such as autism spectrum disorder (see page 430) or secondary to child abuse (especially neglect or emotional abuse).

Clinical features

The presentation of developmental delay depends on the domains affected and on its extent and severity. Failures to achieve specific milestones by certain ages are considered 'red flags' (**Table 17.3**) that warrant more detailed assessment (see page 426).

The milder learning difficulties may not become evident until school age, and may present with disruptive behaviour or struggling to keep up with the class.

Relevant information in the history includes any developmental regression, family history of developmental delay or genetic disorders and consanguinity. Other features that should be sought are:

- dysmorphic features
- inadequate growth and unkempt appearance, which may suggest neglect and therefore lack of stimulation
- anaemia
- Head circumference
- birthmarks
- unusual behaviour, such as lack of eye contact

A multidisciplinary clinical assessment, for example including input from physiotherapists for children with cerebral palsy, is carried out.

Investigative approach

Investigation of developmental delay depends on the specific concern identified. The primary aim is early identification of any treatable cause, such as iron deficiency anaemia or hypothyroidism. Appropriate investigations are shown in **Table 17.4.**

> **Hearing is tested** in all children presenting with delayed speech.

Management

Management of developmental delay depends on the underlying diagnosis made and the specific delay it causes. Support is given to enable the child to reach their full potential. Children with complex disabilities require a multidisciplinary approach, the overall coordination being managed by a community paediatrician. The community paediatrician also treats any associated medical problems.

To address problems at school, the child may be assessed by an educational psychologist; any required additional classroom assistance is supplied. Children with more complex needs are educated in special schools, with a curriculum tailored to their abilities.

> **Cochlear implants are recommended for children who have profound bilateral sensorineural hearing loss and in whom the auditory (cochlear) nerve is functioning normally.** The best results are obtained if the cochlear implants are inserted before the age of 18 months.

Developmental delay: investigations	
Investigations	Underlying condition or typical clinical features
First line	
Full blood count	Anaemia
Ferritin level	Iron deficiency anaemia
Vitamin B$_{12}$ level	Anaemia
Creatinine kinase level	Muscular dystrophy
Thyroid function tests	Hypothyroidism
Urine metabolic screen (amino acids and organic acids)	Inborn errors of metabolism
Array comparative genomic hybridisation (molecular karyotype)	Genetic conditions
DNA test for fragile X syndrome	Fragile X syndrome
Second line	
Metabolic screen (blood and urine)	Family history, consanguinity, developmental regression, acute encephalopathy, recurrent vomiting, organomegaly, coarse features, hypotonia
Neuroimaging (MRI and CT)	Abnormal head size, seizures, focal neurological signs
EEG (consider 24-h EEG)	Speech regression, seizures, neurodegenerative disorder
Genetics referral (consider skeletal survey)	Dysmorphism, abnormal growth, unusual behaviour associated with attention deficit hyperactivity disorder or autism spectrum disorder, consanguinity, family history
Blood lead level	Pica, old house (lead from old paint), family from a low- or medium-income countries
EEG, electroencephalography.	

Table 17.4 Investigations in a child presenting with developmental delay

Behavioural disorders

Common behavioural disorders include attention deficit hyperactivity disorder (ADHD) and autism spectrum disorder. The main features of both commence in the child's first few years, and become more noticeable when circumstances change, such as starting school. Children with ADHD or autism spectrum disorder also often have other mental health conditions (**Table 17.5**).

The diagnosis is often initially suspected by the child's parents, school or nursery staff or a health visitor. Formal assessment is carried out by a child psychiatrist, community paediatrician or learning disability specialist. It includes the use of formalised questionnaires for completion by parents and teachers.

Attention deficit hyperactivity disorder

Attention deficit hyperactivity disorder is the term for a group of symptoms that include inattentiveness, hyperactivity and impulsiveness. It is not just part of a developmental disorder or a 'difficult phase'. It is the most common behavioural disorder in developed countries, affecting 5–8% of school-age children. Boys are more likely to be affected than girls (ratio, 3:1). However, ADHD may be underdiagnosed in girls, in whom the less noticeable symptom of inattentiveness is most common.

The exact cause of ADHD is unknown, but it can be familial and is more likely to affect

Conditions associated with ADHD or autism spectrum disorder	
Condition	**Description**
Anxiety disorder	Worry and anxiety
	May also cause physical symptoms of panic attacks (tachycardia, sweating and dizziness)
Autism spectrum disorder	Impairments in social interaction, communication and behaviour
Conduct disorder	Tendency towards highly antisocial behaviour (e.g. stealing, fighting, vandalism and harming people or animals)
Learning difficulties	For example dyslexia
Sleep problems	Difficulty getting to sleep at night, and irregular sleeping patterns
Oppositional defiant disorder	Negative and disruptive behaviour, particularly towards authority figures such as parents and teachers
Depression	Low mood
Tourette's syndrome	A combination of involuntary noises and movements (tics)

Table 17.5 Conditions often associated with attention deficit hyperactivity disorder or autism spectrum disorder

children born before term or with low birthweight, or to mothers who drank alcohol or misused drugs during pregnancy. It is more common in children with intellectual disabilities, such as Down's syndrome.

> **Many children have restless or inattentive phases.** The presence of symptoms in at least two different settings, e.g. home and school, make it more likely that there is ADHD rather than a simple lack of parental control or a reaction to certain teachers.

Clinical features

The symptoms of ADHD are divided into two categories:

- inattentiveness, i.e. the child has a short attention span or is easily distracted
- hyperactivity and impulsiveness, manifesting as restlessness, constant fidgeting or overactivity

Most but not all children with ADHD have problems in both categories. Either category can result in underachievement at school, poor social interaction or problems with discipline.

Diagnostic approach

The diagnosis is based on observation rather than investigation results, and includes a set of clear criteria in which six or more specific symptoms of both inattention and hyperactivity must be present. They must also:

- be continuous for ≥ 6 months
- occur before the age of 12 years
- occur in at least two different settings
- affect the child's relationships with other people or academic achievement

Management

Mild or moderate ADHD is managed with several behavioural strategies applied in parallel, using an approach tailored to the individual child. Children with severe ADHD may be treated with central nervous system stimulants, such as methylphenidate, usually under specialist guidance. The symptoms of ADHD usually improve with age, but up to 60% continue to experience symptoms as adults.

Autism spectrum disorder

Autism spectrum disorder impairs social interaction and communication, with restricted or stereotyped behaviours. There is a wide spectrum of severity. In the UK, it is estimated to affect 1% of the population. The exact cause is unknown; it is a complex condition caused by interactions between genetic and environmental factors.

Clinical features

Autism spectrum disorder causes a wide range of symptoms, which are grouped into two categories:

- problems with social interaction and communication
- restricted and repetitive patterns of thought, interests and physical behaviours

Specific examples are given in **Table 17.6** Features of autism are often recognised by parents, nursery teachers or other professionals involved with the child before the age of 3 years and become more noticeable with age.

Children with Asperger's syndrome have fewer problems with speech and are usually of average or above average intelligence. They do not have the learning disabilities associated with autism, but they may have ADHD.

> **Parental concern about a child's social development should prompt assessment of their behaviour.** In most cases, the concern is justified.

Diagnostic approach

There is no individual test to confirm a diagnosis of autism spectrum disorder. Assessment combines information from nursery or school staff and a detailed clinical observation of the child to evaluate their use of language, behaviour, cognitive ability and interaction with others.

Management

There is no medication for the core symptoms of autism spectrum disorder, but medication is available to treat some of the related symptoms or conditions, such as melatonin for disordered sleep. Various techniques are used to help improve communication skills, social interaction and the ability to build relationships; these include the use of:

- visual aids: objects, line drawings or picture cards that plan a daily routine,

Autism: features	
Area of impairment	Examples
Social interaction	Preference for playing alone
	Poor eye contact
	Lack of understanding of non-verbal social cues
	Problems understanding and being aware of other people's emotions and feelings
Communication	Delayed speech development (various degrees)
	Echolalia (repetition of words or phrases)
Pattern of interests and behaviours	Lack of imaginative play
	Repetitive behaviours (e.g. hand flapping, opening and closing doors)
	Distress on change to everyday routines

Table 17.6 Features of autism

introduce new activities or situations, or manage behaviour

- picture exchange communication system (PECS): used in children with little or no verbal communication skills. Picture cards are exchanged for a desired item
- Makaton (see box)
- toys, e.g sensory toys, toys that help develop fine motor skills or games that help develop social skills

About 50% of children with autism spectrum disorder also have learning disability and may require additional care and assistance to live independently as adults.

> **Makaton is a simplified 'language' comprising signs, speech and graphics to help people who have difficulty communicating.** In developmental delay it helps patients overcome the frustration of not being able to communicate.

Neglect, abuse and non-accidental injury

Child abuse is the maltreatment of a child. It can take the form of physical, emotional or sexual abuse, or neglect (**Table 17.7**). The most common form of abuse is neglect.

Because of under-reporting, there are no precise figures for the prevalence of child abuse. UK estimates are that about one in five children suffer from abuse at some point during childhood, and one child per week dies as a result of maltreatment.

Abuse is usually committed by someone known to the child. Risk factors that make children more susceptible to abuse include factors relating to:

- the child, for example prematurity or physical and learning disabilities
- the parents, for example mental health problems, alcohol or drug misuse, a history of abuse as a child
- the family, for example domestic violence, poor housing and social deprivation

Clinical features and diagnosis

Detection of abuse can be difficult; physical injuries are the easiest to identify. No injury is pathognomonic of abuse, but some are highly suspicious (**Table 17.8** and **Figure 17.4**).

> **Child safeguarding is the responsibility of all professionals, including teachers, who come into contact with children and their families.** They should remain vigilant at every encounter.

Physical abuse

A high index of suspicion is required in the case of any child presenting with physical injuries. The history is as informative as the examination. Consider the following.

- Has there been a delay in seeking medical attention?
- Is the history consistent with the injury observed and the developmental age of the child?
- Has the history been changing?

Forms of child abuse	
Type	Example
Physical	Any physical act causing pain or harm to the child (e.g. hitting or scalding)
Emotional	Repetitive behaviour leading to emotional harm or low self-esteem in a child
Sexual	Any sexual act including the participation of a child, regardless of whether physical contact is involved
Neglect	Lack of care or failure to attend to a child's basic needs (e.g. provision of food, hygiene, supervision and love)

Table 17.7 Different forms of child abuse

Injuries likely to be non-accidental	
Visible injury	Mechanism
Bruise or fracture in an immobile baby	Rough handling or excessive force in normal handling of baby, or deliberate hitting
Fractured ribs	Shaking
Retinal haemorrhages	Shaking
Torn frenulum	Blow to mouth or force-feeding
Injuries of different ages	Repeated episodes of abuse
Spiral fracture of the humerus	Twisting
Metaphyseal fractures	Twisting
Bruising behind the ear	Blow with hand
Small circular bruises	Fingertip marks
Ring of bruises	Human bite
Small circular burns	Cigarette burns
Burns or scalds to both feet or buttocks, especially with a 'tidemark'	Held in hot water

Table 17.8 Physical injuries raising a high suspicion of non-accidental injury

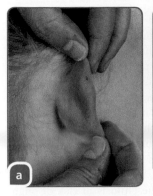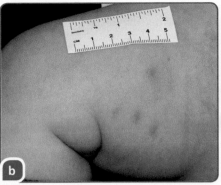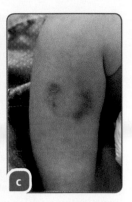

Figure 17.4 Examples of non-accidental injury. (a) Bruising behind the ear; bruising in unusual locations such as this should raise the suspicion of non-accidental injury. (b) Bruising on inner thigh caused by fingertips. (c) Bite marks on lower leg: input from a forensic dentist will help distinguish whether the bite was from an adult or a child.

Be aware that even an older child may be too scared to explain what really happened. Careful examination and detailed notes are essential, because they may be required as evidence in court. Bruises and other injuries must be measured accurately and documented by drawings; medical photographs are also taken, whenever possible.

> Remember, it is not possible to reliably determine the age of bruises from their appearance or colour.

> Consider the age and mobility of a young child when assessing bruises or fractures – 'those who don't cruise rarely bruise'.

Neglect and emotional abuse

These types of abuse are generally harder to detect than physical abuse. Neglect is absence of adequate parental care and supervision. Subtle signs can provide clues indicating the need for further investigation. These include:

- recurrent attendance at the GP clinic or accident and emergency department with accidental injuries
- poor general condition, growth and development of the child

- abnormal parent–child interaction, e.g. lack of empathy or response to cues for attention

Sexual abuse

A child may disclose sexual abuse to a trusted adult or friend. Alternatively, it may be suspected because of the observation of sexualised behaviour (e.g. precocious sexual knowledge) by the child or the finding of physical signs of sexual abuse. Some present with non-specific signs such as self-harm, becoming withdrawn or a change in behaviour. Physical signs include genital discharge or pain, dysuria or underage pregnancy. Clinical assessment of suspected sexual abuse is carried out by specially trained paediatricians.

Fabricated or induced illness

In fabricated or induced illness, a parent or carer (most commonly the child's mother) fakes or induces illness in a child as an attention-seeking behaviour. It is often diagnosed only with the benefit of time and hindsight, and can be difficult to prove. It should be considered when one or more of the following are observed:

- recurrent hospital admission with unusual or unexplained signs or symptoms
- a poor or unexpected response to treatment

- occurence of symptoms only when the child is in the care of a particular person.

Formerly, FII was known as Munchausen's syndrome by proxy.

Investigative approach

Any person who suspects maltreatment of a child has a responsibility to share this concern with the appropriate child safeguarding authority or social services department. This will trigger appropriate examination and investigations, which may include:

- a skeletal survey
- a head CT in babies to look for intracranial bleeds
- fundoscopy to detect retinal haemorrhages
- blood tests to rule out medical causes of any injuries (e.g. thrombocytopenia or coagulation problems)

A fracture in a baby or a young child, especially a rib fracture, may not be immediately apparent on radiography. However, a repeat radiograph 1 week later will show callus formation, making the fracture more obvious (**Figure 17.5**).

Management

Child protection procedures vary from country to country (and different terminology is used for similar procedures), but generally a set procedure is triggered in response to a report of suspected child abuse. In many countries, this uses a multidisciplinary approach that includes consulting with other professionals involved with the family, such as health visitors or school staff. Finally, a decision is made, usually by social services, about whether the child is at risk of ongoing harm. Interventions include placement in foster care, placement with other family members (such as grandparents) or remaining with their parents with support and supervision from social services.

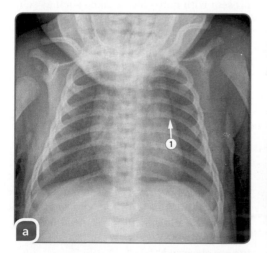
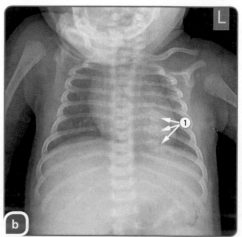

Figure 17.5 Fractures caused by non-accidental injury. (a) Fracture of the 6th rib ①. (b) Further fractures (of the 6th, 7th and 8th rib), apparent as a result of callus formation, 1 week later ①.

Management of minor acute infective illness in the community

An acute febrile illness is the most common reason for a child to the GP especially under the age of 5 years. Most children will have a self-limiting viral upper respiratory tract infection, in which case only reassurance is required. However, serious bacterial infection must be ruled out.

> Fever (pyrexia) in response to infection is a normal, healthy adaptive response. It may be vital in enhancing immune function.

Clinical features

It is essential that any child presenting with symptoms of a minor illness or fever (> 37.5°C) is clinically assessed to detect serious bacterial infection. Features suggestive of a serious illness are listed in **Table 17.9**. Most children with a fever appear miserable and lethargic, but after being given antipyretics they liven up and are able to resume playing, which eliminates the need for admission and investigations.

Diagnostic approach

Minor infections, such as otitis media, tonsillitis and chest infections, are usually diagnosed clinically and can be treated at home without the need for blood tests or microbiological or radiological investigations. The child should be reviewed if the illness persists; investigations may then be appropriate.

Children with fever and no obvious focus of infection should have their urine tested for infection. Microscopy is used for children younger than 3 years, and dipstick urinalysis for older children.

> Not all fevers are a consequence of infection. Inflammatory conditions such as juvenile chronic arthritis can cause fever. In particular, look for signs of Kawasaki's disease in any child with a fever of > 5 days' duration (see page 191).

A child with signs of severe illness or infection requires urgent referral to hospital for appropriate targeted investigations.

Management

A child with signs of severe illness or infection requires urgent referral to hospital for appropriate targeted investigations. However, if no worrying signs are present, the family is given reassurance and provided with advice regarding fluid intake and simple analgesia. Parents may need educating on the inappropriateness of antibiotics in viral illness.

Antibiotics should not be prescribed blindly (i.e. without identifying the infection) except when the child is seriously ill and the results of cultures are awaited. In the latter situation it is acceptable to prescribe a broad spectrum antibiotic; for example a child with a fever and petechial rash requires an intramuscular dose of benzylpenicillin immediately, i.e. before transfer to hospital or blood culture results, because of the possibility of meningococcal sepsis (see page 399).

Features suggesting serious illness in a child
■ Abnormal observations (e.g. tachypnoea and tachycardia)
■ Altered conscious level (e.g. drowsiness, difficulty in waking a sleeping baby)
■ Prolonged central capillary refill time
■ Pale or mottled skin
■ Cool or shut down peripheries
■ Grunting
■ Abnormal cry
■ Bulging or depressed fontanelle in a baby

Table 17.9 Features suggestive of serious illness in a child

Social, educational and legal issues

In paediatrics the challenges presented by the age range are not just clinical ones. There are social, educational and legal practicalites that are unique to the under-18s.

It is necessary to tailor approaches to the child's perceptions and carer's expectations and involvement. Particularly problematic areas include hospital admission, chronic conditions and transition to adult services, as discussed below.

In general terms, medicolegal responsibility for decisions about a child's healthcare rests with parents. However, there are situations when children are competent to make their own decisions to consent to or refuse treatment. Competence can be assessed from a predetermined set of criteria, such as those for assessing 'Gillick competence' (**Table 17.10**), developed as the result of a legal ruling in the UK in 1985 and used widely outside the UK.

Hospital admission

Although many illnesses are managed at home hospitalisation is sometimes unavoidable, for example for:

- elective surgery
- an acute severe illness such as pneumonia
- a chronic illness requiring an intervention such as intravenous antibiotics in cystic fibrosis

Children may be apprehensive about staying in hospital and being separated from their families and their usual activities.

> Children attending for elective surgery are often given an opportunity to visit the ward before admission.

Boredom

To combat boredom, play therapists provide activities for the child to participate in. There is often a playroom on the ward where, children who are is well enough can enjoy activities such as painting. Play therapists also help to distract the child from unpleasant procedures such as venepuncture.

Separation from family

Most paediatric wards impose no restrictions on parental visits, and there is often a relaxed approach towards visits from family and friends. If the child is in a specialist centre a long way from home, parental accommodation is often available.

Chronic conditions

These often require specialist nursing and educational input.

Specialist nurses

Children with chronic conditions, for example epilepsy, asthma and diabetes, receive care from specialist nurses. They are a contact point for the family, and educate the child, the parents and sometimes the school on the condition. They often form a close bond with patients and their families, helping them to manage the condition.

Criteria for Gillick competence
The child must have:
■ An understanding of the illness or condition and its natural history
■ An understanding of the proposed treatment, including the risks, benefits and alternatives
■ An understanding of the consequences of refusing treatment, in both the short and long term
■ An understanding of how the illness or treatment will affect their daily lives
■ Belief in the information given and belief that it applies to them
■ An ability to retain this information for long enough to make a decision

Table 17.10 Criteria for 'Gillick competence', assessing whether a child is competent to make a health decision

> **Specialist nurses may visit schools to educate staff about a child's condition.** For example, an epilepsy specialist nurse would explain the condition and what to do if the child has a seizure at school.

Education

A child with a chronic disease may have frequent and prolonged hospital stays, which may affect their education. Therefore the local education authority may arrange for home tutoring or access to online teaching resources.

Transition to adult services

Children with chronic conditions are transferred to adult services at the age of 16–18 years. This is a huge step for them and their parents. Clinicians should aim to make this transition as smooth as possible.

As an adolescent, the patient is encouraged to start taking responsibility for their health. To help promote independence, the patient may start ordering prescriptions from their GP and seeing their paediatrician without their parents present. To prepare for the move to adult services, there is often a joint clinic at which the adult services physician meets the patient and their paediatrician.

Paediatric palliative care

Paediatric palliative care is the medical care of children with life-limiting conditions, usually but not exclusively children who are not expected to reach adulthood. It is a holistic approach embracing physical, psychological and social elements.

Palliative care is provided in hospital, in the child's home or in a hospice, and is tailored to the needs of the family. Hospices provide respite care, short breaks for families, assistance with end-of-life care, information about disease, 24-hour advice and support, and bereavement counselling.

The prevalence of life-limiting conditions is highest in children younger than 1 year, and decreases with age. In the UK, about 50,000 children and young people under the age of 19 years old live with a life-limiting condition, a prevalence of about 36 per 10,000 children.

Scope of paediatric palliative care

Paediatric palliative care specialists offer services to some children over many years, not only when death is imminent or certain to occur in the near future. **Table 17.11** lists the four groups of children for whom palliative care is considered.

> **Uncertainty over the progress or final outcome of an illness should not preclude provision of palliative care services,** especially if it seems appropriate at the time.

Provision of palliative care

Palliative care services are provided by a team. One of the main aims is control of symptoms, such as pain, nausea, constipation, anxiety and sleep disturbance; this is achieved with pharmacological, psychological and therapy-based treatments. The palliative care team also helps with more practical aspects of day-to-day family life, such as access to government benefits, liaison with education services and arrangement of respite care.

For children whose condition appears to be deteriorating and who are nearing the end of their life, an emergency care plan should be produced. This document aims to communicate the wishes of the child and family with regard to treatment in the event of an emergency, and includes:

- instructions on tailored management of specific problems, such as seizures

Circumstances for considering palliative care	
Group	Examples
Children with conditions for which treatment and cure is possible but not certain	Childhood cancers
	Single-organ failure (e.g. heart or kidney failure)
Children with conditions for which long periods of intensive treatment may prolong life but are not curative, and premature death is still likely	Cystic fibrosis
	Muscular dystrophy
Children with conditions that are progressive, with no curative options	Certain neurodegenerative disorders
	Inborn errors of metabolism
Children with severe neurological conditions that are not in themselves progressive but lead to susceptibility to death from other complications	Severe cerebral palsy (e.g. secondary to a hypoxic event or prematurity)

Table 17.11 Children for whom palliative care should be considered

- wishes regarding the extent of intervention in the event of sudden collapse or life-threatening deterioration
- wishes relating to end of life

The emergency care plan is carried with the child and disseminated to professionals involved in their care. A copy is given to the police and ambulance service so that the information is available in an emergency.

Sudden unexpected death in infancy

Sudden unexpected death in infancy (SUDI) is the unexpected and initially unexplained death of a previously well child under the age of 1 year. A cause of death may be determined on investigation and post-mortem examination, but if the death remains unexplained it is defined as sudden infant death syndrome (SIDS). SIDS is also known as 'cot death'.

Epidemiology and aetiology

Causes of SUDI include infection, metabolic conditions and trauma (non-accidental injury). SIDS is, by definition, of unknown origin. The risk of SIDS is highest during the first 4 months of life; premature and low-birth-weight babies are at greater risk.

The incidence of SUDI varies hugely worldwide and between socioeconomic and ethnic groups within countries. The incidence in many populations has fallen significantly with

the realisation that placing babies on their backs to sleep greatly reduces the risk of SUDI. For example, following a 'back to sleep' campaign and other advice in the UK (see **Table 17.12**) it has fallen by 80% to 0.35 per 1000 live births since the early 1990s.

Clinical features

The child is found to have died in their sleep. Even if an underlying cause is later determined, there are usually no clinical signs on presentation.

Investigative approach

The main aims are to investigate the cause of death and to support the family. The death must be referred to the coroner, and a post-mortem examination carried out. The police are informed and will question the family. Representatives from all agencies involved attend an information-sharing meeting to consider any concerns about the family and

Strategies to avoid SIDS	
Advice to parents	Arrangement of cot
Do not smoke in the same room as the baby	Do not use pillows or duvets
Avoid bed sharing after drinking alcohol or taking drugs	Always place the baby to sleep on their back
Avoid sleeping with the baby on a sofa	Ensure that the baby's feet are at the foot of the cot
Consider breastfeeding, which is protective	Tuck the blanket below the baby's shoulders to avoid covering the head or use a baby sleeping bag
Offer the baby a dummy while they are falling asleep	
*The safest place for a baby to sleep is in a cot in the parents' bedroom.	

Table 17.12 Strategies to avoid sudden infant death syndrome (SIDS)

the possibility of death caused by non-accidental injury.

Consultations and investigations prompted by SUDI must be handled in a sensitive way. The priority is the provision of support for the family, because the majority of cases (90%) are events that could not have been predicted rather than a result of abuse or neglect.

Management and prevention

Families that have experienced SUDI need support during bereavement. If they go on to have another baby, they need help with preventive measures. These two facets may be integrated in a single service, such as the Care of Next Infant programme in England, Wales and Northern Ireland. As well as receiving emotional support, parents are provided with an apnoea monitor and resuscitation training, for example, and their baby is weighed weekly.

Global health

With increased migration for economic reasons and displacement of populations by war and poverty, problems that may once have been considered those of the developing world may present in developed countries. Consequently, an understanding of global health has become more important. This includes knowlege of cultural practices and traditions that are encoutered in or have an influence on medical practice.

Detailed discussion of global health is beyond the scope of this book but following subsections introduce five of the most prominent aspects.

Communication

Effective communication relies on language and an understanding of the patient's cultural beliefs. Consultations carried out via a third party, whether a professional interpreter or a family member are fraught with difficulties; information may be lost or changed during translation, and there is unavoidably a breach of confidentiality.

Beware of using family members as interpreters when trying to communicate bad news. For example, if you are explaining a very poor prognosis for a sick newborn, relatives may try to 'protect' the mother by withholding the full facts. As a result, when the baby dies this is even more devastating.

Female genital mutilation

Female genital mutilation (FGM) is a traditional practice carried out in certain countries. The term covers a variety of procedures that intentionally remove or alter parts of the female genitalia (**Table 17.13**). It is done at any time from infancy into the teenage years.

The motivation for FGM is social, cultural or religious; there are no medical reasons for FGM, no benefits and much harm. Long-term consequences include recurrent urinary and pelvic infections, chronic pain, menstrual problems, physical and psychological difficulties with sexual intercourse, and complications during childbirth.

Female genital mutilation is illegal in most high-income nations. However, even in these nations many girls whose families originate from countries in which FGM is practised are at risk of being taken abroad for FGM to be carried out.

All medical practitioners should be aware of FGM and be able to identify girls who are at risk. They must take responsibility for keeping themselves informed as to local or national guidelines on action to take when an at-risk girl is identified or when a child is found to have undergone FGM. Often, however, FGM does not present until adulthood (in pregnancy).

> In the UK, all healthcare workers who identify FGM are legally bound to record this in the patient's clinical notes and ensure it is reported to the police within 1 month.

Child trafficking

All health care professionals who deal with children need to be aware of child trafficking and of the signs that a child may be a victim of trafficking. Child trafficking is a form of child abuse in which children, often separated from their families, are recruited and transported with the intention of exploitation in the form of slavery and forced labour, criminal activity and engagement in sexual acts. The child suffers neglect and emotional, physical and sexual abuse.

It is difficult to obtain reliable estimates for the number of children trafficked, because of

Terms in female genital mutilation	
Type	Description
1a	Removal of clitoral prepuce only
1b	Removal of clitoral prepuce
	Partial or total removal of clitoris
2	Clitoris removed
	Partial or total removal of labia minora
3	Partial or total removal of labia minora
	Labia majora sewn together to cover the urethra and vagina, with only a small hole remaining for the passage of urine and menstrual blood
4	All other harmful non-medical procedures on the female genitalia, including tattoos and piercings

Table 17.13 Types of female genital mutilation

the covert and criminal nature of the practice. An estimated 300 children are trafficked to the UK every year.

Trafficking victims are often lured by false promises, so they may not easily trust others. They may also be fearful of people in authority, including medical staff. They may believe that their life or the lives of their family members are at risk if they escape or inform others.

Physical or psychological trauma is another sign that a child may be a victim of child trafficking. They may also show signs of low self-image, self-harm or an eating disorder.

Nutritional deficiencies

In some immigrant communities children are at higher risk of several nutritional deficiencies (see page 216) as the result of a variety of factors such as:

- ethnicity (e.g. a darker skin children raise the risk of vitamin D deficiency)
- diet (e.g. a vegan diet)
- poverty

These should be born in mind during history taking and diagnosis.

Infectious disease

Many immigrant children are at increased risk of infectious disease because of factors such as overcrowded accommodation and depressed immunity secondary to malnutrition. In addition, the clinician should be alert to a higher likelihood of infectious diseases that are uncommon to the host country but common in the country of origin, for example tuberculosis or HIV.

Answers to starter questions

1. Rib fractures are difficult to identify on chest X-ray when they are new. However a week later, callus formation at the healing fracture site is easily identifiable. Therefore, if there is a high index of suspicion a repeat X-ray after a week is useful, even if the original was normal.

2. Parents and healthcare professionals are often unduly worried about fever in children: this is 'fever phobia'. Children with fever should always be assessed, however serious complications are actually rare and often treatment for the fever is not indicated. Using antipyretics to prevent serious complications, such as febrile convulsions, is also a common misconception and is not indicated.

3. The paediatric palliative care team provides care to children with life-limiting illnesses, whether they are likely to die in the near future or live for years, because these children face many of the same issues that occur in palliative care. Their services include symptom control, respite care, emotional support and assistance with family finances.

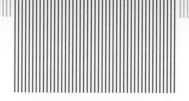

Chapter 18
Self-assessment

SBA questions

Neonatology and perinatal medicine

1. A 2-month-old boy attends for his first set of immunisations. This is the mother's first baby. He is fully breastfed. His birth weight was on the 50th centile and is now between the 25th and 50th centile. He is jaundiced but is feeding well, contented, has no vomiting and his bowels open once a day with a pale-coloured, formed stool.
What is the single most appropriate next action?

 A Arrange for the mother to have further breastfeeding advice
 B Give immunisations and reassure mother regarding breast milk jaundice
 C Request full blood count and film
 D Request split bilirubin blood test
 E Send stool for culture and sensitivities

2. A 6-hour-old girl born at term, birth weight 2.71 kg is admitted with tachypnoea. Her respiratory rate is 65 breaths/minute. Her heart sounds are difficult to hear because she is grunting. Her temperature is 35.8°C and blood glucose 1.4 mmol/L. She is placed in a heated incubator. Her oxygen saturation, measured by pulse oximetry, is 92% in air, increasing to 98% in 2 L of oxygen.
What is the single next best step?

 A Give intravenous bolus of 10% dextrose
 B Give surfactant
 C Perform an echocardiogram
 D Request a chest radiograph
 E Start continuous positive airway pressure (CPAP)

3. A 3-day-old preterm boy (24 weeks' gestation) has an intraventricular haemorrhage that extends extensively into the brain parenchyma (grade IV) on a routine cranial ultrasound scan. He has been stable since admission but remains on a ventilator. He is the mother's first baby. Which is the single best statement to tell the parents?

 A A neurosurgical opinion needs to be sought
 B Intensive care should be withdrawn
 C Nothing as the parents do not need to know about this
 D The baby is likely to have neurological sequelae
 E The baby will need to be investigated for haemophilia

4. A 27-week gestation boy infant is 7 days old. He is ventilated and receiving nasogastric feeds of maternal expressed breast milk. He has been stable for the last 48 h but over the past 6 h he has had two bile stained aspirates and has just passed a bloody stool with some mucous. On examination his abdomen is distended but not discoloured. His capillary refill time is 5 s.
What is the single most appropriate next action:

 A Stop feeds and arrange for an abdominal US scan
 B Stop feeds and check the baby's clotting profile
 C Stop feeds and put the mother on a cows' milk free diet
 D Stop feeds and send a stool sample for culture
 E Stop feeds, take blood cultures and start antibiotics

5. A boy is born at term with thick meconium in the liquor. He is white, floppy with no respira-

tory effort and has a heart rate of 30 bpm at the first assessment. There is no meconium on inspection of the oropharynx. He is given five inflation breaths by mask and chest movement is seen. His heart rate remains at 30 bpm.
What is the single most appropriate next step?

A Give mask ventilation and commence cardiac massage
B Intubate with an endotracheal tube and ventilate
C Obtain venous access and give adrenaline
D Perform a two-person jaw thrust and repeat the five inflation breaths
E Turn off the overhead heater and start cooling

6. A girl born at 25 weeks' gestation is due to go home on oxygen for chronic lung disease. She had a relatively uneventful stay on the neonatal unit. She had normal cranial US scans. She developed early retinopathy of prematurity (ROP) that has not progressed. There is no family history of note. The parents are non-smokers. What single complication is she most likely to have over the next few years?

A Bronchiolitis
B Cerebral palsy
C Severe visual impairment
D Sudden infant death syndrome (SIDS)
E Type 2 diabetes

Respiratory and ENT disorders

1. A 6-month-old boy has coryza, cough and tachypnoea. It is November. His respiratory rate is 60 breaths/min and heart rate 110 bpm. His oxygen saturations are 95% in air. He has moderate recession, bilateral widespread crackles and occasional wheeze. There is no stridor.
What is the single most appropriate treatment?

A Amoxycillin
B Antihistamine
C Bronchodilator inhaler
D Dexamethasone
E Supportive treatment

2. A 6-year-old boy with cough and wheeze on running has been using a bronchodilator via a metered dose inhaler and large volume spacer, after sufficient training from his mother. At review 3 months later he responds to the inhaler and needs to take it at least once every day.
What is the single most appropriate next step?

A Change the bronchodilator to a dry powder device
B Give the child a nebuliser
C Start a long acting beta 2 agonist

D Start a leukotriene receptor antagonist
E Start regular low dose inhaled steroid

3. A 4-month-old girl has a 6-week history of noisy breathing. The breathing is getting louder and is particularly noticeable when she is upset or lying on her back. In clinic she has obvious stridor at rest and her weight has fallen from the 25th to the 2nd centile. The girl has two cutaneous strawberry naevi.
What is the next single most appropriate step?

A Non-invasive ventilation (NIPPY)
B Give oral dexamethasone
C Perform a laryngo-bronchoscopy
D Undertake a sleep study
E Watch and wait

4. A 7-year-old boy with cystic fibrosis feels generally unwell, has a productive cough and feels breathless. His appetite is reduced. On examination his oxygen saturation is 94% in air, his respiratory rate is 30 bpm and he has no recession. He has crackles in both bases.
What is the single most useful investigation to perform?

A Bronchodilator reversibility
B Cough swab
C Lung function tests
D Sweat test
E Vitamin A, D and E serum levels

5. A 9-year-old girl has a 6-week history of cough. The cough is worse at night; in the day she has a sudden onset of prolonged coughing bouts, often triggered by laughing or exercise, when she looks frightened and has trouble getting her breath. She has mild asthma managed with low dose inhaled steroid via a spacer. Her teacher wonders if it is habitual. The episodes are becoming less frequent. She has no respiratory distress and her chest is clear. Her peak expiratory flow rate (PEFR) is at the upper range. Her full blood count and urea and electrolytes are normal.
What is the single most useful next step?

A Arrange for a contrast swallow
B Change her inhaler device
C Increase the dose of inhaled steroid
D Reassure her with supportive treatment
E Request a psychologist's assessment

6. A 7-year-old boy with cystic fibrosis has unexpectedly developed weight loss over the past 4 months despite maintaining his high fat and high calorie diet. His stools are normal for him and he is taking his pancreatic enzyme supplements. He says his chest is no worse than normal and there is no change in his lung function tests. His chest radiograph looks similar to the one taken 9 months ago.

What is the single most useful investigation to perform?

A Serum IgE test
B Blood glucose test
C DEXA scan
D Echocardiogram
E Stool fat analysis

Cardiovascular disorders

1. A 2-year-old boy is brought to casualty. He has been off his food for 24 hours and becoming more lethargic. He is pale, tachycardic and has a weak pulse. His chest is clear. An ECG trace confirms a regular rhythm with a rate of 230 bpm.
   What is the single most appropriate action?

   A Cardiac massage
   B Chest X-ray
   C Intravenous adrenaline
   D Intravenous adenosine
   E Synchronised direct current (DC) shock

2. A 3-year-old girl has a 10-day history of fever and rash. She has cervical lymphadenopathy, red eyes (conjunctival injection) and erythema of the hands with some skin peeling of her fingers.
   What is the single most useful investigation to perform?

   A ASO (antistreptolysin O) titres
   B Electrocardiogram
   C Echocardiogram
   D Eye swab for culture
   E Skin scrapings for microscopy

3. A 14-year-old girl has a 6-week history of severe headaches. She has no past medical history of note. She is on no medication. She has normal peripheral pulses and no radio-femoral delay. Her blood pressure is 180/110 mmHg. There is no papilloedema. She has no cardiac murmur and her chest is clear.
   What is the single most useful investigation to perform?

   A Cranial CT scan
   B Chest X-ray
   C Electrocardiogram
   D Echocardiogram
   E Renal ultrasound scan

4. A 3-month-old boy is on daily oral diuretics for a ventricular septal defect. He is taking longer to feed and becomes 'sweaty'. His weight has fallen from the 25th to the 9th centile.
   What is the single most appropriate next step?

   A Auscultate the lung bases
   B Compare his femoral and radial pulses

C Inspect his jugular venous pressure
D Measure his blood pressure
E Palpate his abdomen

5. A 14- year-old boy is brought to the emergency department, following a brief collapse during a 5 km run. A few weeks earlier he had upper chest discomfort after playing a football match soon after a meal. His grandfather died aged 36 years with a 'heart attack'. On examination he is alert and orientated. His blood pressure is normal, heart rate 86 bpm, with normal heart sounds and no murmur. His ECG is normal apart from mild left ventricular hypertrophy. His PEFR is good.
   What is the single most appropriate next step?

   A Arrange a 24-hour electrocardiogram with normal exercise
   B Arrange for an echocardiogram and referral to a cardiologist
   C Arrange for an electroencephalogram and referral to a neurologist
   D Arrange for an exercise test to assess lung function
   E Referral to a geneticist

6. A 3-year-old girl has a viral upper respiratory tract infection. She is usually well and is thriving. She has been unwell for 36 hours with mild fever and cough. Her temperature is 38°C, she is flushed, miserable and has a runny nose. Auscultation reveals clear lung fields but a grade 2/6 mid-systolic murmur at the lower left sternal edge. There is minimal radiation of the murmur and it becomes quieter when she is lying down compared with sitting, but persists. Her peripheral pulses are normal.
   What is the single most appropriate next step?

   A Chest X-ray
   B Electrocardiogram
   C Echocardiogram
   D Full blood count
   E Reassure

Gastrointestinal and liver disorders

1. A 2-year-old boy has a 48-hour history of vomiting (at least 10 times/day), along with frequent, loose, offensive stools. He is lethargic and has dry mucous membranes. His heart rate is 120 bpm. His mother has tried giving him small amounts of oral rehydration solution over the last 2 hours but he is refusing to take it.
   What is the single most appropriate next step?

   A Administer fluids intravenously
   B Insert a nasogastric tube and give oral rehydration fluids

C Prescribe antibiotics
D Send bloods to check urea and electrolytes
E Send the child home with advice on effective hand washing

2. A 5-year-old girl has a 3-month history of diarrhoea. She has been following the 25th weight centile since birth but recently her weight has dropped by two centiles. She has been healthy and has not had any previous hospital admissions. Around 4 months ago she had viral gastroenteritis. On examination she looks pale and thin and has a slightly protuberant abdomen with wasted buttocks.
What is the single most appropriate next step?

A Blood test for anti-tTG (anti-tissue transglutaminase) antibodies while on a gluten-free diet
B Blood test for anti-tTG antibodies while on her normal diet
C Blood test for the cystic fibrosis gene
D Reduce the amount of fructose in her diet
E Watch and wait, no investigations are currently indicated

3. A 2-week-old boy has evidence of bilious vomiting over the last 24 hours. Otherwise, he looks well. His observations are stable and examination is normal. His bowel motions are normal.
What is the single most appropriate investigation to perform?

A Barium meal and follow through
B pH study
C Plain abdominal X-ray
D Test feed
E Ultrasound scan

4. A 2-year-old girl has severe constipation. She only opens her bowels once every 7 days. All investigations performed are normal, therefore she is diagnosed with idiopathic constipation. On examination there is a large amount of palpable faeces in the left iliac fossa.
What is the single most appropriate treatment?

A Glycerine suppositories
B Increase fluid intake
C Macrogol regime for disimpaction
D Manual disimpaction
E Osmotic laxative

5. A 14-year-old boy has a 3-month history of weight loss, intermittent abdominal pain and loose bloody stools. He had been on holiday to Thailand prior to onset of symptoms. On examination he looks pale and thin. He has mouth ulcers and a red rash on his shins.
What is the single most likely diagnosis?

A Coeliac disease
B Crohn's disease

C Meckel's diverticulum
D Traveller's diarrhoea
E Ulcerative colitis

6. A 6-week-old boy has projectile, non-bilious vomiting but no diarrhoea. He appears hungry. He is formula fed. He is fed on arrival, which he promptly vomits with rippling of his abdominal wall, but is looking to feed again. He looks thin and has reduced skin turgor. An intravenous line is inserted to administer fluids.
His blood results show: haemoglobin 112 g/L; white cell count 12.6×10^9 /L; urea 5.1 mmol/L; sodium 134 mmol/L; potassium 3.6 mmol/L; bicarbonate 30 mmol/L.
What is the single most likely diagnosis?

A Cows' milk protein allergy
B Intussusception
C Pyloric stenosis
D Raised intracranial pressure
E Renal salt-losing condition

Urogenital disorders

1. A 6-year-old boy, who is fully immunised, has a sudden onset of testicular pain while running around at school. He is taken straight to the emergency department where he is found to have a swollen, painful left testicle. As the child is so distressed with the pain the doctor is unable to establish whether the cremasteric reflex is present.
What is the single most appropriate next step?

A Apply ice to the scrotum
B Arrange an out-patient scrotal ultrasound
C Dip test the urine
D Obtain blood sample for mumps IgE
E Request an urgent surgical review

2. A 4-year-old boy has a non-blanching rash over his lower legs and buttocks. He is complaining of some joint pain, but is generally well. Observations are stable, he is afebrile. On examination there is palpable purpura over his legs and buttocks. Blood pressure is normal. There is also evidence of bilateral ankle swelling. He is given analgesia.
What is the single most appropriate next step?

A Give an intravenous bolus of normal saline and start broad spectrum antibiotics
B Send him home with reassurance
C Start oral steroids
D Take an ankle radiograph
E Take bloods to test for renal function

3. A 7-year-old boy has just started to wet the bed after being dry at night for 3 years. His father recently passed away unexpectedly.

He is referred by his GP to the nocturnal enuresis clinic. His mother feels he has lost some weight although she can't quantify this. On examination he looks tired and slim and you think there is some thrush in his mouth. His mother is struggling to manage his enuresis.
What is the single most appropriate next step?

A Dip test his urine
B Give an enuretic alarm
C Refer him to the child and adolescent mental health team
D Start desmopressin
E Start oxybutynin

4. An 8-year-old boy has a 1-week history of periorbital swelling that is worse on waking in the morning. He suffers from eczema and has hayfever and takes a daily antihistamine. The family bought a new dog 3 months ago. He has gained 500 g in 2 weeks. On examination he has mild periorbital oedema. You note when examining his feet that there is a mark on his ankle where his sock elastic has been.
What is the single most appropriate next step?

A Advise the family to rehome the dog
B Dip test his urine
C Give dietary advice
D Prescribe a new antihistamine
E Reassure parents that no action is needed

5. An 8-month-old girl, who is known to have a left hydronephrosis and vesico-ureteric reflux, has a 24-hour history of temperature, vomiting and lethargy. She is on prophylactic trimethoprim. On examination she is miserable. She is febrile and tachycardic. She has cool peripheries. ENT examination is normal. Her fontanelle is not bulging. She vomited once during the examination.
What is the single most appropriate next step?

A Arrange for an urgent renal ultrasound
B Give intravenous antibiotics immediately
C Obtain a clean catch urine and start intravenous antibiotics
D Obtain a clean catch urine and start oral antibiotics
E Refer her to the surgeons

6. A 3-year-old boy has a 48-hour history of being unwell with vomiting, severe colicky abdominal pain and bloody diarrhoea. He has not passed much urine in the past 24 hours. He was previously fit and well and is not on medication. On examination he is pale and jaundiced.
Urine dipstick shows 3+ blood and 2+ protein. His other result show: haemoglobin 78 g/L; white cell count 11.3 x 10⁹; platelets 20 x 109; urea 14 mmol/L; creatinine 140 mmol/L; normal clotting profile.

What is the single most likely diagnosis?

A Disseminated intravascular coagulation (DIC) from sepsis
B Haemolytic uraemic syndrome
C Intussusception
D Urinary tract infection
E Viral gastroenteritis

Neurological disorders

1. A 12-year-old girl has had a generalised tonic clonic seizure. It lasted nearly 3 minutes and stopped spontaneously without treatment. She was initially in a post-ictal state but now has a Glasgow coma score of 15/15 and a normal examination. She has been otherwise well and has never previously had a seizure. Her tests show: heart rate 84 bpm; respiratory rate 16 breaths/minute; capillary refill time <2 seconds.
Which is the single most appropriate next step?

A Admit for observation
B Arrange an electroencephalogram
C Arrange an MRI of her head
D Perform an electrocardiogram then discharge
E Start sodium valproate

2. A 3-year-old boy has a temperature of 38.8°C. He has been vomiting and had loose stools over the last few hours. He is complaining of a headache, general myalgia and dislikes the light. His heart rate is 150 bpm; respiratory rate 30 breaths/minute; capillary refill time <2 seconds.
What is the single most appropriate next step?

A Give 50 mL/kg of dioralyte over 4 hours
B Give a bolus of 20 mL/kg of normal saline
C Give paracetamol and observe
D Send stool for culture
E Take a blood culture and start cefotaxime

3. A 15-year-old girl has recurrent headaches. They have been occurring weekly for the past 2 months, usually in the afternoon. She describes a pressure all over her head. There is no nausea, vomiting or photophobia. Her examination, including fundi, is normal. She is worried as the headaches are preventing her from revising for her exams.
What is the single most appropriate next step?

A Arrange an urgent CT of her head
B Arrange an MRI of her head
C Fasting blood glucose
D Perform a lumbar puncture with measurement of opening pressures
E Reassure, no investigations are necessary

4. A 3-year-old boy has a waddling gait, and has to use his hands to help stand up from the floor.

He first walked at 17 months of age. Examination of his legs show symmetrical findings of proximal weakness and hypertrophied calves. His tone is normal but reflexes are diminished. There is a full range of movement at the hips. Examination of his upper limb, cranial nerves and other systems are normal.

What is the single most appropriate investigation to perform?

A CT of his head
B MRI of his spinal cord
C Muscle biopsy
D Nerve conduction studies
E Serum creatine kinase test

5. A 5-year-old boy has had odd behaviour over the past 24 hours. His parents are not aware of any recent head injury. He has vomited three times in 24 hours. On examination his temperature is 38.5°C. He is not very verbal and appears confused, frequently falling asleep. He has mild papilloedema so a CT scan is carried out before proceeding to a lumbar puncture. The CT scan shows cerebral oedema and inflammation especially of the temporal lobes.

What single feature would you expect the cerebrospinal fluid to show?

A Cloudy appearance
B Low glucose levels
C No organisms
D Raised white blood cells, predominantly neutrophils
E Very high protein

6. A 2-year-old boy has a history of possible fit. He was well in the morning but became quiet around lunchtime and had an episode of loss of consciousness and rhythmic jerking of all four limbs, witnessed by his mother. The jerking lasted 5 minutes and he was disorientated for a few minutes, then back to his normal self 30 minutes later. His mother felt he was hot and gave him some paracetamol. On arrival to the emergency department his temperature is 38.5°C, he is flushed, and his capillary refill time is < 2 seconds. He has no rash and starts playing with the toys. He has a left red bulging tympanic membrane, but no other findings.

What is the single most appropriate investigation to perform?

A CT scan
B Electroencephalogram
C Lumbar puncture
D None
E Urine metabolic screen

Musculoskeletal disorders

1. A 3-year-old girl is unwell with a 6-day history of high fevers, abdominal pain and painful knees and feet. On examination her temperature is 39.5°C. She has a widespread pink macular rash and cervical lymphadenopathy. Her knees, fingers and toes are swollen – there is no redness but the swelling appears warm to touch. Passive and active movement of her knees and fingers is reduced. She also has splenomegaly.

What is the single most likely diagnosis?

A Henoch–Schönlein purpura
B Kawasaki's disease
C Rheumatic fever
D Systemic onset juvenile idiopathic arthritis
E Transient synovitis

2. A 14-year-old boy has sudden onset of a limp and pain of his right hip and knee. He is otherwise well. On examination his weight is on the 98th centile and his height is on the 50th centile. His right leg is mildly externally rotated and he has reduced range of movement of his right hip with pain on both active and passive movement. There is no swelling or tenderness of his right knee.

What is the single most likely diagnosis?

A Osgood–Schlatter disease
B Perthes' disease
C Polyarticular juvenile idiopathic arthritis
D Slipped upper femoral epiphysis
E Transient synovitis

3. A 7-year-old boy has a high fever and a painful left knee. His is normally fit and well with no significant past medical history. On examination his knee is red, hot and swollen and exquisitely painful with movement. A full blood count shows: haemoglobin 135g/L; white cell count 36 x 10⁹/L; platelets 365 x 10⁹/L; C-reactive protein 80 mg/L. Blood cultures are taken along with aspiration and irrigation of the joint.

What is the single most important next step?

A Anti-inflammatory analgesics
B Intravenous antibiotics for group B *Streptococcus*
C Intravenous antibiotics for MRSA
D Intravenous antibiotics for *Salmonella sp*
E Intravenous antibiotics for *Staphylococcus aureus*

4. An 11-year-old boy presents with a week's history of pain and swelling of his right knee. There

is no history of recent trauma, but he does have intermittent heel pain following treatment for an ankle sprain a few weeks previously. He is otherwise well with no fever, rash or bowel symptoms. There is no family history of joint problems. On examination his right knee is swollen, warm and tender at the insertion of the patellar ligament. Flexion is limited to 90°. All other joints are normal apart from decreased lumbar flexion.

His full blood count is normal. His erythrocyte sedimentation rate (ESR) is 36 mm/hour. A radiograph of the knee is normal.

What is the single most appropriate investigation to perform?

A HLA (human leukocyte antigen) typing
B Mantoux test
C Slit lamp examination of the eyes
D Rheumatoid factor
E Skeletal survey

5. A 14-year-old girl is going through her growth spurt. Her mother is concerned on watching her on the beach that she has 'curvature of the spine'. She is an active child with no back pain or other joint pain. On examination she is on the 50th centile for height. She has no skin stigmata. When asked to bend forward with arms hanging loosely down there is a mild 'rib hump'.

What is the single most likely diagnosis?

A Adolescent idiopathic scoliosis
B Leg length discrepancy
C Marfan's syndrome
D Neurofibromatosis
E Spinal tumour

Allergy, immunology and infections

1. A 4-year-old boy is seen in the emergency department having developed a rash 10 minutes after eating a chocolate bar. He is usually well and is not on any medication. There is an obvious urticarial rash. There is no swelling of his lips but he complains of some tingling of his tongue. His respiratory rate is 30 breaths/min and his heart rate is 90 bpm. The rest of his examination is normal.

What is the single most appropriate next step?

A Adrenaline pen training
B Advise not to eat chocolate again
C Advise to stay off school for the next few days
D Arrange for serum-specific IgE for mixed foods
E Suggest the family change their clothes washing powder

2. An 8-year-old boy has had fever, malaise and pharyngitis for 24 hours. He has just developed a widespread pruritic vesicular rash. He is on regular oral steroids for severe asthma. His chest is clear.

What is the single most appropriate treatment?

A Aciclovir
B Antihistamines
C Penicillin V
D Supportive treatment
E Zoster immunoglobulin

3. A 3-year-old girl has a 4-day history of a cough. She has previously been admitted on two occasions with right upper lobe pneumonia, and responded well to antibiotics. Her respiratory rate is 35 breaths/min. There is no recession. On auscultation she has crackles on the right upper chest. A chest radiograph shows shadowing in her right upper lobe.

What is the single most appropriate investigation to perform?

A CT scan of the chest
B Flexible bronchoscopy
C Immunoglobulins test
D Mantoux test
E Rigid bronchoscopy

4. A 2-month-old boy is miserable and grizzly all the time. He has several small vomits each day and a frequently distended abdomen. He has regular loose stools. He is formula fed. He is following the 9th centile for weight. His abdomen is soft.

What is the single most appropriate treatment?

A Antireflux medication
B Change the type of milk
C Introduce solids
D Oral rehydration fluid
E Thicken the milk

5. A 4-year-old boy is pale with a respiratory rate of 45 breaths per minute. He has had three episodes of pneumonia in the past year. *Haemophilus influenza* has been cultured on two occasions. He was born at term and is fully immunised. He has had a few episodes of severe otitis media and discharging ears and conjunctivitis. His height and weight are on the 3rd centile. He has no clubbing and no chest deformity. Auscultation reveals reduced breath sounds on the right.

What is the single most likely underlying condition?

A Cystic fibrosis
B Immunoglobulin deficiency
C Neutrophil defects
D Normal childhood infections
E Severe combined immunodeficiency (SCID)

Genetic disorders and dysmorphology

1. Immediately at birth a term baby girl is noted to have swelling of her hands and feet. Apart from some loose skin around her neck the examination is otherwise normal. Her weight is on the 25th centile and she is feeding well.
   What is the single most appropriate investigation to perform?

   A Echocardiogram
   B Hearing test
   C Karyotype test
   D MRI of her head
   E Renal ultrasound

2. A 6-hour-old newborn boy, born at term, is not feeding well. On examination he is hypotonic. He has a large anterior fontanelle and a posterior fontanelle. His eyes are upslanting and he has epicanthic folds. His tongue appears to be quite large and there is a simian crease on the left hand.
   What single classification best describes this baby's likely genetic condition?

   A Mitochondrial disorder
   B Sex chromosome abnormality
   C Single gene disorder
   D Trisomy
   E X-linked disorder

3. An 18-month-old boy developed severe swelling of the knee following a minor fall. Investigation reveals a haemarthrosis. Further investigation shows a prolonged activated partial thromboplastin time (APTT) and factor VIII activity of 3%. He has a newborn baby sister.
   What single statement best describes the likelihood of his sister having the same condition (and transmitting it to her offspring)?

   A She has a 50% chance of suffering from the condition
   B She has a 1 in 4 chance of suffering from the condition
   C She will not be affected by the condition
   D She will not have the condition but may transmit it to her sons
   E She will not have the condition but has a 50% chance of transmitting it to her children

4. A 6-hour-old newborn baby girl on newborn examination is noted to have the ends of her toes missing and a constriction mark around her ankle. Her mother had an uneventful pregnancy and her scans were all normal. The baby is spontaneously moving her legs fully. The remainder of her examination is unremarkable.

   What is the single most appropriate next investigation?

   A A skeletal survey
   B An echocardiogram
   C Karyotype test
   D Hip ultrasound scan
   E No investigations indicated

5. A 14-year-old girl has shortness of breath and a sharp right-sided chest pain after a netball match. She is normally fit and well, has a tall and slim athletic build and is a county netball player. On examination she has shallow breaths limited by pain: respiratory rate 50 breaths/minute; heart rate 90 bpm. Auscultation is unremarkable. Oxygen saturation is 98% in air. A chest radiograph shows a large pneumothorax on the right side. This is managed with a chest drain.
   What is the single most appropriate investigation to perform?

   A CT of chest
   B Echocardiogram
   C Exercise test
   D Lung function tests
   E No investigations required

6. A 7-year-old boy with Down's syndrome presents with worsening constipation. His mother gives him daily stool softeners but he is straining to open his bowels. His mother has no other concerns – he has settled in junior school well with better behaviour than in infant school. His weight has gone from the 50th to 75th centile. On examination firm stool is palpable on the left side of his abdomen but it is non-tender.
   What is the single most appropriate investigation to perform?

   A Blood anti-tTG (anti-tissue transglutaminase) antibody test
   B Blood thyroid function test
   C Lower bowel contrast study
   D Plain abdominal X-ray
   E Rectal biopsy

Endocrine disorders

1. An 8-year-old boy has a 1-week history of polydipsia and polyuria. He has no other symptoms. His blood sugar is 13.8 mmol/L. Urine dip test shows glycosuria and 1+ketones. His mucous membranes are moist. Other tests show: heart rate 100bpm; respiratory rate 20 breaths per minute; capillary refill time <2 seconds. Blood gas shows pH 7.34; pCO_2 4.6 kPa; bicarbonate 20.3 mmol/L; base excess -1.
   What is the single most appropriate next step?

A Give appropriate dietary advice
B Give subcutaneous insulin with an infusion of intravenous 0.9% saline with added potassium.
C Start continuous intravenous insulin with an infusion of 0.9% saline with added potassium
D Start subcutaneous insulin with normal oral fluid intake
E Undertake a 24 hour urine collection

2. A 12-year-old girl has not started menstruating. She is fit and well. Her height is on the 9th centile for her age. Pubertal assessment shows breast stage 3 and pubic hair stage 2. Her mother reached menarche at 14 years.
What is the single most appropriate investigation to perform?

A Blood LH, FSH and estradiol levels
B Blood karyotype
C No intervention required
D Pelvic ultrasound
E Start oestrogen therapy

3. A mother is concerned that her 7-year-old son is short. He is otherwise fit and well and she has no other concerns about him. His height is on the 2nd centile for age, and weight on the 9th centile. His mid-parental is on the 9th centile for height. He is pre-pubertal.
What is the single most appropriate next step?

A Blood test for coeliac screen
B 6-month follow-up appointment
C Radiograph for bone age
D Start growth hormone therapy
E Thyroid function tests

4. A 12-year-old girl has had loose stools for 2 weeks, but has not been vomiting. She has a very good appetite and plenty of energy. Her height is on the 91st centile and weight on the 75th. Test results include: heart rate 120 bpm; respiratory rate 20 breaths/minute; capillary refill time <2 seconds. On examination there is a systolic murmur heard throughout the precordium.
What is the single most appropriate next step?

A Anti-tTG (anti-tissue transglutaminase) antibodies test
B Arrange an echocardiogram
C Collect stool for microscopy, culture and sensitivity
D Thyroid function tests
E Urea and electrolyte blood test

5. A 6-hour-old baby, initially thought to be a girl, has an enlarged clitoris raising concerns of ambiguous genitalia. Her birthweight is on the 25th centile, she is feeding well and there are no other concerns. The examination is otherwise normal.
What is the single most appropriate next step?

A 17-hydroxyprogesterone test
B Blood glucose test
C Karyotype
D Ultrasound of pelvis
E Urea and electrolyte test

Skin disorders

1. A 1-month-old baby boy has a raised irregular, strawberry red lesion on its left thigh. It has been present for 2 weeks and is getting bigger. The baby is well and other than the skin lesion measuring 1 cm by 1 cm, examination is normal. The baby's parents wish for the lesion to be removed.
What is the single most appropriate next step?

A Reassure parents, no treatment is needed
B Refer for a biopsy
C Refer for laser surgery
D Refer to a plastic surgeon
E Start propranolol

2. A 2-week-old Asian baby girl has a 2 cm by 2 cm dark blue lesion on the skin at the top of her left buttock. The mother says it was there at birth but she doesn't have her maternity notes to confirm this. Otherwise examination of the baby is normal. She wants to know what the lesion is.
What is the single most appropriate next step?

A Contact social services
B Obtain birth notes to check mark was noted at birth
C Perform a full blood count and coagulation screen
D Reassure the mother it is a café au lait spot
E Reassure the mother it a congenital melanocytic naevi

3. A 6-year-old girl has small fleshy dome shaped lesions with umbilication of the centre, on her neck and trunk. She suffers from eczema, which has recently flared up. Other than these lesions and some dry skin over the flexures, examination is normal. The child is very conscious of them and wants them treated.
What is the single most appropriate next step?

A Cryotherapy
B Explain no treatment is indicated
C Refer to a dermatologist
D Start oral antibiotics
E Start oral antivirals

4. A 6-month-old girl has large patches of red-dened dry skin on both cheeks and smaller annular patches over her limbs and trunk. They have been present for 2 months. She is other-wise well, is formula fed and on no medication. There is a family history of asthma.
    What is the single most appropriate next step?

    A Advise not to bath every day
    B Apply emollients liberally
    C Apply steroid cream to all lesions twice a day
    D Commence a cows' milk free diet
    E Use anti-allergy bedding

5. A 6-year-old girl has been taking erythromy-cin for 36 hours for a chest infection as she is thought to have an allergy to penicillin. She then develops pink macular lesions which evolve into lesions with pale centres and a pink outer ring. Her cough has greatly improved.
    What is the single most likely diagnosis?

    A Erythema multiforme
    B Erythema toxicum
    C Erythromycin drug allergy
    D Stevens–Johnson syndrome
    E Urticaria

6. A 4-hour-old newborn boy is noted to have a red area on his forehead in a typical trigeminal distribution on his newborn examination. It has clear demarcated edges. He is reviewed in out-patients a few weeks later and the area has deepened in colour, is non-blanching and non-raised.
    What is the single most appropriate next step?

    A Arrange for an ophthalmology assessment
    B Arrange for a brain MRI scan
    C Blood culture and commence antibiotics
    D Refer for laser treatment
    E Refer to genetics

Haematology

1. A 3-year-old boy has had a rash for 24 hours. He is generally well although he has had a nose bleed earlier in the day and has a large bruise on his knee after a fall in the garden. On examina-tion he has a widespread petechial rash over most of his body and a large bruise on his left knee. There is no organomegaly. Observations (heart rate, respiratory rate, blood pressure and temperature) are stable.
    What is the single most appropriate investiga-tion to perform?

    A Bone marrow biopsy
    B Full blood count
    C Haemophilia screen

D Meningococcal polymerase chain reaction (PCR) test
E Urea and electrolytes

2. An 11-month-old boy has a painful swollen knee after falling against a piece of furniture. He is normally fit and well and has seen his general practitioner on one other occasion when his thigh became swollen after routine immunisa-tion. The doctor performed a range of blood tests including a full blood count which was normal. The APTT was prolonged.
    What is the single most appropriate investiga-tion to perform?

    A Bone marrow biopsy
    B Factor VIII levels
    C Platelet function test
    D Skeletal survey
    E Von Willebrand factor levels

3. A 2-year-old Caucasian girl has a 2-month history of poor appetite and lethargy. The only thing her mother can persuade her to take is cows' milk. On examination she is extremely pale, there is no evidence of organomegaly. A soft systolic murmur is heard. There are no signs of heart failure. A full blood count reveals hae-moglobin of 75 g/L with a low mean corpuscu-lar volume and low ferritin. A blood film shows a microcytic hypochromic picture.
    What is the single most appropriate next step?

    A Blood transfusion
    B Bone marrow biopsy
    C Echocardiogram
    D Plasma electrophoresis
    E Start iron supplementation

4. A 6-year-old girl has cough, dyspnoea and chest pain. She has a diagnosis of sickle cell disease. On examination she is tachypnoeic and tachycardic. Her pain is 10/10 in severity. Her saturation is 91% on air.
    What is the single most likely diagnosis?

    A Acute chest syndrome
    B Cardiac chest pain
    C Community acquired pneumonia
    D Splenic sequestration crisis
    E Vaso-occlusive crisis

5. A 3-year-old boy presents with a 24-hour his-tory of anorexia, lethargy, pallor and dark urine. Born at term he became jaundiced within 24 hours, was treated with double phototherapy and settled. His mother is Greek, his father English. He is not taking medication. He has spent the weekend with his grandmother, who is an organic farmer. On examination he is pale and slightly jaundiced. He is well perfused with a heart rate of 105 bpm, and a soft ejection

murmur at the apex. Examination is otherwise normal.

Further investigations show: haemoglobin 62 g/L; mean corpuscular volume 82 fl; white cell count 10.3 x 10⁹/L; platelets 280 x 10⁹/L; reticulocytes 18%; blood film – polychromasia, red cell fragments and cremated cells; no spherocytes; U&E normal. Urinalysis shows urobilinogen and haemoglobin.

What is the single most likely diagnosis?

A   G6PD deficiency
B   Haemolytic uraemic syndrome
C   Hereditary spherocytosis
D   Infective endocarditis
E   Iron deficiency anaemia

Childhood cancer

1. A 3-year-old girl has not been herself for a few months. Her mother reports nonspecific lethargy and she seems to have picked up more infections recently that take her a long time to recover from. She has experienced some gum bleeding when cleaning her teeth. On examination she appears pale. Her observations are stable. Examination of her abdomen reveals hepatomegaly and splenomegaly.
    What is the single most likely diagnosis?

    A   Acute lymphoblastic leukaemia
    B   Acute myeloid leukaemia
    C   Hodgkin's lymphoma
    D   Non-Hodgkin's lymphoma
    E   Wilms' tumour

2. A 5-year-old boy has a 1-month history of waking with headaches, occasionally associated with vomiting. His mother has kept him off school for the last week as his condition is worsening. On examination there is bilateral papilloedema with no other notable neurology.
    What is the single most appropriate investigation?

    A   Cranial ultrasound scan
    B   CT of his head
    C   Lumbar puncture
    D   MRI of his head
    E   Ophthalmology assessment

3. A 2-year-old boy has a 1-month history of abdominal pain and abdominal distension. He is pale and lethargic. He appears to have lost weight. He takes a laxative for constipation. On examination he has a firm 5 cm by 5 cm mass over the left side of the abdomen.
    What is the single most appropriate next step?

    A   Increase laxative dose
    B   Measure anti-TTg antibodies

C   Perform colonoscopy
D   Perform ultrasound scan of abdomen
E   Urine culture

4. A 4-year-old boy is referred with a lump in his neck. This has been present for several months increasing and decreasing in size. His mother is Caucasian and his father Asian. On examination he is on the 75th centile for height and weight. He is not clinically anaemic. He has a mobile 2 cm sized lump in his left cervical area. Ear and throat examination is normal. His teeth seem in good condition. His chest is clear.
    What is the single most appropriate next step?

    A   Chest radiograph
    B   Full blood count
    C   Mantoux test
    D   Needle biopsy of the lump
    E   Reassurance

Emergencies

1. A 7-year-old girl has a 1-week history of polydipsia and polyuria. She is now vomiting. Her blood sugar is 23.1 mmol/L. Urine dipstick shows glycosuria and 3+ ketones. Her consciousness level is normal. Her mucous membranes are dry. Other results show: heart rate 140 bpm; respiratory rate 35 breaths per minute; capillary refill time 3 seconds. Blood gas shows pH 7.19; pCO_2 3.1kPa; bicarbonate 12.1 mmol/L; base excess -12.
    What is the single most appropriate next step?

    A   Give a bolus of 0.9% saline followed by a maintenance infusion with potassium
    B   Give an intravenous bicarbonate correction
    C   Give an intravenous bolus of short-acting insulin
    D   No fluid bolus, start an infusion of 0.9% saline with potassium
    E   No insulin bolus, start continuous intravenous insulin in conjunction with 0.9% saline with potassium

2. A 2-year-old boy has a 3-hour history of stridor, which was present when he awoke in the middle of the night with difficulty in breathing. He is also coryzal and has a barking cough. There are intercostal recessions but air entry is satisfactory throughout his lung fields.
    Test results show: temperature 37.8°C; heart rate 130 bpm; respiratory rate 35 breaths/minute; capillary refill time <2 seconds; his saturation is 97% on air.
    What is the single most appropriate treatment?

    A   Face mask oxygen
    B   Intramuscular adrenaline

C Nebulised adrenaline
D Nebulised salbutamol
E Oral dexamethasone

3. A 4-year-old girl has a temperature of 38.9°C. She has been vomiting and is now developing a purpuric rash. She is lethargic but responds to her mother's voice and is crying. Her peripheries are cool to touch.
   Test results show: heart rate 160bpm; respiratory rate 28 breaths/minute, capillary refill time 4 seconds; saturation is 98% on air; capillary blood sugar 3.4 mmol/L.
   What is the single most appropriate initial treatment?

   A Bolus of 20 mL/kg of normal saline
   B Bolus of 2 mL/kg of 10% dextrose
   C Intravenous cefotaxime
   D Intubate and ventilate
   E Per rectum paracetamol

4. An 8-year-old boy is short of breath. He had been coryzal since the previous day and then became breathless while playing football. He took four puffs of his salbutamol inhaler which gave some relief to his symptoms. He is using his accessory muscles but can speak in short sentences. There is widespread wheeze throughout his chest.
   Test result show: heart rate 120 bpm; respiratory rate 30 breaths/minute; saturation is 94% on air.
   Which is the single most appropriate treatment?

   A 10 puffs of salbutamol via spacer device
   B Intravenous hydrocortisone
   C Nebulised salbutamol
   D Nebulised ipratropium bromide
   E Oral prednisolone

5. A 12-year-old girl has difficulty breathing while eating a Chinese takeaway. She also feels itchy and is complaining of a burning sensation in her throat. Her lips and tongue are swollen and she has obvious stridor. There is widespread wheeze on auscultation of her chest.
   Test results show: heart rate 130 bpm; respiratory rate 35 breaths/minute; saturation is 94% on 10 L of oxygen; blood pressure 98/66 mmHg.
   What is the single most appropriate treatment?

   A Intramuscular adrenaline
   B Intravenous adrenaline
   C Intravenous hydrocortisone
   D Nebulised salbutamol
   E Oral prednisolone

6. A 6-year-old girl has had open heart surgery 2 weeks ago for correction of an atrial septal defect. She presents to the clinic with breath-

lessness. She is conscious and talking. Test results show: heart rate 95 bpm (normal), with weak pulses and a blood pressure of 65/30 (low for her age); capillary refill time is 2 seconds. The doctors are unable to get intravenous access.
What is the single most appropriate next step?

A Adrenaline via intraosseous access
B Chest radiograph
C Direct current (DC) shock
D Echocardiogram
E Electrocardiogram

Community paediatrics

1. A 2-year-old girl has a fever with a temperature of 39.4°C and has had a non-bilious vomit. She is coryzal, miserable and refusing fluids. Her tonsils are enlarged and erythematous, but no exudate is seen. Her chest is clear, abdomen soft and there is no rash present.
   Test results show: heart rate 140 bpm; respiratory rate 30 breaths/minute; capillary refill time <2 seconds. You prescribe paracetamol.
   What is the single most appropriate treatment?

   A Alternating paracetamol with ibuprofen
   B Analgesic throat spray
   C Encourage oral fluid intake
   D Intravenous bolus of 20 mL/kg normal saline
   E Oral antibiotics

2. A 10-week-old boy has a small bruise on his cheek. His mother reports that he rolled onto a toy his sister had left on the floor. His examination is otherwise normal, with a weight on the 25th centile. He is not on the child protection register and the family are not known to social services.
   What is the single most appropriate next step?

   A Admit the baby and await a review from social services
   B Admit the baby for skeletal survey, CT of head and fundoscopy
   C Allow the baby to go home, with advice regarding safety in the home
   D Allow the baby to go home with social services to review the following day
   E Arrange an emergency foster placement while investigations are performed

3. A mother is concerned that her 15-month-old boy is still not walking. He can crawl and pull himself up to stand. He has a good pincer grasp with no hand preference. He can spoon feed himself and uses six words with meaning.
   What is the single most likely diagnosis?

A Cerebral palsy
B Developmental dysplasia of the hip
C Development is within normal limits
D Global developmental delay
E Gross motor developmental delay

4. A 2-month-old boy has attended for his first
    routine vaccinations. He was born at 36 weeks
    but had no complications and has been well. He
    has had a runny nose and occasional cough for
    the last couple of days but has not been febrile.
    His mother has epilepsy.
    Which is the single most appropriate next step?

    A Delay vaccinations for 1 month as the baby
       was 4 weeks premature
    B Delay vaccinations for 1 week as the baby is
       unwell at present
    C Give the vaccination as planned
    D Omit all vaccinations due to the family his-
       tory of epilepsy
    E Omit the pertussis vaccine due to the family
       history of epilepsy

5. An 18-month-old boy has 'slow development'
    compared with twin sister. He is a "good baby",
    and placid compared with his sister. He rolled
    at 5 months, sat unaided from 11 months
    and now he can crawl, pull to stand and walk
    around furniture but is not walking unaided.

He builds a tower of two bricks, responds to his
name but speaks no recognisable words. He is
thriving (in terms of both weight and height),
prone to constipation, and not dysmorphic.
What is the single most appropriate next step?

A Advise an increase in stimulation at home
B Chromosome analysis
C Creatine kinase test
D Thyroid function test
E TORCH screen

6. A 6-year-old boy is referred to the community
    paediatric team as his mother is concerned with
    his behaviour. He was born at 26/40 gestation
    but has achieved his development milestones.
    He has frequent tantrums, which result in him
    throwing objects about and he occasionally hits
    his mother. She is a single mother and he is an
    only child. His school is complaining that he is
    disruptive and has poor concentration.
    What is the single most appropriate next step?

    A Arrange for a statement of special educa-
       tional needs
    B Arrange for an electroencephalogram
    C Complete parent and school behavioural
       questionnaires
    D Enrol mother in parenting classes
    E Start methylphenidate

SBA answers

Neonatology and perinatal medicine

1 D

The pale stools suggest an obstructive liver cause for the jaundice, which will be identified by a split bilirubin blood test. The most urgent pathology to exclude is biliary atresia. In breast milk jaundice the stool is a 'seedy yellow'. The fall in weight centiles is within normal limits, bowel infections result in watery or bloody diarrhoea, and haemolysis causes early neonatal jaundice.

2 A

The most urgent problem is the hypoglycaemia as this can cause seizures and affect neurodevelopment, giving 10% dextrose is therefore the correct answer. The baby will need a chest radiograph and may go on to need CPAP depending on the work of breathing and oxygen requirement, but the oxygen saturation is good at the moment. Surfactant is usually needed for preterm babies (with respiratory distress syndrome) and can only be given if the child requires intubation. The next step would be intravenous antibiotics.

3. D

The baby is likely to have a hemiplegia on the opposite side to the haemorrhage. He may also have other developmental delay, especially due to the extreme prematurity. This is not sufficient grounds to withdraw intensive care, unlike bilateral grade IV haemorrhage. Such haemorrhages, common in preterm infants, do not usually reflect underlying bleeding tendencies and are not amenable to neurosurgery, unless hydrocephalus develops.

4 E

This baby has most likely developed necrotising enterocolitis. Discolouration of the abdomen will be a later sign. The management is to stop feeds and start antibiotics to include cover for anaerobic organisms. A blood culture should be taken before any antibiotic is started. An abdominal radiograph rather than an US scan will help confirm the diagnosis if air is seen in the bowel wall. The bloody stool is due to the sloughing of the bowel wall lining and not due to abnormal clotting. Cow's milk protein intolerance can present with bloody stools but the triad of bile aspirates, abdominal distension and bloody mucous stool along with clinical deterioration (increased capillary refill time) makes this unlikely. Usually no organism is cultured on stool samples in necrotising enterocolitis.

5 A

The baby's chest is moving but the heart rate has not increased. The next step is cardiac compression. As the chest is moving, further airway manoeuvres such as a two-person jaw thrust is not indicated. Intubation has no advantage over mask ventilation, and drugs are only given after cardiac compressions. Although the baby may be developing hypoxic ischaemic encephalopathy (HIE) cooling is usually not started until 10 mins of resuscitation.

6 A

All extremely preterm infants but especially those with CLD are likely to contract bronchiolitis in their first winter. SIDS is a risk, but the incidence is low and reduced here by the parents not smoking. With the normal cranial US scans any neurological consequence such as CP is unlikely, although delayed development can occur. Resolved ROP will not result in severe visual impairment. Type 2 diabetes is a much later complication.

Respiratory and ENT disorders

1. E

The infant most likely has bronchiolitis at this time of the year with these symptoms and signs. The wheeze will not respond to bronchodilators or dexamethasone. Pneumonia is less likely and croup or allergy very unlikely.

2. E

The use of the bronchodilator every day indicates more severe asthma and so commencing regular low dose inhaled steroid is the next step up the treatment ladder. The mdi and large volume spacer is an appropriate device for this age.

3. C

The stridor is chronic and likely to be caused by laryngomalacia or a haemangioma in the larynx. As the stridor is worsening, present at rest and associated with faltering growth the larynx needs to be examined with laryngo-bronchoscopy. Dexamethasone is the treatment for acute croup. A sleep study and NIPPY are treatments for obstructive sleep apnoea.

4. B

A productive cough suggests bacterial infection. A cough swab will identify the pathogen and guide antibiotic treatment. Lung function tests may indicate the severity of the infection, and bronchodilators may help but are not the most important treatment. The boy already has a diagnosis of cystic fibrosis so a sweat test is not needed. Vitamin levels are routinely performed at the annual review but do not help in managing acute exacerbations.

5. D

The history is very suggestive if whooping cough. Vaccination as an infant is no longer very protective at this age. Her normal PEFR and clear chest makes deterioration in her asthma unlikely. She has presented too late for the typical lymphocytosis to be detected on the FBC (Also at this stage her pernasal swab culture is likely to be negative).

6. B

Diabetes is a complication of CF. It usually presents insidiously. No deterioration in lung function or symptoms makes allergic bronchopulmonary aspergillosis (identified by raised IgE) unlikely. The other investigations would not be indicated by the history.

Cardiovascular disorders

1. D

The child has SVT which usually responds to a rapid iv bolus of adenosine. Synchronised DC shock is used if adenosine is unsuccessful or there is no circulation. The child has a cardiac output so cardiac compression is not indicated. Adrenaline is the treatment for asystole.

2. C

Kawasaki's disease is a likely contender here, particularly with the desquamation. The most worrying sequel is due to coronary aneurysms, seen on Echo, and their presence supports the diagnosis. The aneurysms would not be detected on an ECG. The desquamation and conjunctival injection are not due to direct infection so skin scrapings and eye swabs are negative.

3. E

The commonest cause of hypertension in a teenager is renal. A renal ultrasound is quick and easy to perform. Here it is likely to show small kidneys. Raised intracranial pressure is still a possibility even with no papilloedema but less common and should be considered especially if the renal ultrasound is normal. Coarctation of the aorta is less likely with the normal cardiovascular examination (apart from the hypertension).

4. E

This baby is showing increased signs of heart failure. In this age group this is most easily monitored by the presence and degree of hepatomegaly. Crepitations and peripheral oedema are unreliable signs for heart failure in infants. The JVP is impossible to clinically assess in infants.

5. B

Syncope and chest pain can indicate a risk for sudden cardiac death and should be investigated, especially with a family history. Mild ventricular hypertrophy can occur with intense training but is less likely at this age. It would be unwise to allow further exercise until he has been investigated. Genetic screening is non-urgent, although it may be prudent to consider restricting exercise on other family members until the Echo has been undertaken.

6. E

The murmur has typical characteristics of an innocent flow murmur, likely to be audible at the moment because of the increased heart rate with the pyrexia. The child is also of typical age for such murmurs so it may persist even after the URTI has settled but does not need investigation. Severe anaemia may cause such murmurs but is unlikely with a thriving child and normal examination.

Gastrointestinal and liver disorders

1. B

Inserting a nasogastric tube is the most appropriate next step in management. The child is not shocked therefore does not need intravenous fluids. Antibiotics are not routinely given in gastroenteritis. Blood tests are not usually indicated in gastroenteritis. Advice regarding hand washing should be given to caregivers but the child has signs of dehydration therefore should not be sent home.

2. B

Loose stools can persist after gastroenteritis but only for a few weeks. Falling two centiles is a red flag and always needs investigation therefore E is not appropriate and toddler diarrhoea excluded. The history suggests coeliac disease and testing should be performed whilst the child is on a diet that contains gluten. Cystic fibrosis is diagnosed on a sweat test and the child would likely to have suffered with chest infections.

3. **A**

Bilious vomiting in a young baby is a red flag and malrotation should be excluded with a barium study. Pyloric stenosis causes obstruction proximal to the duodenum therefore no bile in the vomit. Duodenal atresia presents during the first few days of life and the baby would not have normal bowel movements. The baby is too young for an intussusception. Gastro-oesophageal reflux is not associated with bilious vomiting.

4. **C**

Increasing fluid intake will help with constipation but the presence of a large amount of impacted stool means that macrogol treatment is the most successful. Manual disimpaction is performed as a last resort in children mainly if they have failed medical treatment. Suppositories are unpleasant and not generally given to children. Lactulose (osmotic laxative) is usually given for maintenance therapy rather than disimpaction.

5. **B**

There are multiple causes of bloody stools in children. The age of the patient and weight loss and loose bloody stool suggests inflammatory bowel disease, the presence of ulcers should lead you to the diagnosis of Crohn's disease. Coeliac disease doesn't tend to cause bloody stools unless it is severe. Travellers' diarrhoea would not persist for this long. Meckles diverticulum tends to present in the toddler age group and is not associated with mouth ulcers or pyoderma gangrenosum (the rash on the shins).

6. **C**

Pyloric stenosis results in dehydration and hypochloraemic alkalosis as indicated by the high bicarbonate. Chloride is not routinely measured – it has to be specifically requested. Variable sodium and potassium losses occur. A test feed will show peristaltic waves (and also a mass on palpation).

Urogenital disorders

1. **E**

A painful swollen testicle could be a testicular torsion and needs urgent surgical review because there is a window of only 6 hours to reverse the torsion by surgical means. UTIs do not usually present with testicular swelling. Mumps can present with painful testicular swelling (although bilateral in up to 40%) but is associated with parotid swelling, which this patient doesn't have. A urine dip test should be performed if there is bilateral testicular swelling to identify urinary protein suggestive of nephrotic syndrome. An ultrasound is appropriate if the swelling was painless to identify a hydrocele.

2. **E**

This child has HSP. The management is supportive and the child can be send home with analgesia and reassurance after the baseline bloods have been performed including renal function. There must be a plan in place for regular monitoring of urine dip testing and blood pressure. A is not appropriate as the child is well and afebrile. Swelling of joints is common in HSP and therefore x-rays are not appropriate. Palpable purpura is not a feature of nephrotic syndrome so there is no indication to commence steroids.

3. **A**

This child has a new onset of nocturnal enuresis. Alarm systems are used prior to starting medication. Some may consider the nocturnal enuresis to be secondary to bereavement but referral to CAHMS is not appropriate until organic problems are excluded. Weight loss suggests there may be an underlying cause. It is appropriate to exclude diabetes or a urinary tract infection. In this case the urine dip showed glucose and ketones a blood glucose was checked and it was 24mmol/L. The cause of the nocturnal enuresis was type one diabetes. A high blood glucose is associated with the development of oral thrush.

4. **B**

Peri-orbital oedema can be secondary to allergy. However, although this child is atopic the dog is unlikely to be the cause as it has been in the household for a while. Periorbital swelling worse in the morning does not tend to be a picture of allergy, therefore trying a new antihistamine is unlikely to help. The history of the periorbital swelling along with the presence of pitting oedema (as evidenced by the sock marks) and weight gain suggests nephrotic syndrome. Dietary advice on weight loss and reassurance is not appropriate, the child's urine needs to be tested for the presence of protein.

5. **C**

The clinical picture given is that this child is not well. We know she has a diagnosis of hydronephrosis and VUR which can predispose her to UTIs, even if she is on prophylactic medication. Antibiotics should not be commenced until a urine sample is obtained. A clean catch sample is the best method. As she is vomiting and clinically unwell it would be most appropriate to commence IV antibiotics. A renal ultrasound would have little to add. Urgent surgical referral is not indicated and elective surgery is only considered if the child has several breakthrough infections.

6. **B**
This boy has haemolysis, low platelets and acute renal failure. The most likely cause is haemolytic uraemic syndrome (HUS) from *E. coli* 0157 contaminated meat. DIC can cause haemolysis but also results in abnormal clotting. The other causes do not cause haemolysis (resulting in anaemia and jaundice) or low platelets.

Neurological disorders

1. **D**
This child has fully recovered from her first uncomplicated seizure. There is no indication for any further investigation at present, apart from an ECG to rule out long QT syndrome. Anti-epileptic medication is not usually commenced after a single seizure.

2. **E**
This boy has features of meningitis (raised temperature, headache and photophobia) which needs treatment with antibiotics (cefotaxime). He has no features of shock at present, as his heart rate, respiratory rate and capillary refill time are within normal limits. Therefore he does not require fluid resuscitation (a bolus of normal saline). He may require dioralyte if the loose stools persist (as long as he tolerates oral fluids) but this is not the most appropriate next step.

3. **E**
This history is suggestive of a tension headache. There are no red flag symptoms, such as early morning headache, nausea and vomiting, visual changes and/or an abnormal neurological examination to suggest an intracranial pathology, and no associated symptoms of migraine such as vomiting, visual disturbances and photophobia.

4. **E**
Duchenne muscular dystrophy is the most likely diagnosis in this case. Serum creatine kinase (CK) is a simple minimally invasive test to support this

diagnosis. More invasive or specialist tests such as a muscle biopsy and genetic testing can be used later to confirm the diagnosis. If the CK is normal the diagnosis is not muscular dystrophy and further investigation is required. There are no upper motor neurone signs therefore CT head and MRI brain are not indicated.

5. **C**
The history and CT scan result point to viral encephalitis. The CSF would be clear, with raised WC predominantly lymphocytes, normal glucose and normal or high protein. Bacterial or TB meningitis has cloudy CSF, all have raised WCs, bacterial predominantly neutrophils with TB mixed. A very high protein is seen in TB meningitis.

6. **D**
He has had an uncomplicated febrile convulsion, at a typical age, with an obvious focus of infection (otitis media). No further investigation is required. He requires oral amoxicillin and can be discharged home.

Musculoskeletal disorders

1. **D**
Systemic onset juvenile idiopathic arthritis is commonest in under 5 year olds. Systemic features are usually more prominent at presentation but the joints can be involved. Hepatosplenomegaly can cause abdominal pain. This rash is not typical of rheumatic fever. HSP is less likely as although associated with joint pains and abdominal pain the rash is purpuric and distributed over the buttocks and legs, with no fever. Transient synovitis can be associated with a viral rash but usually only a low grade fever and larger joints. Kawasaki's disease does not have joint involvement, only finger redness and swelling.

2. **D**
A slipped upper femoral epiphysis (SUFE) of his right leg is the most likely due to the sudden onset in a typical overweight adolescent boy, and painful hip which is externally rotated on inspection. SUFE can lead to referred pain to the knee. Osgood–Schlatter disease has knee pain only and Perthes disease is usually painless and occurs in younger children. Polyarticular JIA although affecting children of this age, needs to involve four or more joints, is not usually of sudden onset and would have less mild symptoms at onset. Transient synovitis (irritable hip) usually affects younger children, associated with symptoms of an URTI.

3. **E**

This child has septic arthritis. *Staphylococcus aureus* is the most likely organism in a child who was previously well. MRSA would need to be considered in a child previously hospitalised, and salmonella in a child with sickle cell disease. Group B *Streptococcus* is a cause of septic arthritis in neonates. Whilst pain relief is important, and can be given orally, giving antibiotics is the priority.

4. **C**

This boy most likely has an enthesitis-related arthritis (ERA), a subtype of JIA, characterised by onset of arthritis in an older boy, often later developing sacrolitis. The mildly raised ESR is consistent with this diagnosis. It is associated with anterior uveitis, which may be asymptomatic, therefore regular screening with a slit lamp examination is indicated to prevent permanent damage to the eye. ERA is strongly associated with HLA-B27 but this is not a diagnostic test and therefore not urgent. Septic arthritis is unlikely with only mild tenderness but would need to be excluded. TB arthritis is also usually more painful and long standing but needs to be considered. Malignancy would be expected to cause more systemic features and osteolytic lesions. Seropositive rheumatoid arthritis affects older children and mainly girls. ERA is usually rheumatoid factor negative.

5. **A**

Adolescent idiopathic scoliosis is the most likely cause of her scoliosis. Leg length discrepancy would not result in a rib hump. She is unlikely to have Marfan's syndrome with her height. Neurofibromatosis is unlikely at this age with no skin manifestations. A spinal tumour is rare and likely to cause other symptoms but needs to be excluded.

Allergy, immunology and infections

1. **D**

The most likely cause at this age is cross contamination of the chocolate with nuts. He is likely to have eaten chocolate before but may not have had nuts. This will be identified by serum-specific IgE for mixed foods. In the absence of respiratory or circulatory compromise and no history of asthma, an adrenaline pen is not indicated at this stage. The timing with eating the chocolate makes other causes of urticaria such as washing powder or infection unlikely.

2. **A**

The most likely diagnosis is chicken pox. This can cause severe illness in immunosuppressed children, such as those on regular oral steroids. Acyclovir may control the infection. Zoster immunoglobulin is only effective if given on exposure, before symptoms develop.

3. **B**

The girl most likely has a structural abnormality of her right upper lung such as a narrowing of the right upper bronchus, which is best visualised with a flexible bronchoscopy. A rigid bronchoscope would not reach this distally into the lung. The abnormality would not be easily seen on a CT scan. The child is thriving and well in between episodes making immunodeficiency and tuberculosis unlikely.

4. **B**

This cluster of symptoms points towards cow's milk allergy. This would settle with a change to cow's milk protein free milk formula. Gastro-oesophageal reflux is a less likely cause for all these symptoms and he is too young for introduction of solids. Oral rehydration fluid is the treatment for gastroenteritis.

5. **B**

The most likely cause is immunoglobulin deficiency (hypogammaglobulinaemia), which often doesn't start until 18 months due to protective maternal factors. SCID is unlikely to present this late. The ear and eye infections in addition to lung suggests generalised immunodeficiency rather than CF. Neutrophil defects are unlikely as usually the patient also gets skin sepsis, mouth ulcers/gingivitis and suppurative cervical lymphadenopathy. Recurrent ear infection is common in childhood but purulent ear discharge at this age is unusual.

Genetic disorders and dysmorphology

1. **C**

Lymphoedema in a female baby at birth should raise suspicions for Turner's syndrome, but the diagnosis needs to be confirmed by karyotype before screening for associated problems (cardiac and renal anomalies and later hearing problems). There is no abnormality of the brain therefore MRI of the head is not indicated.

2. **D**

This baby has several features of Down's syndrome which occurs due to a trisomy of chromosome 21.

3. **D**

This child has Haemophilia A, which is an X-linked recessive disorder. This means that he has inherited the condition from his mother, who is a carrier but not affected. Any future brothers he may have will also be affected but his sister will not be affected, but she will be a carrier capable of transmitting the condition to her sons.

4. **E**

The most likely cause of the anomaly is amniotic bands preventing normal development of the toes. This is supported by the presence of the constriction mark. This isolated finding is not associated with any chromosomal or other skeletal anomaly and the parents can be reassured.

5. **B**

This girl has suffered a spontaneous pneumothorax. The most important diagnosis to exclude is Marfan's syndrome which is associated with aortic root dilatation, which could lead to aortic dissection and sudden death. An Echo will show up this complication.

6. **B**

The most likely cause of his constipation, weight gain and better behaviour is hypothyroidism, which has a higher chance of developing in Down's syndrome. Hirschsprung's disease and duodenal atresia would be present from birth. Coeliac disease usually presents with faltering growth.

Endocrine disorders

1. **D**

This child has a new diagnosis of diabetes mellitus but does not fit the criteria for diabetic ketoacidosis. He is not vomiting therefore there is no indication for intravenous fluids and subcutaneous insulin in a basal bolus regime is most appropriate. Type 1 diabetes does not respond to diet alone.

2. **C**

The first sign of puberty in girls is breast bud development therefore this girl with breast stage 3 and pubic hair stage 2 has already entered puberty and menarche will normally follow around 2 and a half years later.

3. **B**

This child is most likely to have familial short stature. This is a clinical diagnosis therefore no investigation is required. However it would be prudent to monitor the growth for a period of

time as interpretation of a growth chart on the basis of one measurement is not possible.

4. **D**

The most likely unifying diagnosis for all these signs and symptoms is hyperthyroidism. Whilst assumptions regarding growth cannot be made based on one measurement a height on the 91st centile implies that growth is good (or excessive), the opposite of what may be found with chronic illness, infection or coeliac disease. The murmur is likely to be secondary to increased flow due to the tachycardia, and will resolve when the hyperthyroidism is treated.

5. **B**

The most common cause of cliteromegaly in a newborn girl is congenital adrenal hyperplasia. Although a full work-up for ambiguous genitalia including all the investigations mentioned should be performed, the immediate priority is to check the blood glucose as hypoglycaemia may be an early complication. Urea & electrolytes should also be monitored closely but salt wasting usually occurs in the first few days rather than hours

Skin disorders

1. **A**

The infant has a small capillary haemangioma. Typically no treatment is indicated unless the haemangioma is very large or is obstructing vision or breathing, when a referral to a dermatologist and treatment with propranolol would be appropriate. Here the size and location does not warrant anything other than reassurance.

2. **B**

The appearances suggest a Mongolian blue spot. These typically occur in Asian children and are present from birth. They can be mistaken for bruises. It is helpful to confirm its presence from birth to exclude a bruise as any bruise in a non-mobile child requires careful evaluation. Café au lait spots are light brown or tan in colour.

3. **B**

The fleshy dome shaped lesions are suggestive of molluscum contagiosum. No treatment is indicated for molluscum. Antibiotics and antiviral may be appropriate if the eczema was secondarily infected however this is not the case. Dermatologists do not need to see these children.

4. **B**

The baby most likely has eczema. Although the skin is dry, bathing every day removes the dead skin and is recommended. Steroid creams should not be applied to infant faces. Eczema is not usually due to cows' milk allergy and anti-allergy bedding may be useful for allergic respiratory disease but not eczema.

5. **A**

The described 'target lesions' are typical of Erythema multiforme (EM). In this case it is most likely due to *Mycoplasma pneumonia*. Some drugs including antibiotics can precipitate EM but not usually erythromycin, and it is a drug reaction rather than allergy. Erythema toxicum is a neonatal skin rash. In Stevens–Johnson syndrome the child is very unwell and has blisters.

6. **A**

This is a port wine stain. In this distribution it may be associated with Sturge–Weber syndrome but the most important assessment is to monitor for glaucoma. It can be treated with laser therapy but this is not started until at least 6 months of age. It is not inherited.

Haematology

1. **B**

Easy bruising and bleeding associated with a petechial rash could be consistent with a leukaemia or immune thrombocytopenia purpura. A patient with leukaemia is not as well as this child appears so ITP is the most likely diagnosis and the appropriate investigation is a full blood count. A bone marrow biopsy would only be performed if there was a suggestion of leukaemia on the full blood count. The distribution of the rash is not consistent with HSP therefore U&E is not indicated. A well child with a non-blanching rash is unlikely to have meningococcal septicaemia.

2. **B**

This child has a haemarthrosis secondary to a bleeding disorder. The most likely cause would be haemophilia A. It would be sensible, in view of the history and prolonged APTT to take factor VIII levels. The picture is not that of leukaemia. There is no prolonged PT so platelet function and von Willebrand tests are not required. There is no suggestion of non-accidental injury.

3. **E**

This child has iron deficiency anaemia secondary to poor dietary intake. This is often seen in children who drink excessive amounts of milk. There is no sign of heart failure so blood transfusion is not indicated. The murmur is likely to be secondary to the anaemia and will resolve when treated. A bone marrow biopsy would only be indicated if the blood film was suggestive of leukaemia. The child needs iron supplementation and dietary advice.

4. **A**

This girl has symptoms consistent with an acute chest crisis of sickle cell disease. These severe symptoms would not be expected in community acquired pneumonia. There is no suggestion of cardiac disease in this girl. Vaso-occlusive crises tend to result in pain and swollen joints. Splenic sequestration crisis causes hypovolaemia rather than pain and chest symptoms.

5. **A**

The sudden onset of anaemia with jaundice, reticulocytes in the blood and urobilinogen in the urine indicate an acute haemolytic episode. In this case it is most likely G6PD deficiency, the acute episode triggered by ingestion of broad beans or infection. There is no renal failure and normal platelets excluding HUS. The blood film excludes spherocytosis. The murmur is due to the anaemia. The normal MCV excludes iron deficiency anaemia.

Childhood cancers

1. **A**

This child has features of leukaemia. The features of pallor, easy bleeding and increased infections suggest bone marrow infiltration of leukaemic cells. The most common in this age group is acute lymphoblastic leukaemia. Both Hodgkins and non-Hodgkins lymphoma present with lymphadenopathy and night sweats which this patient doesn't have. Wilms tumours present with abdominal masses not hepatosplenomegaly.

2. **B**

This child has features of raised intracranial pressure so the possibility of a brain tumour must be considered. The most appropriate investigation is a CT scan and if it reveals a mass this can be evaluated further by an MRI. A cranial ultrasound scan cannot be performed in a child of this age as the anterior fontanelle has closed. A lumbar puncture should not be performed if there is a suspicion of raised intracranial pressure. Ophthalmology assessment would be indicated after the CT scan.

3. **D**

A firm abdominal mass on a background of weight loss and abdominal distension is very worrying and malignancy should be ruled out. An abdominal ultrasound scan is the initial investigation of choice. Although constipation causes abdominal pain and distension, palpable faeces are not typically hard. Coeliac disease is not associated with abdominal masses.

4. **E**
This is reactive lymphadenopathy with the lymph node changing in size with viral URTIs, supported by the node not being fixed to surrounding tissues and a well child. This is a very common finding in children but causes great parental anxiety.

Emergencies

1. **A**
This child has diabetic ketoacidosis (DKA). She is dehydrated and shocked. Therefore a fluid bolus should be given before commencing an infusion of fluid replacement. A smaller than usual bolus is given to reduce the risk of cerebral oedema. Intravenous insulin will be required but should not be started until the intravenous fluids have been running for at least an hour to avoid a very rapid fall in blood glucose levels. Bicarbonate is not given in DKA.

2. **E**
This child has croup, the treatment of which is steroids. Dexamethasone is the usual choice because there is some evidence to suggest that a single dose of dexamethasone is more effective against croup than a single dose of prednisolone. In this particular scenario there are no features of severe croup, which would be an indication for nebulised adrenaline. Giving face mask oxygen is not indicated with this saturation and may upset the child precipitating worsening stridor.

3. **A**
This child is shocked, most likely as a result of meningococcal sepsis. Therefore the first priority is a fluid bolus to boost the circulating volume. Antibiotics are important and should follow closely but the fluid bolus will have a more rapid effect initially. Although the airway is the usual priority in the management of a sick child, this girl is still able to maintain her airway. Addressing circulatory issues therefore takes priority, although she is likely to need intubation and ventilation eventually. The blood sugar is in the normal range.

4. **A**
This boy has an acute exacerbation of asthma. There are no features of a severe attack and his oxygen saturations are above 92%. He therefore does not require oxygen. The most appropriate initial treatment is 10 puffs of salbutamol via a spacer device to provide bronchodilation and rapid relief. Steroids should be given as soon as possible following bronchodilation to reduce background lung inflammation and quicken symptom resolution.

5. **A**
This girl has anaphylactic shock. The immediate treatment is IM adrenaline as it is the only fast acting treatment for this life-threatening situation. Nebulised salbutamol and IV hydrocortisone would be appropriate supplementary medications to help alleviate her symptoms. Intravenous adrenaline is only used in severe shock resistant to IM adrenaline or cases of cardiac arrest.

6. **D**
The weak pulses and low BP suggest a pericardial effusion which can occur post cardiac surgery. If present this will need to be drained urgently under ultrasound guidance as tamponade is starting to occur. The child is likely to require urgent intubation, both to enable drainage of the tamponade without distressing the child and in anticipation of a deterioration which can occur quickly. Adrenaline is not indicated at the moment although it should be available.

Community paediatrics

1. **C**
This child is febrile and miserable but otherwise stable and observations are within normal limits. She is most likely to have a self-limiting viral upper respiratory tract infection so antibiotics are not indicated. Administration of paracetamol is reasonable to make the child feel better but should not be given with the sole intention of reducing the temperature and will not prevent a febrile convulsion.

2. **B**
Any bruise in a non-mobile baby must be thoroughly evaluated. The explanation given here does not correlate with the developmental age of the baby (this baby is too young to roll) and the observed injury. Admit to a place of safety whilst investigations for further injuries or underlying pathological conditions are performed. Social services decide further action.

3. **C**
Most babies are walking by 15 months but walking is not considered to be delayed until the

baby is 18 months old. No investigation or intervention is indicated here unless an abnormality is found on examination or there are other concerns. A thorough examination of the hips is vital to rule out missed developmental dysplasia of the hip. The other milestones mentioned for this baby are also within normal limits.

4. **C**

Vaccinations should be delayed if a child is unwell with a febrile illness but are not contra-indicated during a mild viral illness. Premature babies should be vaccinated according to their chronological age. A family history of epilepsy or epilepsy in the child is not a contraindication for vaccination, including pertussis, (which can now only be given as part of a combined vaccine anyway).

5. **D**

Hypothyroidism causes developmental delay and slow 'quiet' children. Thyroid function (TSH) tested at birth does not exclude central congenital or acquired hypothyroidism. With delayed fine motor as well as gross motor skills Duchenne muscular dystrophy is less likely. He is expected to have normal home stimulation with the normal development of his twin. A chromosome problem is less likely with no dysmorphism. Congenital infection is very unlikely.

6. **C**

This boy may have ADHD, which is known to be of higher incidence in ex-preterm infants. However he requires full assessment, including completion of standard questionnaires in at least two different settings before managing with a MDT and possibly starting medication.

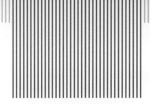

Index

Note: Page numbers in **bold** or *italic* refer to tables or figures, respectively.